Lasers in Cutaneous and Cosmetic Surgery

Lasers in Cutaneous and Cosmetic Surgery

Gary P. Lask, MD

Clinical Professor
Division of Dermatology
University of California, Los Angeles
    UCLA School of Medicine
Director of Dermatologic Surgery
Mohs Surgery and the Dermatology Laser Center
Los Angeles, California

Nicholas J. Lowe, MD

Clinical Professor of Dermatology
University of California, Los Angeles
    UCLA School of Medicine
Los Angeles, California
Senior Lecturer and Honorary Consultant in Dermatology
    University College London
Director, Cranley Clinic for Dermatology
London, England

Churchill Livingstone
A Division of Harcourt Brace & Company
Philadelphia   London   Toronto   Montreal   Sydney   Tokyo   Edinburgh

CHURCHILL LIVINGSTONE
A Division of Harcourt Brace & Company

The Curtis Center
Independence Square West
Philadelphia, Pennsylvania 19106

Library of Congress Cataloging-in-Publication Data

Lask, Gary P. (Gary Philip)
Lasers in cutaneous and cosmetic surgery / Gary P. Lask, Nicholas
J. Lowe.—1st ed.

     p.   cm.

ISBN 0-443-07639-1

1. Skin—Surgery.　2. Lasers in surgery.　3. Surgery, Plastic.
I. Lowe, N. J. (Nicholas J.)　II. Title.
[DNLM: 1. Skin Diseases—surgery.　2. Skin—surgery.　3. Laser
Surgery—methods.　4. Lasers—therapeutic use.　5. Surgery, Plastic.
WR 650 L345L 2000]
RD520.L374　2000　　617.4′77059—dc21

DNLM/DLC　　　　　　　　　　　　　　　　98-7037

LASERS IN CUTANEOUS AND COSMETIC SURGERY　　　　　　　　　　　ISBN 0-443-07639-1

Churchill Livingstone® is a registered trademark of Harcourt Brace & Company.

⟊ is a trademark of Harcourt Brace & Company

Printed in the United States of America.

Last digit is the print number:　9　8　7　6　5　4　3　2　1

CONTRIBUTORS

Lisa Airan, MD
Fellow Dermatologic Surgery, Division of Dermatology, Washington University School of Medicine, St. Louis, Missouri
Hypertrophic Scars and Keloids

Reza Babapour, MD
Resident, Dermatology, University of California, Los Angeles, UCLA School of Medicine, Los Angeles, California
Low-Energy Laser Systems

Sterling Baker, MD
Oculoplastic Surgery, Oklahoma City, Oklahoma
Blepharoplasty

Kathleen Behr, MD
Assistant Clinical Professor, University of California, Los Angeles, UCLA School of Medicine, Los Angeles, California

Peter Burrows, MD
Clinical Fellow, Clinical Research Specialists, Santa Monica, California
Benign Pigmented Lesions

Vladislav Chizhevsky, MD
Clinical Fellow, Clinical Research Specialists, Santa Monica, California
Benign Cutaneous Lesions; Vascular Lesions; Tattoos; Benign Pigmented Lesions; Facial Acne Scars

Julene E. Cray, RN
President, Aesthetic Laser Consultants, Laguna Beach, California
Endoscopic Laser Surgery of the Aging Face

Richard H. Epstein, MD
Associate Professor of Anesthesiology, Jefferson Medical College of Thomas Jefferson University, Philadelphia; Director of Pediatric Anesthesia, Thomas Jefferson University Hospital, Philadelphia, Pennsylvania
Anesthesia for Cutaneous Laser Surgery

Edward Glassberg, MD
Clinical Assistant Professor, University of California, Los Angeles, UCLA School of Medicine, Los Angeles; Chief of Dermatology, Long Beach Memorial Medical Center, Long Beach, California
Low-Energy Laser Systems; Tattoos

Bill Halmi, MD
Private Practice, Phoenix, Arizona
Anesthesia for Cutaneous Laser Surgery

Christopher Ho, MD
Resident, Dermatology, University of California, Los Angeles, UCLA School of Medicine, Los Angeles, California
Skin Resurfacing; Hair Transplantation with Carbon Dioxide and Er:YAG Laser Donor Incisions

Robert W. Hutcherson, MD
Associate Clinical Professor of Surgery, Division of Head and Neck Surgery, UCLA Hospital and Clinics, University of California, Los Angeles; Associate Medical Director, Head and Neck Surgical Oncology, John Wayne Cancer Institute, Santa Monica, California
Endoscopic Laser Surgery of the Aging Face

Gregory S. Keller, MD
Clinical Associate Professor of Surgery, Division of Head and Neck Surgery, University of California, Los Angeles, UCLA School of Medicine, Los Angeles, California
Endoscopic Laser Surgery of the Aging Face

Donna Ko, MD
Clinical Assistant Professor, University of California, Los Angeles, UCLA School of Medicine, Los Angeles, California
Hair Removal

Gary P. Lask, MD
Clinical Professor, Division of Dermatology, University of California, Los Angeles, UCLA School of Medicine; Director of Dermatologic Surgery, Mohs Surgery and the Dermatology Laser Center, Los Angeles, California
Low-Energy Laser Systems; Anesthesia for Cutaneous Laser Surgery; Benign Cutaneous Lesions; Vascular Lesions; Telangiectasias of the Legs; Tattoos; Benign Pigmented Lesions; Skin Resurfacing; Hair Transplantation: with Carbon Dioxide and Er:YAG Laser Donor Incisions; Facial Acne Scars; Hypertrophic Scars and Keloids; Hair Removal

Patrick K. Lee, MD
Assistant Clinical Professor of Medicine/Dermatology, University of California, Los Angeles, UCLA School of Medicine, Los Angeles, California
Telangiectasias of the Legs

Nicholas J. Lowe, MD
Clinical Professor of Dermatology, University of California, Los Angeles, UCLA School of Medicine, Los Angeles; Clinical Research Specialists, Santa Monica, California; Senior Lecturer and Honorary Consultant in Dermatology, University College London; Director, Cranley Clinic for Dermatology, London, England
Laser Physics for Clinicians; Benign Cutaneous Lesions; Vascular Lesions; Tattoos; Benign Pigmented Lesions; Skin Resurfacing; Hair Transplantation with Carbon Dioxide and Er:YAG Laser Donor Incisions; Facial Acne Scars; Hypertrophic Scars and Keloids; Hair Removal

Philippa Lowe, MB, ChB
Senior House Officer, Department of Medicine, University of Liverpool, Aintree Hospital, Liverpool, England
Skin Resurfacing; Facial Acne Scars

C. Anne Maxwell, MB, ChB
Dermatology, Cranley Clinic, London, England
Skin Resurfacing

Quan Nguyen, MD
Resident, Dermatology, University of California, Los Angeles, UCLA School of Medicine, Los Angeles, California
Skin Resurfacing

Bernard I. Raskin, MD
Assistant Clinical Professor, Division of Dermatology, University of California, Los Angeles, UCLA School of Medicine, Los Angeles, California
Vascular Lesions

David Sawcer, MB, ChB, PhD, MRCP
St John's Institute of Dermatology, London, England
Laser Physics for Clinicians; Benign Pigmented Lesions

Walter P. Unger, MD
Private Practice, Toronto, Ontario, Canada
Hair Transplantation: An Overview

Joshua Wieder, MD
Clinical Assistant Professor, Division of Dermatology, University of California, Los Angeles, UCLA School of Medicine, Los Angeles, California
Benign Pigmented Lesions

PREFACE

Since lasers were first used in medicine in the early 1960s, there has been a dramatic expansion in their variety and clinical application. Much of the expansion has occurred over the last decade, and we now have, as laser physicians and surgeons, a wide choice of laser systems. Nowhere is this more evident than in the lasers now available for treating the skin and a growing number of skin diseases and problems.

The technology of cutaneous lasers changes so quickly that lasers and the parameters of treatment change from one year to the next. We have, with this book, tried to reach a balance in discussing clinical experience, guidelines, and predictions of the efficacy and complications of different lasers. With the need to provide up-to-date information, several of the chapters were being rewritten and updated almost as we went to press. We hope that we have provided our readers with a useful text with which to continue to explore this dynamic and challenging therapeutic area.

Gary P. Lask
Nicholas J. Lowe

ACKNOWLEDGMENTS

We thank our publisher for the patience, support, and encouragement to complete this book. I (NJL) would like to thank my wife, Pamela, and daughters, Nicholas and Philippa, for their support, advice, and patience. To the patients and my staff in California and England, thank you for your loyalty and trust. I (GPL) would like to thank my office staff at UCLA and Encino and my family for their consistent support. We also owe a debt of thanks to our contributing authors, who have given their unique experience and wisdom to this book, and to many of the laser companies, without whom we would not have the multiplicity of therapeutic lasers.

CONTENTS

1

LASER PHYSICS FOR CLINICIANS

David Sawcer
Nicholas J. Lowe

Since they were first introduced in 1960, lasers have frequently been considered "a solution looking for a problem." Their use in research in many fields is widespread, and their application in areas as diverse as fusion physics and compact disk players is now commonplace. Medicine and surgery are no exceptions to this. Various procedures, both diagnostic and therapeutic, that use lasers are available in many specialties, including dermatology, ophthalmology, gynecology, otolaryngology, and endoscopy. Dermatologic applications of the laser were among the first medical uses, and the technology has continued to be fully applied in this area. Furthermore, research in dermatology has been and will continue to be a major contributor to advances in laser medicine and photobiology.

During the past three decades, dermatologic laser technology has flourished. There now exists a wide spectrum of dermatologic laser systems, with a large variety of beam properties, such as wavelengths and energy-delivery parameters. A similar expansion has been seen in beam-delivery devices, and complete laser systems have become smaller, more reliable, and less expensive. Technology is moving rapidly onward, with new lasers appearing at an ever-increasing rate. Understanding of the photobiology involved in the laser–tissue interaction is also progressing. In fact, many new systems are no longer solutions in search of problems but have been designed with specific purposes in mind. Advances in laser technology now permit physicians to provide treatment for a large variety of cutaneous disorders for which no therapy, or only ineffective forms of therapy, previously existed. Much work remains, however, to optimize therapeutic regimens for use of existing systems on specific conditions, to extend understanding of the laser–tissue interaction, and to develop new goal-specific systems.

To make the most effective use of available technology (clinically or for research purposes), modern dermatologists must maintain an up-to-date understanding of the laser systems available and of the conditions to which each can be successfully applied. Also, they must be aware of new developments in this rapidly expanding field and of the trends and direction of current research, in terms of both applications and the technology itself. To achieve these goals, a basic understanding of lasers, of the terminology used in connection with them, and of the fundamentals of laser–tissue interaction is necessary.

Electromagnetic Radiation

Electromagnetic radiation forms a continuous spectrum ranging from low to high energy or, equivalently, long to short wavelength. Many bands within this continuum (often overlapping) are labeled with names in common use: radio waves, microwaves, infrared light, visible light (a relatively small band of wavelengths), ultraviolet light, x-rays, gamma rays, and cosmic rays, from low to high energy, respectively.[1-4]

A variety of comparable terms are used to identify a point (or band) in this spectrum, such as *energy,* and *frequency,* and *wavelength.* These terms are interrelated and stem essentially from the dichotomous nature of radiation itself. At any given point in the spectrum, radiation exhibits both properties of discrete particles—*photons,* which are characterized by energy and are continuously propagating electric and magnetic fields, and *waves,* which are characterized by frequency and wavelength.[1, 3, 4] Either description is acceptable, and the terms are interchangeable in many cases, although occasionally one is more appropriate than the other.

The most complete description of laser theory requires an explanation in terms of the photon or *quantum* nature of radiation. However, with minimal loss of understanding (and a considerable simplification of the mathematics), the wave or classical theory, can also be used, which is more intuitive and in some instances more enlightening. For the following description, elements of both theories are used, for a "semi–quantum mechanical" theory.

Fundamental Phenomena

The fundamental phenomena on which all lasers are essentially based were first described by Albert Einstein in the early 1900s. Einstein proposed three basic processes by which electromagnetic radiation can interact with matter (an atom or a molecular or crystal system). These purely quantum mechanical processes are *absorption, spontaneous emission,* and *stimulated emission.*[1–5]

All matter is composed of protons, neutrons, and electrons. The protons and neutrons form clusters, nuclei, and the electrons associate with these nuclei in "orbits" (in the case of atoms and molecules) or "bands" (in the case of crystals). In either case, the electrons are said to exist in *energy levels* or *states.* The energy states present are determined by the structure of the system at an atomic level. Importantly, they are not continuous; only certain energy states are possible for each electron and therefore for the system as a whole.

Under resting conditions, electrons occupy lower energy levels, and the electrons are said to be in their *ground state,* Eg. If energy is supplied to the system, an electron may be promoted from its ground state to one of higher energy. Such an electron is said to have undergone a *transition,* or, more specifically, *excitation,* and the system/electron is said to be in an *excited state,* Es. Such processes are governed by quantum mechanical rules. Stated most simply, these rules require an excitation to occur between two energy states, Eg to Es, and the system must absorb precisely the required energy (Es minus Eg); any fraction or multiple thereof will not result in a transition.

The process of *absorption* is said to occur when a photon of an appropriate energy interacts with a material in such a manner that the photon is annihilated and its energy transferred to the material, producing an electron transition to an excited state (Fig. 1–1).

Compared with the excited state, the ground state is an inherently more stable situation, since it is a lower-energy configuration. Quantum mechanics predicts that after a period of time, a material in an excited state tends to spontaneously return to the ground state, and in doing so releases the excess energy in the form of an emitted photon; such a transition is termed a *decay.* This is the process of *spontaneous emission.* The photon produced in this manner is of the same energy as that which formed the excited state in the first instance and therefore has the same frequency and wavelength (provided the decay occurs between the same two states, Es to Eg). It is released independently of any stimulus, however, and is in no other way related to the exciting photon or to photons emitted at other sites in the

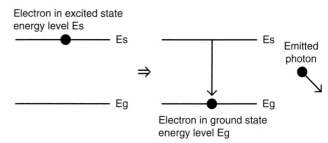

Figure 1–2. Spontaneous emission.

overall system. Radiation emitted in this manner is termed *noncoherent* (Fig. 1–2).

The final process Einstein described, that of *stimulated emission,* involves the interaction of a material already in an excited state with a second photon of the same energy as that which caused the initial excitation. When this interaction occurs, there is a finite probability that the material will be stimulated to decay to the ground state and in so doing will emit a further photon of identical energy. In this case, however, the emitted photon and the stimulating photon are related; they are both spatially and temporally *coherent* in that they travel in the same direction, are in phase, and have the same energy (frequency or wavelength) (Fig. 1–3).[1, 3] The laser exploits all three of these phenomena.

The Model Laser

Under normal circumstances, most electrons in a material are in the ground state because this is a more inherently stable situation. An appropriate photon flux (number of photons) incident on such a material results predominantly in absorption. In fact, all three interactions occur, but absorption is the most statistically likely at first, and the incident photon flux therefore suffers net losses or, more correctly, is attenuated.

When there are more electrons in an excited state than in the ground state, a *population inversion* is said to exist (this is the "inverse" of the normal situation). A population inversion can be created in a variety of ways, including by the absorption of other electromagnetic radiation. A material that can contain and be maintained in a population inversion is termed an *active medium.*[1, 3, 5, 6] An appropriate photon flux incident on an active medium in population inversion results predominantly in stimulated emission, which is the most statistically likely process under those conditions. This results in coherent amplification of the photon flux (Fig. 1–4). An active medium in population inversion represents a fundamental radiation amplifier; the degree of amplification is termed the *gain.*

When the energy of the photons to be amplified is in the microwave band (wavelength 1 mm to 10 cm), the system is termed a *maser,* an acronym for *microwave amplification by stimulated emission of radiation.* The first maser was developed in 1954 by Townes at Columbia University.[7] When

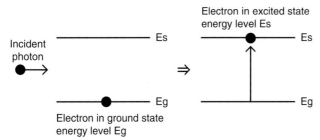

Figure 1–1. Absorption.

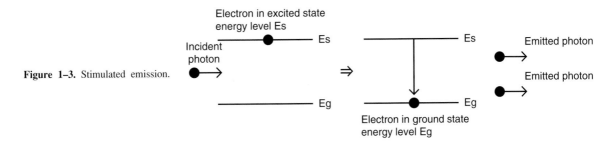

Figure 1–3. Stimulated emission.

the energy is in the visible band of the electromagnetic spectrum (wavelength 400 to 750 nm), it is termed a *laser,* an acronym for *l*ight *a*mplification by *s*timulated *e*mission of *r*adiation. The term *laser* is also applied to systems operating in both the infrared (wavelength 750 nm to 1 mm) and the ultraviolet (wavelength 100 to 400 nm) bands also. The first laser, a ruby laser, was developed by Maiman of Hughes Aircraft Company in 1960, and many other designs and systems soon followed.[7–13]

The Practical Laser

All practical lasers can be divided into five major sections[1, 4, 5, 9] (Fig. 1–5):

1. Lasing material (also called active medium, laser medium)
2. Optical resonance cavity (also called optical resonator, laser cavity). The lasing material and the optical resonance cavity together provide amplification and output coupling.
3. Pumping system—creation and maintenance of the population inversion
4. Laser beam delivery devices—external optical elements guiding laser to the treatment site
5. Elements for creating pulses

Several elements for controlling the laser are present in modern systems, including a means of adjusting the output parameters of the laser beam and elements necessary for power supply, cooling, and so forth.

Lasing Material

The laser medium represents the heart of the laser system, and lasers are usually named according to their active medium.[3, 5, 9, 12] Choice of the lasing material is of prime importance.[4] In a practical sense, choosing the laser material for existing systems is equivalent to choosing the function of the device. Most lasers operate at a single wavelength, and it is the wavelength that largely determines the clinical properties of the laser. The same is true for lasers that produce several wavelengths such as tunable dye lasers, with the difference being increased flexibility of function by choice of an alternative wavelength. With wavelength fixed, the conditions that can be successfully treated are also essentially set unless a new application is conceived. In either case, developmental or practical, it is usually the desire to treat a specific condition or subgroup of conditions that in practice determines choice of lasing material and laser.

Optical Resonance Cavity

Photons passing through an active medium in population inversion are amplified by stimulated emission. However, they also suffer losses or attenuation (e.g., absorption interactions that result in nonlaser decays or heating). The net amplification or gain of a single pass through the active medium is rarely enough to produce a significant, usable output of laser energy (except for a few pulse laser designs). As its name suggests, the optical resonance cavity is a positive feedback element that guides photons traveling

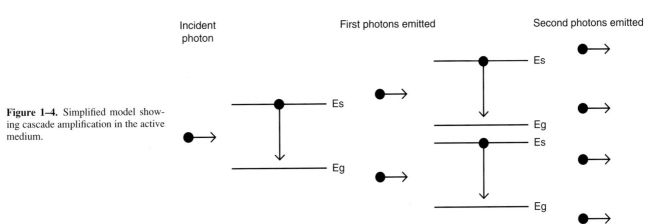

Figure 1–4. Simplified model showing cascade amplification in the active medium.

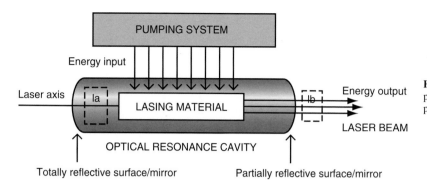

Figure 1–5. The practical laser system. 1a indicates position of the Q-switching element, and 1b shows the position of the mechanical shutter gating element.

parallel to its axis back and forth through the active medium, allowing for repeated amplification and, therefore, potentially a more significant output. Systems are designed so that the population inversion is maintained (by the pumping system) and a simple threshold condition is met: the round trip gain within the cavity (left to right and back, equivalent to two passes through the active medium) is greater than the round trip losses. In such a cavity, coherent photon energy builds up by repeated amplification, being limited on the whole only by rate of input of energy and the amount of energy removed in the laser beam.

The usual optical resonance cavity consists simply of two reflective surfaces, typically plain or curved mirrors, placed at either end of the active medium and aligned precisely so that their axes are parallel and are along the axis of the laser medium (see Fig. 1–5). One of the surfaces is 100% reflective, but the other is only 90% to 95% reflective. It is through the partially reflective surface that the laser energy emerges as the laser beam, which is sometimes referred to as the *output coupling*.[1, 4, 5]

In addition to providing positive feedback amplification, the arrangement of the cavity determines some of the properties of the output beam. Classical wave and quantum mechanical solutions to the arrangement described here for a cavity predict that only certain standing waves will oscillate back and forth constructively (without canceling each other out), that is, will "resonate" in the cavity. These resonating *modes* have almost exactly the same wavelength (negligible differences in practical terms) but differ in cross-sectional appearance. The output beam of most systems is a composite of several modes determined by the design of the optical resonance cavity (see later section on Cross-Sectional Power Density).

Pumping System

Pumping systems supply energy to the lasing material to create and maintain a population inversion within it. They vary in type (and efficiency) between different lasers. The mechanism of energy transfer is chosen and tailored to suit the particular laser. Even with careful design consideration, however, efficiency of pumping is usually low, varying from a fraction of a percentage in most systems up to 30% in a

few cases.[4] Primarily because of such inefficiency, cooling systems (to deal with the nonuseful energy produced by the pump) and large power supplies are necessary and are incorporated in many systems.

Common pump sources in current use include optical devices, flashlamps, other lasers and electrical discharges, direct current (DC) excitation, and radio frequency (RF) excitation. Other forms less often encountered in medical systems include chemical pumping (using the energy of a suitable chemical reaction) and gas dynamic pumping (using a supersonic gas expansion).[1, 5]

Most optical pumping involves the use of a powerful light source with broad-spectrum noncoherent output such as a flashlamp. This is directed onto the lasing material, where a proportion of its output is absorbed by the appropriate energy levels to result in the necessary excited state. Discharge characteristics of the flashlamp are adjusted to create and maintain the population inversion in the face of continuous losses within the cavity. Optical pumping is particularly suited to solid-state (e.g., ruby, alexandrite, neodymium:yttrium-aluminum-garnet [Nd:YAG])[4, 5, 14, 15] and liquid (e.g., dye)[13, 14, 16, 17] lasers. In these materials, the energy levels are broadened by a variety of mechanisms (e.g., crystal effects, thermal broadening) into narrow bands rather than single precise energy levels. Such bands can efficiently absorb a greater proportion of the broad-spectrum emission of the flashlamp, thereby increasing the overall efficiency.

Lasers themselves (e.g., argon, nitrogen [N_2], Excimer, kromium fluoride [KrF], xenon fluoride [XeF]) can be used for optical pumping, and such systems are among the most efficient. Perhaps more importantly, lasers can be used to create a population inversion between levels for which it was previously impossible to do so, allowing many new lasers to be developed, for example, the argon pumped dye laser.[13, 18] (The pump laser excites to a higher energy state than that of the lasing transition. From this state, there is a rapid spontaneous decay to the upper laser level and subsequent decay to the ground state during stimulated emission.)

Electrical pumping is probably the most common form of pumping used in medical systems. Such a method is most suited for use with gas lasers (e.g., carbon dioxide [CO_2], argon, copper vapor, Excimer, helium-neon lasers),[4–6, 12, 19–21] for which the minimally broadened energy levels do not lend themselves to efficient optical pumping. DC excitation is achieved by applying a direct intermittent high voltage (15 to 20 kV) across the lasing gas. This results in an electrical discharge within the gas and, following energy transfer by collisions, production of the required population inversion. This arrangement has several problems, however, including low efficiency and degradation of the gas (requiring gas flow or a built-in catalyst system to restore function). More recently, low-voltage RF excitation systems have been developed. In these devices electrical discharge produces the population inversion, but many of the other difficulties mentioned with DC excitation are eliminated. Furthermore, noticeable advantages during the pulsed mode of operation may be possible (e.g., Coherent Medical Ultrapulse™ technology).[19, 22, 23]

Evolution of the Laser Beam

When the laser is switched on, most electrons of the lasing material are in the ground state. The pumping system is activated, and a proportion of these electrons is excited to the upper laser level (either directly or indirectly by means of higher energy states followed by rapid spontaneous decay), creating a population inversion in the lasing material. Spontaneous decay to the ground state results in emission of numerous, but incoherent, photons moving at random orientations and with no phase relationship. Some of these, moving parallel to the cavity axis, begin to oscillate back and forth. These oscillating photons have a statistically greater probability of causing stimulated emission as they pass repeatedly through the active medium.

Repeated or continuous activation of the pumping system maintains the population inversion, and in a very short time (light travels exceptionally fast), there is a large buildup of oscillating photons as a result of coherent amplification by stimulated emission. Energy is continually supplied by the pumping system and emerges from the resonance cavity through the output coupling (partially reflective surface) as the laser beam.

Properties of the Laser Beam

The output of the optical resonance cavity is considered a uniform collimated beam of coherent monochromatic radiation. However, this statement needs some qualification.

Monochromaticity

Monochromatic radiation is radiation of a *single* wavelength. The monochromaticity, or "spectral purity," of most lasers is very great; for example, the argon ion laser, wavelength 488 nm, typically has a "line" or "bandwidth" of output around 0.004 nm in most systems.[4, 13] This high degree of purity of output can be explained as follows: Theoretically, only the single wavelength of the lasing transition should be amplified because all elements in design are chosen to ensure population inversion and decay between two chosen levels each of a unique energy. However, line broadening mechanisms (e.g., crystal effects, thermal effects) allow amplification of a wider band of wavelengths centered on that value by separating the unique energy of the two laser levels into two narrow bands of energy. Not all of these possible wavelengths are amplified, however, as the optical resonance cavity enhances spectral purity by the nature of its design. Only certain wavelengths can efficiently oscillate, or resonate in the cavity; the remainder cancel out because of slight phase differences and interference. The net effect is that only resonant wavelengths within the amplifiable band are present, and the output spectral purity is very great.

In medical systems and for most clinical applications, the bandwidth of the output beam is so small as to be negligible, and these lasers can reasonably be referred to as operating at a single wavelength—as monochromatic.

Collimation

A truly collimated beam of radiation travels in a *single direction* with a *constant* cross-sectional diameter. As with the monochromaticity, the collimation of the laser beam is not absolute. All laser beams have a small but significant divergence centered around a given direction. The inherent divergence of the beam is due primarily to diffraction at the output coupling or at the output of any fiber optic or other external beam-handling device that is present. Optical elements, such as lenses, can significantly alter the beam divergence and are present in many systems. A converging lens results in a minimum beam diameter or *spot size* at approximately the focal length of the lens. At this point the beam is said to be *focused*. At distances from either side of the focal point, the spot size increases, and the beam is said to be *defocused*[1, 3, 12, 19, 22] (Fig. 1–6).

Collimation of the output beam from medical laser systems is sufficiently great to allow the clinician to direct the beam with ease. Precise directionality is utilized in many modern delivery devices. The divergence of the beam is also important clinically, particularly if lenses are present, because variations in spot size can significantly alter the effects produced within a treatment area. The spot size of a divergent beam increases with increasing distance from the point of origin. A larger spot size in general covers a greater area in a smoother, more uniform manner and is therefore desirable. As the spot size increases, however, power density (irradiance) and energy density (or fluence) both decrease, and only small changes in spot size can result in significant changes in these parameters (they are inversely proportional to the square of the beam diameter).

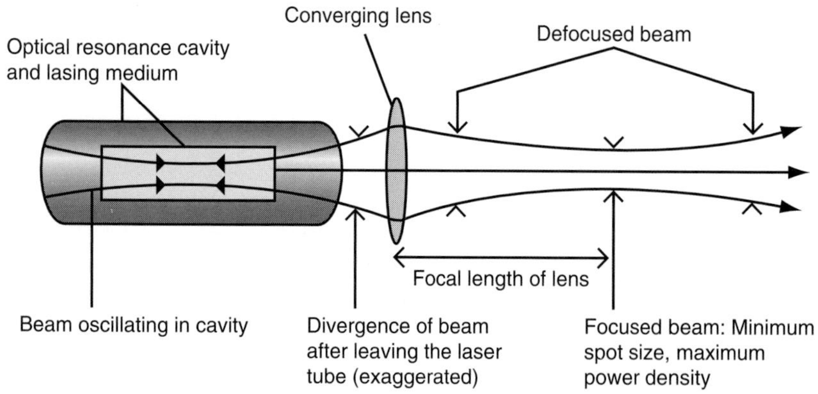

Optical resonance cavity
and lasing medium

Converging lens

Defocused beam

Beam oscillating in cavity

Divergence of beam
after leaving the laser
tube (exaggerated)

Focal length of lens

Focused beam: Minimum
spot size, maximum
power density

Figure 1–6. Divergence of a laser beam and the effect of a converging lens.

Energy Density (Fluence) and Power Density (Irradiance)

Energy density or fluence is the total energy of the beam divided by its cross-sectional area (spot size). Equally, it may be thought of as the product of the power density and exposure time during treatment (joules per square centimeter). Its importance is that it reflects the total energy delivered to the tissue, which is directly related to the volume of tissue that will be treated; a fixed energy is needed to treat a fixed volume. In principle, any suitable combination of power density and exposure time could be used to supply the necessary energy to treat a given region. When dissipation of heat by conduction within a tissue is considered, however, limiting the duration of treatment (exposure time) is seen to be a critical factor.

Power density or irradiance is the rate of energy delivery (power) divided by the cross-sectional area of the beam (watts per square centimeter). Power density is the primary determinant of the rate of tissue treatment. Increasing power density allows sufficiently rapid treatment to keep the exposure time to a minimum while still delivering the required total energy to treat the region concerned.

As mentioned, both the fluence and irradiance depend on spot size and therefore on beam divergence. Varying the distance to the treatment site or focusing and defocusing a beam can therefore produce significantly different tissue responses. A skilled clinician can use this to achieve a desired effect.[1, 3, 5, 12, 19, 22, 23] In most clinical situations, however, to evaluate or reproduce any therapeutic effect, the spot size, power density (or an equivalent energy delivery parameter), and exposure time must be known at an *operating distance* (usually the focal length of the lens if present). Modern systems are supplied with a range of data from the manufacturers specifying the various possible operating distances (and whether the beam is focused or defocused at that point) and allowable energy delivery parameters (depending on the laser type) at each distance. Away from the manufacturers' specified operating distance, these parameters are not normally known, so care must be taken.

Cross-Sectional Power Density

The power density referred to here relates to an average power over the cross-sectional area of the laser beam that is taken to be uniform. A closer examination of the beam across its transverse diameter reveals it is not usually uniform but is in fact made up of several components, notably transverse electric modes (TEMs). These TEMs are the result of the allowable oscillation patterns within a given cavity, resonating waves. Each mode has its own unique cross-sectional power density pattern or energy fingerprint. Several TEMs are possible, and most lasers produce at least the lower two or three modes when operating; hence the term *multimode output*. The lowest-order mode, TEM00, has a relatively uniform (gaussian) cross-sectional power density pattern, but higher-order modes are far less uniform (e.g., TEM01, an annular pattern). Careful cavity alignment and maintenance of the laser helps eliminate most higher-order modes.[1, 4] In addition to the predictable nonuniformities produced by the TEMs, there is almost always a degree of irregularity in the cross-sectional profile of the beam, which is random. This has various causes, both within the cavity and outside it, such as the hot spots or peaks in power density produced by articulated arm–type delivery devices or those of the Q-switched ruby laser.[15] In either case the effect is the same.

During therapy the clinician aims to deliver energy uniformly over the treatment site. This goal is achieved in the first instance by good clinical technique. Scattering and reflection in the tissue and spatial mode mixing in any fiber optic delivery device result in a more homogeneous beam cross section and improved uniformity of energy deposition. Robotic and computerized handpieces add an even greater degree of precision to delivery. The TEMs and other irregularities present in the output beam theoretically may become important constraints limiting uniformity of energy delivery, particularly with lasers with low tissue scattering, such as the far infrared lasers, or those with high tissue absorption, such as ultraviolet and erbium (Er):YAG lasers, for obvious reasons.

Temporal Mode of Output

There are two broad categories of temporal modes in which lasers operate—*continuous-wave* (CW) and *pulse*. As their name suggests, CW lasers produce an uninterrupted beam of radiation; examples are argon and CO_2 lasers. Energy is delivered at some mean level (power density, spot size) continuously for as long as the operator desires[1, 3, 4] (Fig. 1–7A). This mode of energy delivery can be mimicked by lasers whose output consists of a high-frequency (high–repetition rate) train of pulses (e.g., copper vapor lasers).[13, 21] In such cases, the pulses are so close together that the laser behaves as though the beam were continuous. With CW lasers, a great deal of operator skill is required to deliver energy uniformly at the required dose over the area to be treated, but larger areas can be treated rapidly.[5, 12, 13, 24]

A variety of lasers operate in a truly pulsed manner, the effects of each pulse being discrete and identifiable.[1, 3, 4, 21–23] The mechanisms for achieving pulsed output differ depending on the laser and even between identical lasers but different manufactured systems. The most simple method is a gated system, which can produce pulses or pulse trains with a width of the order of 0.1 msec to 0.1 seconds, each pulse having the same peak power as the ungated CW laser's mean power. Most CW lasers can be gated (see Fig. 1–7B). The gating is usually achieved by a simple mechanical shutter system, effectively cutting the continuous beam on and off to form the pulses.

True pulses can be produced by other processes, including mode-locking, Q-switching, and controlled pumping and discharge. Mode-locking produces ultrashort-duration (picosecond) and ultrahigh–peak power (gigawatt) pulses, and is not used currently in clinical systems. Q-switching is a technique for producing short pulses (of the order of tens of nanoseconds) with high peak powers (of the order of megawatts), such as with Q-switched ruby and Q-switched Nd:YAG lasers (see Fig. 1–7C). The Q refers to the quality factor of the laser cavity, a factor directly related to the overall gain (but independently of size population inversion). When Q is high, the photons remain in the cavity for long periods, so gain is high; the opposite is also true. Techniques of Q-switching are varied, but in most cases, it is achieved by introducing a saturable absorber into the laser cavity. When such an absorber is desaturated, it decreases the photon lifetime in the cavity, reducing Q and therefore the gain. In this state, while Q is low the population inversion reaches a high level. However, when the absorber becomes saturated, Q instantly becomes higher, as does the gain. At this point, all of the energy stored in the accumulated population inversion is released in a single, short, high-energy pulse, and the absorber is then desaturated again. The process can be repeated to create further pulses. Pulsed systems allow more flexible control over energy delivery, compared with CW operation with improved delivery of a uniform dose of radiation across the treatment area, but the treatment itself can be more time-consuming.

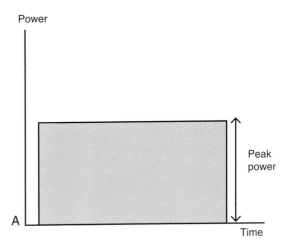

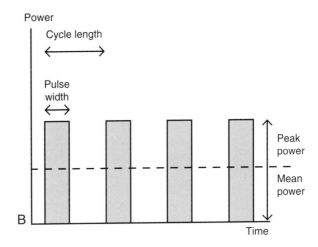

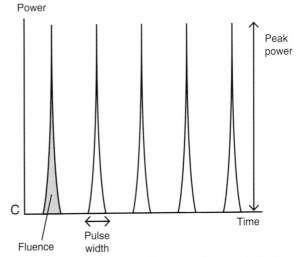

Figure 1–7. Energy delivery in various temporal modes. *A,* Continuous-wave operation. *B,* Pulsed operation, gated. *C,* Pulsed operation, Q-switched.

The power profile of a pulse over time can be important in determining some of the tissue effects it produces. The area under a time-power profile is the total energy and therefore reflects the volume of tissue that can be treated by the pulse. An example of the importance of the pulse profile can be seen by comparing the effect of pulse from an Ultrapulse CO_2 laser (Coherent Medical, Inc., Santa Monica, CA)—which is more rectangular with a slightly higher peak power but similar duration—with the pulse produced by a typical superpulsed CO_2 laser. The energy delivered with each Ultrapulse pulse is sufficient to result in vaporization, whereas that of most superpulsed pulses is insufficient to ablate tissue unless repeated pulses are used.[23]

Beam-Delivery Systems

The laser beam emerges from the output coupling and is manipulated thereafter using standard optical elements—mirrors, lenses, fibers, and so forth. To create a system sufficiently flexible for clinical use, the beam must be delivered to a highly mobile handpiece or down an endoscope, microscope, or other device, depending on the application. An *articulated arm* is a series of coupled hollow tubes along which the beam is guided by reflection at precisely aligned mirrors or prisms contained within the tubes. Initially, articulated arm systems were cumbersome to use, and the mirror alignment often required constant adjustment. This is no longer true, however. Modern systems are flexible and easy to use and require little maintenance. The CO_2 laser wavelength (10,600 nm) cannot be transmitted through any available fiber optic material and is usually delivered by means of an articulated arm system. More recently, rigid wave guides have been developed for use with CO_2 lasers in endoscopic systems. These guides are hollow tubes, coated internally with ceramic materials, along which the laser beam is guided by a series of total internal reflections.[1, 5, 8, 19, 22]

Fiber optic delivery systems are more popular because of their ease of use, despite their minor disadvantages, such as a slight reduction in the power delivered to the output and mild increase in divergence. The fibers are made of quartz or glass and the beam is guided along their length by total internal reflection as with the wave guides. All visible wavelengths and the near infrared spectrum can be transmitted through suitable fibers.[1, 3, 4, 8, 13, 14, 20, 21] However, many Q-switched lasers (e.g., ruby, Nd:YAG) are also transmitted by means of articulated arm systems to avoid the problems of high-power pulse transmission in these fiber optic guides.

The final element in delivery is a handpiece, tip, or micromanipulator. Most dermatologic lasers in current use use noncontact handpieces; that is, only the laser beam itself is allowed to interact directly with the tissue. Contact delivery systems, or *hot tips*, contain elements, crystals or sculptured fiber ends coated with absorbing material, that absorb the laser light and are heated by it. The tips are placed into contact with the tissue to be treated, and energy is transferred to it by conduction.[1, 3, 4, 8, 22] In *noncontact* systems, the handpiece is typically a simple handheld lightweight device that contains only a converging lens system (focusing the beam to one or more spot sizes at the operating distance) and a pointing guide, which aids the surgeon in controlling the distance between the handpiece and the target tissue. More complicated handpieces are available, each designed for a specific purpose, usually improving uniformity of energy delivery. One example is the Hexascan system used with CW lasers, which incorporates both a converging lens and a microprocessor-controlled element to actively scan a given area uniformly.[13, 25, 26] Other computerized pattern generators are for use with pulse laser systems. The Sharplan SilkTouch flashscan system modifies the output of a conventional CO_2 laser to produce a spiral scan pattern in a manner such that the dwelling time at any given site is kept below a critical limit to minimize residual tissue damage. Micromanipulators allow extremely precise directional control of the laser beam at small spot sizes during microscopic surgical procedures. (They are seldom required in dermatology.)

Optical Properties of the Skin

In general, the skin is a multilayered medium that is optically both variable (site to site, person to person) and dynamic (changing with time). Several models have been developed to represent its optical properties with varying degrees of complexity, but none are completely satisfactory. Most simply, it can be considered a two-layered structure—the stratum corneum/epidermis and the dermis—the optics of each layer being noticeably different.[27–30]

The stratum corneum (10 μm) and epidermis (100 μm) form an optical barrier because of absorption, which is high across a wide band, including the wavelengths of most lasers. Major absorbing *chromophores* (substances in the skin that significantly absorb radiation) include the following, by wavelength absorption:

Less than 300 nm—Melanin, peptide bonds, aromatic amino acids, nucleic acids, urocanic acid

More than 320 nm (to 1500 nm)—Melanin

More than 1100 nm—Water

Each chromophore has a strong wavelength-dependent absorption spectrum, characterized by an *absorption coefficient* (Fig. 1–8). The stratum corneum/epidermis is composed of a matrix of chromophores that vary in type and concentration from point to point. For a particular wavelength, the net absorption depends on the absorption coefficient and concentration of all chromophores present. This net absorption is characterized by an *absorption length,* the distance light of a certain wavelength travels before its intensity falls by 63% solely because of absorption (stronger absorption, shorter absorption length). Scattering of radiation occurs but has been shown to be of less importance in the epidermis than in the dermis, so that most light entering this layer is absorbed or transmitted unscattered to the dermis.

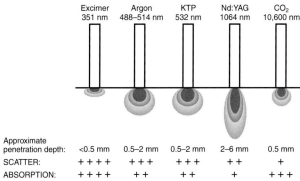

	Excimer 351 nm	Argon 488–514 nm	KTP 532 nm	Nd:YAG 1064 nm	CO$_2$ 10,600 nm
Approximate penetration depth:	<0.5 mm	0.5–2 mm	0.5–2 mm	2–6 mm	0.5 mm
SCATTER:	+ + + +	+ + +	+ + +	+ +	+
ABSORPTION:	+ + + +	+ +	+ +	+	+ + +

Figure 1–8. Effects of absorption and scattering on the irradiated volume.

The dermis (3 mm) also forms an optical barrier, but within this layer both scattering and absorption are of equal importance in determining the optical properties. Absorption is by dermal chromophores, which include most of those in the epidermis (with the possible exception of melanin) and also hemoglobin in its various states (e.g., oxygenated hemoglobin [HbO$_2$] and methemoglobin), as well as blood-borne chromophores such as bilirubin. Again, the net absorption at a given wavelength depends on the absorption coefficient and concentration of all chromophores present. Scattering is due to inhomogeneities in the skin's structure, such as molecules, organelles, cells, or larger tissue structures. The spatial distribution and intensity of scatter depends on the size and shape of the inhomogeneities compared with wavelength and the distribution of these inhomogeneities, which results in variations in refractive index (n). In the dermis, scattering has been shown to occur predominantly from inhomogeneities whose size is of the order of the wavelength or slightly larger (e.g., collagen fibers). It therefore appears to act as a turbid matrix in which scattering is an approximately inverse function of wavelength (shorter wavelength, greater scattering).

The main effect of scattering is to modify the region in which radiation is absorbed. In general, a greater degree of scatter results in a reduced *depth of penetration*. This is because on average a photon must have traveled further to reach a certain depth if it has undergone several scattering events beforehand; and because, all else being equal, the probability of being absorbed depends on distance traveled, increased scattering must result in reduced depth of penetration. *Depth of penetration* is a parameter similar to absorption length but that reflects the effects of both absorption and scatter. An increase in either results in a decrease in depth of penetration. It is defined as the average distance into the skin at which the intensity has fallen by a certain percentage (e.g., 50%). In addition, scattering alters the cross-sectional profile of the beam, producing a more homogeneous and diffuse beam across its cross-sectional diameter. When the spot size is large compared with the absorption length, the effect of scatter on the cross-sectional diameter is minimal; that is, there is insignificant deposition of energy outside the incident beam diameter. When the spot size is reduced to the absorption length or less, however,

scattering, if marked, can result in a significant amount of energy's being deposited outside the incident diameter, and the depth of penetration is also further reduced. Finally, a small but significant amount of backscattering occurs, which can contribute to losses and create a potential safety hazard.[27, 28, 30]

Laser–Tissue Interaction

In general, light incident on a surface undergoes *reflection, transmission, scattering, absorption,* or a combination.[1, 3, 6, 27–30] The interactions that occur (a function of the laser used, angle of incidence, and properties of the skin) determine the following:

1. The light leaving the tissue (reflection, scattering)
2. The irradiated volume (transmission, scattering, absorption)
3. The therapeutic effects (absorption)

Light Leaving the Tissue

When a laser beam is incident on the surface of the skin, a certain proportion of the radiation is reflected. This occurs because there is an abrupt change in refractive index at this interface: n = 1 for air and n = 1.55 for stratum corneum. The proportion reflected depends on the angle of incidence but is relatively independent of wavelength (250 nm to over 3000 nm) and skin type. It may be dependent on disrupting skin pathology, such as psoriasis, which increases reflection.[27] Some reflection is unavoidable, but it can be minimized by ensuring the angle of incidence is zero; that is, the beam should be at right angles to the skin surface. In this case, 5% to 10% of incident light is reflected.

Transmitted light is scattered or absorbed. Scattering in the dermis (and epidermis) is predominantly forward. However, a proportion is backscattered from smaller objects, and this contributes to radiation's leaving the tissue. Normally, about 10% to 20% of the incidence light leaves the skin unabsorbed, being reflected or backscattered. Such radiation serves no clinical use and in fact creates a significant safety hazard to the operator, patient, and others in the vicinity, as well as decreasing the dose available for therapeutic effect. All personnel in the treatment area should therefore be provided with appropriate protective eyewear, and access to the area must be controlled while the laser is in operation.[5, 14, 22, 31]

Irradiated Volume

The energy not reflected or backscattered is absorbed with or without scattering in a volume of tissue referred to here as the irradiated volume. The extent of this volume (depth of penetration, cross-sectional profile) and pattern of energy deposition within it are directly related to clinical effects. It is impossible to predict this information in detail, and in reality the pattern of energy distribution changes with subsequent conduction. Here we consider the irradiated volume produced by an instantaneous pulse of radiation before conduction occurs.[14, 27–30]

Below 300 nm (e.g., Excimer lasers), absorption is so great at typical concentrations of epidermal chromophores that almost all energy is deposited in the first few microns. With a penetration depth of microns, the entire irradiated volume lies within the stratum corneum/epidermis. The cross-sectional features of this volume reflect those of the incident beam (e.g., mode profile, irregularities). These features are modified, however, by the uneven nature of the skin's surface and by any scattering that occurs, both of which tend to cause diffusion of the beam's profile.

Between 320 and 1200 nm (e.g., argon, copper, ruby, alexandrite, dye, and Nd:YAG lasers), melanin is the principal absorbing chromophore of the epidermis. (Significant absorption by water begins with a small peak of absorbance around 950 nm.) Over this band, absorption by melanin decreases with increasing wavelength (see Fig. 1–8). At 1200 nm irrespective of skin type, over 90% of incident energy is transmitted across the epidermis, whereas at 400 nm only 50% is transmitted for fair-skinned individuals and 20% for dark-skinned individuals. Absorption in the epidermis can significantly alter the dose of radiation that reaches the dermis. In general, this dose depends on wavelength and skin type as well as incident intensity.

In the dermis, scattering occurs from collagen fibers as an inverse function of wavelength (increasing with decreasing wavelength). The major dermal chromophores include the hemoglobin derivatives, notably HbO_2. The absorption coefficient for HbO_2 decreases gradually over this range (320 to 1200 nm), but there are two or three peaks at which absorbance is significantly increased—418 and 542/577 nm (there is also a smaller broader peak around 900 nm; see Fig. 1–8).

Considering the effects of scattering and absorption in the dermis, combined with the absorption in the epidermis, it is apparent that the most penetrating wavelengths are in the range of 650 to 1200 nm, the red to near-infrared radiation (ruby, alexandrite, and Nd:YAG lasers). For these wavelengths, scattering is less than is seen at shorter wavelengths but may become important when spot size approaches absorption length (e.g., spot size approximately 3 mm for the Nd:YAG laser). From 320 to 650 nm, penetration gradually increases with wavelength. Because of the peaks in the HbO_2 absorption spectrum, however, this increase is not uniform and some sharp reductions in depth of penetration are seen around the peaks; for example, 535-nm radiation is more penetrating than that of wavelength 577 nm. The greater scattering at the shorter wavelengths produces more diffuse beam cross sections, but smaller spot sizes are possible before concerns over scatter outside the original beam diameter are necessary.

Above 1200 nm (e.g., holmium [Ho]:YAG, erbium:YAG, and CO_2 lasers), absorption by water becomes important, increasing steadily with increasing wavelength but being punctuated by prominent peaks in absorbance (see Fig. 1–8). The absorption occurs first in the epidermis and then in the dermis. The Ho:YAG (2140 nm) laser beam penetrates to the dermis and is significantly absorbed in both layers. Above 2500 nm, however, little if any radiation reaches the dermis. The CO_2 laser (10,600 nm) has a penetration depth of 20 μm and the whole irradiated volume therefore lies in the epidermis. Wavelengths corresponding to the peaks of absorbance are particularly rapidly absorbed, such as wavelength 2940 nm of the Er:YAG laser. This wavelength coincides precisely with the largest absorption peak of water and thus its depth of penetration is 0.5 to 1 μm! Scattering is present at all wavelengths, but its effects are minimal except in rare cases in which spot size approaches absorption length.

The irradiated volume can be altered by changing incident power density as well as by the effects mentioned above. In principle, the higher the incident power density, the greater the depth of penetration. The tissue and its absorption characteristics can be significantly altered, however, by being irradiated in a manner dependent on those very parameters. For example, above a certain power density, the superficial tissue may be ablated, removed, or desiccated. Thus, care must be exercised if one is attempting to alter the volume of irradiated tissue by increasing or decreasing incident power density, since unwanted effects on the tissue may result.

Therapeutic Effects

Absorption results in all of the therapeutic effects produced by a laser, either directly or indirectly (following conduction). It is important to appreciate, however, that the subsequent response of the tissue to these initial changes can also be important in determining the ultimate results seen clinically, particularly with pulsed lasers.[32–37]

Radiant energy is absorbed in a tissue by chromophores, which can be endogenous as described earlier, or exogenous, as a result of the pigments of amateur or professional tattoos or drugs or prodrugs used in photodynamic therapy. The absorption of photons by skin tissue occurs in a manner similar to what happens in the laser tube: a photon interacts with tissue and is absorbed, resulting in movement or separation of charge, with the energy of the photon being invested in the chromophore. The energy of the laser is thereby imparted to the tissue.[5, 6, 8, 14, 18, 22, 28–30, 32, 38]

These excitations ultimately manifest in several forms—photochemical reactions, heating, or mechanical damage. The energy of photons in the ultraviolet/visible bands is sufficient to excite the electron transitions responsible for chemical reactions (e.g., photosynthesis, carcinogenesis, vitamin D metabolism) and fluorescence. The use of photosensitizers in this waveband is commonplace (e.g., ultraviolet phototherapy with psoralens). Longer-wavelength photosensitizers (red and near-infrared) are being studied in photodynamic therapy of tumors. Excitations that do not result in a chemical reaction can decay with the release of energy in a variety of other ways. Notably, internal conversion of energy through thermal interactions (molecular, atomic, vibrational, or rotational states) results in heating and/or mechanical damage. Mechanical injury is seen when ultrarapid heating follows very high–peak power, short-duration exposures, such as occur with pulsed laser irradiation. The rate of heating is so great that tissue structures are torn apart by pressure waves, cavitation (expansion and collapse of a steam bubble), or rapid differential expansion.

Laser-induced heating occurs at any wavelength or photon energy and is the most important manner in which energy is imparted to the tissue. The effect of heating depends on the absolute temperature, duration of heating, and the rate of heating with mechanical injury. At elevated temperatures, typically between 40° and 90°C, proteins *denature,* that is, lose function as they physically unravel or deform (e.g., fibrillar type 1 collagen of the dermis denatures at 60° to 70°C). Thermal denaturing is a rate-dependent process in which higher temperatures increase the rate of denaturation. But at a given temperature, a certain duration of heating is required before denaturation occurs. For denaturation of most proteins, temperature must increase by 10° to 20°C for each decade decrease in heating time required. When large concentrations of denatured proteins are present, the process becomes irreversible and *coagulation* occurs. The same temperature–time combination governs coagulative thermal damage. The effects observed include cell necrosis, hemostasis, and distortion of the extracellular matrix over much of the irradiated volume. In essence, this laser-induced thermal coagulation injury represents a partial-thickness burn. As with any burn, it can result in scarring if it is marked or extensive.

Heating to temperatures above 100°C results in vaporization (boiling) or *ablation* of tissue. Ablative patterns of tissue damage vary between two extremes. At one end is *localized* ablation with minimal residual thermal damage (coagulation injury) or charring. At the other end, ablation is associated with an extensive area of desiccation or charring and marked residual thermal damage (i.e., poorly localized injury). The former pattern is achieved when sufficient energy is delivered to a superficial layer of tissue for a short period of time. "Sufficient energy" implies that enough energy is supplied to heat a significant proportion of the irradiated volume to boiling. The fluence required to achieve this is approximately proportional to the depth of penetration and is also related to tissue characteristics, such as specific heat capacity for water. Similarly, "short period of time" implies that the exposure time should be equal to or less than the *thermal relaxation time (Tr)* for the region concerned, which is the time it takes for a tissue to cool to 50% of its initial temperature, immediately after exposure. The magnitude of relaxation time is also related to the depth of penetration, squared (for nonselective absorption in a planar structure, such as a layer of irradiated skin). Estimates of relaxation time are $Tr = 325$ msec for pure water

and on the order of $Tr = 695$ msec for human skin. Under these conditions, a volume of tissue roughly equal to the spot size multiplied by the depth of penetration is rapidly vaporized (taking most of the generated heat away in the debris and steam). The remaining energy (sub–vaporization threshold radiant heating) and any energy conducted away from the irradiated volume result in a region of residual thermal damage, typically on the order of two to four times the depth of penetration. Because heating is brief, there is no desiccation or charring.[19, 23]

Such a pattern of highly localized ablation can be achieved with pulsed irradiation provided appropriate values for pulse width and fluence are chosen (e.g., CO_2 laser superpulsed at fluences of 5 J/cm^2 or more and pulse durations of 700 msec or less). It can also be achieved with CW lasers scanned across the tissue surface sufficiently fast so that the net exposure time at any given site is less than or equal to the relaxation time (provided the irradiance is sufficient to deliver the required energy during exposure). Using CW lasers is usually far less reliable, even with a skilled operator, unless the treatment area is scanned by machine (e.g., CO_2 laser or Sharplan SilkTouch flashscan device).

Any heating at supravaporization threshold levels (fluences and durations sufficient to produce temperatures above 100°C) results in ablation. When the duration of heating exceeds the relaxation time (or repeated heating occurs at a rate less than the relaxation time), however, heat accumulates in the irradiated area. The additional energy supplied is conducted away from the irradiated volume or causes vaporization in deeper layers. This results in desiccation of local tissues with subsequent carbonization and charring, which can interfere with healing. Furthermore, the charred layer, which does not evaporate, can be heated to temperatures in excess of 200°C, which significantly enhances the temperature gradient for conduction of energy to other sites. Conducted energy results in an extensive area of residual thermal damage (coagulation necrosis), which can increase the incidence of scarring. Not surprisingly, CW lasers typically result in this pattern of poorly localized ablation. For example, a CW CO_2 laser used to ablate tissues typically results in a layer of coagulation injury of about 1 mm as well as significant desiccation and charring of the treated area. Pulsed lasers can also cause a similar pattern of heating with certain parameters (e.g., high repetition rates or wide pulse widths).

In general, energy must be delivered at a therapeutic level to produce the desired heating and hence effect at all points within the treatment area. Uniform deposition of energy over a site in a manner that does not cause undue charring or excessive coagulation injury is the aim of laser therapy. This goal can be achieved by manipulating the energy delivery parameters (irradiance, fluence, spot size, repetition rate, and possibly operating distance) and by ensuring that the exposure time at all points within the treatment area is the same and appropriate. To achieve the latter, the clinician must have a good delivery technique, aided on occasion by intelligent delivery devices. Uniform energy delivery is typically easier with pulsed lasers than with CW lasers, since some pulsed lasers operate with pulse widths less than the thermal relaxation time.

Thus far, this description has been concerned primarily with nonspecific absorption. The tissue acts as a relatively homogeneous optical medium (with regard to its absorption characteristics). Energy is deposited throughout the irradiated volume in a reasonably uniform manner, being absorbed by many chromophores or in a ubiquitous chromophore (e.g., water). Good examples of lasers operating in this manner are the CW argon ion laser (absorbed in hemoglobin melanin) and the CW CO_2 laser (absorbed in water). The predominantly nonspecific absorption of these lasers accounts for their relative success in treating a wide variety of different lesions (e.g., vascular and pigmented lesions) and in surgery. However, it also explains many of their drawbacks, such as the high incidence of side effects seen, including scarring and unwanted pigmentary changes.[5, 6, 12, 13, 23, 24, 33, 39] Improved localization of absorption under these circumstances can be achieved but requires careful energy delivery, particularly by ensuring the exposure time is less than the thermal relaxation time (but not at the expense of sufficient energy delivery). A good example of a laser operating in this manner is the Ultrapulse CO_2 laser.[23]

Selective Photothermolysis

An increase in our understanding of and ability to manipulate the laser tissue interaction, coupled with advances in technology, has added greatly to the success of laser therapy. A particularly interesting and successful area of research and clinical application is embodied in the concept of selective photothermolysis first presented more than 10 years ago.[38] Selective photothermolysis involves the use of pulsed laser light and carefully selected delivery parameters chosen so that energy is absorbed by cellular or subcellular targets, which are selectively destroyed with minimal or no damage to any of the immediately adjacent or surrounding tissue. Several elements are necessary to achieve selective photothermolysis: (1) the presence of a unique structure to act as the target within the lesion to be treated, (2) a wavelength that reaches and is selectively absorbed within these targets, (3) an exposure duration less than the thermal relaxation time of the target (but greater than that of other similar but smaller targets), and (4) a fluence delivering sufficient energy over the exposure time to achieve the desired tissue effect within the targets.[5, 6, 10, 30, 32, 35, 36, 38]

Unlike the situation with nonspecific absorption, in which the tissue being treated behaves as a homogeneous medium, for effective selective photothermolysis inhomogeneities are necessary. It is these inhomogeneities that can be used as target sites. A knowledge of the site and distribution of inhomogeneities within the lesion to be treated allows a suitable target to be chosen. Targets that have been used include melanosomes in pigmented tissue,[14, 15, 17, 21, 34, 35] ectatic microvessels in vascular lesions,[16, 18, 32, 33, 36] and exogenous structures, such as pigment granules in tattoos[14, 15, 17, 21, 32] or photodynamic chemicals accumulated at a desired site.[6, 10, 12] An important property of suitable targets is that they are uniquely distinguishable from neighboring tissue by virtue of their higher absorption of a given wavelength. This property is conferred by the presence of a significantly higher concentration of a chromophore or a unique chromophore within the target itself. A suitable wavelength may then be chosen to coincide with a peak of absorption within such a chromophore. Theoretically, this results in a maximum differential absorption in the target structures compared with the surrounding tissue and potentially, therefore, causes their destruction without damaging adjacent poorly absorbing elements, provided energy spread by conduction can be kept to a minimum. The wavelength used must also have sufficient penetration depth to reach the desired targets; that is, its absorption and scattering must not be so great that insufficient energy remains at the depth of the targets. (As mentioned earlier, increasing the incident fluence or irradiance cannot always be used to increase the dose delivered to a given depth.)

Pulsed irradiation can be used to minimize spread of conducted energy. The ideal pulse duration is determined by the thermal relaxation time of the target: Pulse duration must be shorter than the thermal relaxation time for the target structure to ensure that energy is localized as far as possible within the site of absorption. Similarly, the interval between pulses must be greater than the relaxation time to avoid accumulation of energy in the targets when there is repeated irradiation of the same site. When the pulse duration is less than the relaxation time, the rate of energy delivery is greater than the rate of cooling in target structures during irradiation, which ensures the most selective target heating possible. The relaxation time depends on the size and shape of the target structure. In general, the thermal relaxation time of any structure is proportional to the square of its size. An approximate rule of thumb is that the relaxation time in seconds is equal to the square of the structure size in millimeters, for example, capillaries, diameter 5 μm, Tr = tens of microseconds; small venules, diameter 20 μm, Tr = hundreds of microseconds; large ectatic vessels of port-wine stains, diameter 0.1 mm, Tr up to 5 msec. Also, spherical targets (e.g., melanosomes) cool faster than cylinders (e.g., vessels), which cool faster than planes (e.g., tissue layers). Melanosomes are elliptical organelles (0.5 to 1 μm in length); the precise thermal relaxation time for melanosomes is not known but it is thought to be of the order of 250 to 1000 nsec.[38]

When duration of irradiation (pulse width) exceeds the thermal relaxation time, heating of target structures becomes inefficient. In this case, significant cooling occurs during the period of irradiation. Because thermal relaxation time increases rapidly with size of a structure, there exists the possibility for selecting only larger targets among a group of structures that are otherwise similar in shape and composition (e.g., selective damage to ectatic microvessels with sparing of capillaries). To achieve this, the pulse duration must be set just smaller than relaxation time for the larger target structures, which will be destroyed, but greater than thermal relaxation time for the smaller structures, which will be relatively spared. This approach has yet to be exploited.

The total energy delivered in a pulse depends on its fluence and duration (strictly the power profile with time). Pulse duration is limited by considerations of relaxation time. Fluence is therefore selected to ensure sufficient energy to produce the necessary heating and hence the required thermal damage. A variety of thermally mediated damage mechanisms are possible in selective photothermolysis, such as thermal denaturation and mechanical damage (e.g., cavitation). Several current models of laser–tissue interaction suggest that thermal injury is cumulative over time. If this is correct, it may be possible to use multiple lower fluence pulses, the cumulative effect of which is equally selective and gentler, and possibly may result in a more complete overall response. Again, this approach has yet to be explored.

Conclusion

The evolution of the laser as a medical instrument is a process of continual improvement and refinement. The ability to achieve the desired laser-induced therapeutic effect depends on optimizing intrinsic laser parameters— wavelength, energy delivery (including spot size and temporal mode), and duration and uniformity of exposure for each lesion. Continued evolution in this exciting area of dermatology is certain to provide even greater refinement and better results in an ever-enlarging number of cutaneous disorders.

REFERENCES

1. Ratz JL: Laser physics. Clin Dermatol 1995;13:11–20.
2. Nolan LJ: Laser physics and safety. Clin Podiatr Med Surg 1987;4(4): 26–31.
3. Absten GT: Physics of light and lasers. Obstet Gynaecol Clin North Am 1992;18:407–427.
4. Fuller TA: Physical considerations of surgical lasers. Obstet Gynaecol Clin North Am 1991;18:391–405.
5. Bailin PL, Ratz JL, Wheeland RG: Laser therapy of the skin: A review of principles and applications. Otolaryngol Clin North Am 1990;23: 123–164.
6. Parrish JA: Laser medicine and laser dermatology. J Dermatol 1990; 17:587–594.
7. Choy DSJ: History of lasers in medicine. Thorac Cardiovasc Surg 1988;36:114–117.
8. Viherkoski E: Lasers in medicine. Ann Chir Gynaecol 1990;79:176–181.
9. Groot DW, Johnson PA: Lasers and advanced dermatological instrumentation. Australas J Dermatol 1987;28:32–36.
10. Dover JS, Kilmer SL, Anderson RR: What's new in cutaneous laser surgery. J Dermatol Surg Oncol 1993;19:295–298.
11. Stellar S, Polanyi TG: Lasers in neurosurgery: A historical overview. J Clin Laser Med Surg 1992;10:399.
12. Garden JM, Geronemus RG: Dermatologic laser surgery. J Dermatol Surg Oncol 1990;16:156–168.
13. McDaniel DH: Cutaneous vascular disorders: Advances in laser treatment. Cutis 1990;45:339–360.
14. Stafford TJ, Tan OT: 510nm pulsed dye laser and alexandrite crystal laser for the treatment of pigmented lesions and tattoos. Clin Dermatol 1995;13:69–73.
15. Levins PC, Anderson RR: Q-switched ruby laser for the treatment of pigmented lesions and tattoos. Clin Dermatol 1995;13:75–79.
16. Lask GP, Glassberg E: 585nm pulsed dye laser for the treatment of cutaneous lesions. Clin Dermatol 1995;13:63–67.
17. Grekin RC, Shelton RM, Geisse JK: 510nm pigmented dye laser: Its characteristics and clinical uses. J Dermatol Surg Oncol 1993;19:380–387.
18. Key DJ: Argon pumped tunable dye laser for the treatment of cutaneous lesions. Clin Dermatol 1995;13:59–61.
19. Gloster HM, Roenigk RK: Carbon dioxide laser for the treatment of cutaneous lesions. Clin Dermatol 1995;13:25–33.
20. Geronemus RG: Argon laser for the treatment of cutaneous lesions. Clin Dermatol 1995;13:55–58.
21. Dinehart SM, Waner M, Flock S: The copper vapour laser for the treatment of cutaneous vascular and pigmented lesions. J Dermatol Surg Oncol 1993;19:370–375.
22. Reid R: Physical and surgical principles of laser surgery in the lower genital tract. Obstet Gynaecol Clin North Am 1991;18:429–474.
23. Fitzpatric RE, Goldman MP: Advances in carbon dioxide laser surgery. Clin Dermatol 1995;13:35–47.
24. McBurney EI: Clinical usefulness of the argon laser for the 1990s. J Dermatol Surg Oncol 1993;19:358–362.
25. Rotteleur G, Mordon S, Buys B: Robotized scanning laser hand piece for the treatment of port wine stains and other angiodysplasias. Lasers Surg Med 1988;8:283–287.
26. McDaniel DH: Clinical usefulness of the Hexascan. J Dermatol Surg Oncol 1993;19:312–319.
27. Anderson RR, Parrish JA: The optics of human skin. J Invest Dermatol 1981;77:13–19.
28. Hanina D, Landthaler M: Fundamentals of laser light interaction with human tissue especially in the cardiovascular system. Thorac Cardiovasc Surg 1988;36:118–125.
29. Wan S, Anderson RR, Parrish JA: Analytical modelling for the optical properties of the skin with in vitro and in vivo applications. Photochem Photobiol 1981;34:493–499.
30. Jacques SL, Prahl SA: Modelling optical and thermal distribution in tissue during laser irradiation. Lasers Surg Med 1987;6:494–503.
31. Dover JS: Laser safety in dermatology. Dermatol Q 1990;Fall/Winter:1–3.
32. Nelson JS: Selective photothermolysis and removal of cutaneous vasculopathies and tattoos by pulsed laser. Plastic Reconstr Surg 1991;88:723–731.
33. Tan OT, Carney JM, Margolis R, et al.: Histologic responses of port wine stains treated by argon, carbon dioxide, and tunable dye lasers. Arch Dermatol 1986;122:1016–1022.
34. Taylor CR, Anderson RR, Gange RW: Light and electron microscopic analysis of tattoos treated by Q-switched ruby laser. J Invest Dermatol 1991;97:131–136.
35. Margolis RJ, Dover JS, Polla LL, et al.: Visible action spectrum for melanin specific selective photothermolysis. Lasers Surg Med 1989; 9:389–397.
36. Tan OT, Murray S, Kurban AK: Action spectrum of vascular specific injury using pulsed irradiation. J Invest Dermatol 1989;92:868.
37. Dover JS, Margolis RJ, Polla LL: Pigmented guinea pig skin irradiated with Q-switched ruby laser pulses. Arch Dermatol 1989;125: 43–49.
38. Anderson RR, Parrish JA: Selective photothermolysis: Precise microsurgery by selective absorption of pulsed radiation. Science 1983;220: 524–527.
39. Olbricht SM, Sterm RS, Tang SV: Complications of cutaneous laser surgery: A survey. Arch Dermatol 1987;123:345–349.

2
LOW-ENERGY LASER SYSTEMS

Reza Babapour
Edward Glassberg
Gary P. Lask

Low-energy lasers, by definition, are capable of producing energy density so low that any biologic alterations are the result of direct irradiation (photochemical) effect and not of any thermal damage.[1] In this system, the temperature elevations are limited to less than 0.1° to 0.5°C.[2] Table 2–1 lists some of the available low-energy lasers.

Although low-energy lasers have been available for nearly three decades, their clinical importance has not been fully accepted. In spite of an abundance of basic science data on their biologic effects, clinical studies of low-energy lasers have been conducted under such a wide range of conditions that considerable confusion and controversy have been created. Studies range from rigorous basic science investigations to poorly controlled, incompletely documented animal and human trials. The notion that lasers stimulate the healing process, thus, the term "biostimulation," has gained much attention and prompted mechanistic investigation of various biologic effects of low-energy lasers.

More recently reported and better-documented effects of low-energy lasers include stimulation of collagen synthesis by fibroblasts in vitro and in vivo in various animal models, and increased tensile strength in irradiated healing wounds.[3–8]

Even though the recent studies were carefully controlled and better designed and involved well-defined parameters, much controversy still surrounds conclusions drawn about the biologic effects of low-energy lasers. These conflicts stem from a number of sources, including (1) availability of a number of different types of lasers (see Table 2–1), (2) a wide variety of often poorly specified variables used to determine total dose, and (3) utilization of different target cells and tissues for irradiation.

For the purposes of this chapter, a review of the available literature on the molecular and cellular level is presented first, as these areas have been thoroughly studied and the data have been fairly consistent. This is followed by a review of data on animal models and human trials on the effects on wound healing and modulation of the immune system.

Effects of Low-Energy Lasers on Cell Function

The effect of low-energy lasers on cell function and molecular alterations is perhaps the most developed and best understood area of investigation. As the biologic research of low-energy lasers was evolving, much of the early findings were suggestive of enhanced wound healing. These findings came from a series of studies, mainly from Eastern Europe.[9–15] Not surprisingly, therefore, much attention was paid to the investigation of the mechanisms of wound healing, and detailed study of biochemical and histologic alterations of irradiated tissue specimens. The outcome of these studies suggested that the enhanced wound healing effect of low-energy lasers was due primarily to increased collagen formation.[3, 4, 6, 12, 16, 17] Several studies have used animal models as well as cultured human skin fibroblasts to investigate the mechanism of increased collagen metabolism.

In one study, open skin wounds in rats were irradiated daily with a helium-neon (He-Ne) laser plus an argon laser at a constant power density of 45 mW/cm[2]. A statistically significant increase in collagen synthesis in the wounds (maximum effect at an energy density of 4 J/cm[2]) was observed on the 18th postoperative day.[6] In one in vivo study, experimentally induced wounds of hairless mice were exposed to He-Ne laser at a distance of 0.5 cm from the surface of the skin, providing a beam size of 0.385 cm[2] with corresponding irradiance of 4.05 mW/cm[2]. The wound areas were treated for 300 seconds every other day, resulting in an energy fluence of 1.22 J/cm[2]. Reported collagen concentrations in the wound tissue as measured by radioactive hydroxyproline assay were significantly increased at 2 and 4 weeks after the laser irradiation.[3]

In addition, tensile strength was significantly improved at 1 and 2 weeks after irradiation. The authors concluded that the He-Ne laser stimulated wound healing by enhancing collagen synthesis in the wound, which gave it greater tensile strength.[3]

In another study, fibroblasts of human skin were exposed to low-energy (He-Ne and gallium-arsenide [Ga-As]) laser

Table 2-1. Some Low-Energy Lasers and Their Corresponding Wavelengths

LASER	WAVELENGTH (nm)
Helium-neon (He-Ne)	632.8
Gallium-arsenide (Ga-As)	904
Ruby	694.3
Argon	488, 514.5
Gallium-aluminum-arsenide (Ga-Al-As)	660, 820, 870, 880

irradiation at various energy densities using once or twice daily exposures for several consecutive days.[17] In this study, procollagen production was enhanced by He-Ne laser irradiation, approximately four-fold on average. The greatest enhancement (36-fold) was reported in cultures that initially synthesized procollagen at a relatively low level; a less dramatic effect was noted in cultures that already actively synthesized procollagen.[17]

Based on these in vivo and in vitro studies, the investigators concluded that collagen metabolism plays a central role in low-energy laser-stimulated wound healing. The mechanism of increased collagen production by low-energy laser irradiation is not clearly understood at this time. Studies using He-Ne lasers at the same energy density, which caused marked stimulation of collagen synthesis, have shown no effect on cell proliferation as measured by incorporation into DNA of radioactive thymidine.[17] Furthermore, in the same experiments, Ga-As laser inhibited DNA replication. The investigators concluded that the enhanced collagen biosynthesis cannot be explained on the basis of cell proliferation. Additionally, under the same experimental conditions, no changes in the activities of collagenase and gelatinase, two proteolytic enzymes that control the degradative pathway of collagen metabolism, were detected after low-energy laser exposure.[17] These studies suggest that the increased collagen gene expression may reflect alterations on the transcriptional or translational level.[17]

Another study dealing with the mechanism of enhanced collagen production found that both type I and type III procollagen mRNA levels were markedly increased at days 17 and 28 in full-thickness cutaneous wounds on the backs of pigs treated with He-Ne laser.[5] In this study, type III procollagen mRNA levels increase as early as 10 days after irradiation, whereas at days 17 and 28, a concomitant increase in both type I and type III procollagen mRNA levels was noted. According to the investigators these observations suggest coordinate regulation of the expression of these two procollagen genes and that low-energy lasers may exert their effects on the transcriptional level of gene expression.[5]

Still another proposed mechanism involves posttranscriptional modification of propyl residues during collagen formation. In a study that used human skin fibroblast cultures irradiated with the gallium-aluminum-arsenide (Ga-Al-As) laser, hydroxyproline formation and ascorbic acid uptake by cells were significantly increased after irradiation. Since ascorbic acid serves as a co-factor in hydroxylation of proline, the investigators concluded that the increased uptake of ascorbic acid might stimulate collagen formation after laser treatment.[18]

Effects of Low-Energy Lasers on Wound Healing

As noted above, many of the earlier studies have prompted the observation that low-energy lasers can enhance wound healing. Indeed, wound healing was one of the first areas of low-energy laser investigation. These studies, however, were often ill-designed and lacked matched controls. Subsequent studies, however, concentrated on two different aspects of enhanced wound healing; namely, cell alteration and modification of immune response. The cellular and molecular alteration effects of low-energy lasers have already been discussed. To complete this discussion, different clinical observations after low-energy laser exposure as related to wound healing are reviewed. This is followed by a review of literature on modulation of the immune response after laser irradiation.

It was reported more than two decades ago that low-energy laser irradiation can significantly improve wound healing.[9, 10] Most early studies were conducted on experimentally induced wounds in various species of animals as well as in human skin ulcers.[11] Speculations about the mechanism of improved wound healing range from changes at the molecular level to improved metabolic function of wound tissue, increased collagen synthesis, enhanced cell proliferation, increased tensile strength, and improved proliferation phase of repair.

Accelerated wound healing was reported in one study involving experimentally induced wounds in mice and six cases of human skin ulcers.[10] Accelerated wound healing has also been reported in pigskin,[5] which is used as a model system for human skin because of its similar proportions, and in other species of animals, including rats,[6] mice,[4] and rabbits.[7]

Increased tensile strength was reported in experimentally induced wounds in rats after once daily exposure to He-Ne laser irradiation. The increase in tensile strength was demonstrable on the 5th day of exposure, and on the 8th day the increase was highly significant, but on the 12th day, the increase in tensile strength was reportedly closer to that in the control groups. This study also demonstrated an accelerated rate of wound healing.[12] Increased tensile strength was reported as well in experimentally wounded mice subjected to He-Ne laser irradiation every other day after 1 and 2 weeks' exposure.[4]

In another study, increased tensile strength was reported in skin wounds of rabbits irradiated daily with the He-Ne laser; however, no statistically significant difference was noted in the rates of wound closure or collagen area.[7] Although some investigators have proposed that increased collagen synthesis may contribute to increased tensile strength,[3] this later study suggests that other, as yet unknown, mechanisms might contribute to increased strength of wounds subjected to low-energy laser irradiation.

A recent study investigated the effects of neodymium: yttrium-aluminum-garnet (Nd:YAG) laser irradiation on wound healing in rat skin.[19] The clinical effects of the Nd:YAG laser at different energy parameters (low-energy: 1.75 W and 20 pulses per second [pps]; high-energy: 2.0 W and 30 pps) for a duration of 20 to 40 seconds in rat skin over a 28-day period were evaluated. The results were compared with control incisions made with the conventional scalpel. Immunohistochemical techniques were used to quantify the synthesis of collagen types I and III in the extracellular matrix. The results of this study indicate that low-energy laser treatment caused rapid wound healing without any clinically detectable scar tissue formation, as compared with a slower rate of wound healing in the high-energy laser–treated tissues. The laser-induced lesions reportedly healed through reparative synthesis of the matrix proteins, which led to filling of the tissue defects. According to the authors, the differences in the distribution of matrix proteins during the healing process and the coagulation of tissues exposed to low-energy laser irradiation may explain the minimal scarring, contraction, and pigment alterations in the laser-treated tissue as compared with that incised by conventional scalpel.[19]

The effect of low-energy lasers on human skin wounds has also been investigated. In one such study, accelerated wound healing of skin ulcers was reported in six human subjects after application of low-energy laser.[11] In another study, improvement of venous ulcers was reported in human subjects after exposure to low-energy laser irradiation.[20] These improvements reportedly ranged from complete healing to a significant reduction in ulcer size and increased granulation tissue.

In contrast to these beneficial effects, however, other studies of human subjects demonstrated no improvement in venous ulcers subjected to low-energy laser irradiation.[21, 22] In these studies, human subjects were exposed to the He-Ne or Ga-As laser twice weekly for 12 weeks. When the decrease in ulcer area over time was investigated, no significant difference was noted between the control and treated groups at any stage of the study.[21, 22] It should also be added that, in contrast to the animal studies mentioned earlier, which reported improved wound healing with lower-energy irradiation, other animal studies on rats and pigs did not confirm such beneficial effects.[23–25] The investigators have recommended that further studies be conducted to confirm the effectiveness or ineffectiveness of low-energy laser irradiation on wound healing. It would be of much interest to investigate not only the exposed dermal area but also the systemic effect of laser irradiation as related to wound healing. Until further studies are performed, the potential therapeutic effectiveness of low-energy laser on wound healing remains to be elucidated.

Effects of Low-Energy Lasers on the Immune System

In one early study of the effects of low-energy laser irradiation on wound healing in humans, it was noted that in one patient not only the irradiated ulcer wound healed but also similar lesions on the other parts of the body. It was assumed that laser treatment may improve wound healing by affecting certain systemic immune processes.[14]

To study the effect of low-energy lasers on the immune system, both humoral and cellular immunity were investigated. Alterations in serum complement activity and in immunoglobulin levels were reported in human subjects exposed to He-Ne laser irradiation.[14] When the immunosuppressive action of lasers was studied in directly irradiated human lymphocytes, it was found that the argon laser was more effective in the 488- to 501-nm range than was the He-Ne laser.[15]

Because lymphocytes are a known source of important mediators of wound repair, stimulation or inhibition of certain immune pathways might play an important role in the wound healing enhancement of low-energy lasers. In one in vitro study, cultured human lymphocytes were subjected to Ga-As laser irradiation at energy fluences of 2.17 to 651 mJ/cm^2, and cell proliferation was investigated by means of radioactive thymidine incorporation assay.[26] Marked inhibition of both mitogenic proliferation in response to phytohemagglutinin and spontaneous cell proliferation by the laser irradiation was reported at energy fluences as low as 10.85 mJ/cm^2. Furthermore, a decrease in the functional response of cells to antigen stimulation was also observed in a one-way mixed-lymphocyte reaction as a result of laser irradiation.[26] This in vitro study demonstrated that lower-energy laser irradiation can interface with the immune system, and the investigators speculated that similar in vivo immune modulation could possibly occur in humans exposed to laser irradiation.

Another study investigated the role of macrophages in accelerated wound healing after exposure to low-energy laser. In this study, the macrophage-like cell line U-937 was exposed to various wavelengths of light—660, 820, 870, and 880 nm. Twelve hours after exposure, the macrophage supernatant was removed and placed on mouse fibroblast cultures.[27] Fibroblast proliferation was then assessed over a 5-day period. The results of this study showed that exposure to 660-, 820-, and 870-nm wavelengths caused macrophages to release factors that stimulated fibroblast proliferation above the control levels. In contrast, the 880-nm wavelength either inhibited release of these factors or caused release of some inhibitory factors of fibroblast proliferation.[27] According to the investigators, the increase in fibroblast production can accelerate the proliferative phase of repair. Thus, at certain wavelengths, laser can be therapeutically useful by providing means for either stimulating or inhibiting fibroblast proliferation.[27]

Histologic studies of the rheumatoid synovial membrane

after low-energy irradiation also resulted in significant changes.[28] In one such study, patients with rheumatoid arthritis who were scheduled to undergo knee arthroplasty received multiple doses of low-energy laser irradiation before total knee replacement. The lateral aspect of the knee joint was irradiated with the Ga-Al-As laser (790-nm wavelength and 10 mW of output power) for a total of 8 minutes daily for 6 days. After total knee replacement, specimens of the synovial tissue were collected and studied for histologic changes. A decrease in inflammatory cell infiltrate and lymphoid follicles and alterations in synovial epithelial cells and small blood vessels were reported. The authors concluded that low-energy laser irradiation induced suppression of inflammation in synovial membrane involved by rheumatoid arthritis. This study is further evidence of the immunomodulatory potential of low-energy laser systems.[28]

Effects of Low-Energy Lasers on Skin Grafts

A study was conducted in which skin from inbred mice was allotransplanted to members of a genetically different mouse strain.[29] In this study the excised donor skin and the recipient graft bed on the backs of the animals were exposed to various doses of He-Ne laser irradiation (1 to 10 J/cm^2) immediately before transplantation. Additionally, in one of the experimental groups the animals were given immunosuppressive therapy with antithymocyte serum on days 2 and 5 after transplantation, and the combined effects of laser and immunosuppressive therapy were investigated. More than 50% necrosis in a transplant was considered rejection.

The results of this study showed that at certain doses laser treatment alone had a slight influence on survival, whereas antithymocyte serum much improved graft survival. When combined antithymocyte serum and laser treatment was applied, graft survival improved further. The investigators suggested that the combined application of immunosuppressive and laser treatments has a more marked graft-protective effect on mouse skin allotransplants.[29] Whether this beneficial effect can be extrapolated to human skin heterografts remains to be investigated, but it could provide a viable alternative when autograft donor skin is inadequate.

Summary

A review of the existing literature revealed an abundance of information on the biologic effects of low-energy lasers. Among the most extensive and best understood areas of investigation is the basic science data. The clinical studies of low-energy lasers, however, are generally less rigorous and often lack matched controls. This has aroused considerable controversy and skepticism. In general, the low-energy laser is thought to act through photochemical mechanisms, affecting cellular metabolic migratory and secretory wound-healing processes.[30]

Many of the studies of the clinical usefulness of low-energy lasers have led to the conclusion that lasers stimulate healing. The precise mechanisms of biostimulation of low-energy lasers, however, are not yet clear. Most studies in vitro and in vivo in various animal models have shown an increase in collagen synthesis by fibroblasts as well as an increase in tensile strength in irradiated healing wounds. Studies of the enhanced collagen synthesis suggest that low-energy lasers may be capable of altering collagen gene expression at the transcriptional, posttranscriptional, or translational level.

The effect of low-energy lasers on both humoral and cellular immunity has also been investigated. Some have speculated that stimulation or inhibition of certain immune pathways may play an important role in the enhanced wound-healing effect of low-energy lasers. The finding of macrophage-mediated increased fibroblast proliferation after laser irradiation has led some investigators to conclude that low-energy lasers may enhance wound healing by accelerating the proliferative phase of repair, whereas others' findings appear to contradict this assumption.

Most studies have reported the accelerated wound-healing effect of low-energy lasers, but others did not confirm such beneficial effect. More studies are thus needed to elucidate the potential therapeutic effectiveness of low-energy lasers on wound healing. In addition, because the previous investigations were conducted under such a wide range of conditions, it would be of great interest to develop an optimized and standardized condition for further studies.

REFERENCES

1. Babapour R, Glassberg E, Lask G: Low-energy laser systems. Clin Dermatol 1995;13:87.
2. Basford JR: Low-energy laser therapy: Controversies and new research findings. Lasers Surg Med 1989;9:1.
3. Abergel RA, Lyons RF, Castel JC, et al.: Biostimulation of wound healing by lasers: Experimental approaches in animal models and in fibroblast cultures. J Dermatol Surg Oncol 1987;13:127.
4. Lyons RF, Abergel RP, White RA, et al.: Biostimulation of wound healing in vivo and a helium-neon laser. Ann Plast Surg 1987;18:47.
5. Saperia D, Glassberg E, Lyons RF, et al.: Demonstration of elevated type I and III procollagen mRNA levels in cutaneous wounds treated with the helium-neon laser: Proposed mechanism for enhanced wound healing. Biochem Biophys Res Commun 1986;138:1123.
6. Kana JS, Hutschenreiter G, Haina D, Waidelich W: Effects of low-power density laser radiation on healing of open wounds in rats. Arch Surg 1984;116:293.
7. Braverman B, McCarthy RJ, Ivankovich AD, et al.: Effects of helium-neon and infrared laser irradiation on wound healing in rabbits. Lasers Surg Med 1989;9:50.
8. Enwemeka CS: Laser biostimulation of healing wounds: Specific effects and mechanisms of action. J Orthop Sports Phys Ther 1988;9:333.
9. Mester E, Spiry T, Szende B, Tota JG: Effect of laser rays on wound healing. Am J Surg 1971;122:532.

10. Mester E, Szende B, Spiry T, Scher A: Stimulation of wound healing by laser rays. Acta Chir Acad Sci Hung 1972;13:315.
11. Mester E, Korenyi B, Spiry T, et al.: Stimulation of wound healing by means of laser rays. Acta Chir Acad Sci Hung 1973;14:347.
12. Kovacs I, Mester E, Gorog P: Stimulation of wound healing by laser rays as estimated by means of rabbit ear chamber method. Acta Chir Acad Sci Hung 1974;15:427.
13. Mester E, Bacsy E, Spiry T, Tisza S: Laser stimulation of wound healing. Acta Chir Acad Sci Hung 1974;15:302.
14. Mester E, Nagylucskay S, Döklen A, Tisza S: Laser stimulation of wound healing. Acta Chir Acad Sci Hung 1976;17:49.
15. Mester E, Nagylucskay S, Tisza S, Mester A: Stimulation of wound healing by means of laser rays. Acta Chir Acad Sci Hung 1978; 19:163.
16. Abergel RP, Meeker CA, Lam TS, et al.: Control of connective tissue metabolism by lasers: Recent developments and future prospects. J Am Acad Dermatol 1984;11:1142.
17. Lam TS, Abergel RP, Meeker CA, et al.: Laser stimulation of collagen synthesis in human skin fibroblast cultures. Lasers Life Sci 1986;1:61.
18. Labbe RF, Skogerboe KJ, Davis HA, Rettmer RL: Laser photobioactivation mechanisms: In vitro studies using ascorbic acid uptake and hydroxyproline formation as biochemical markers of irradiation response. Lasers Surg Med 1990;10:201.
19. Romanos GE, Pelekanos S, Strub JR: Effects of Nd:YAG laser on wound healing processes: Clinical and immunohistochemical findings in rat skin. Lasers Surg Med 1995;16:368.
20. Sugrue ME, Carolan J, Leen EJ, et al.: The use of infrared laser therapy in the treatment of venous ulceration. Ann Vasc Surg 1990;4:179.
21. Malm M, Lundeberg T: Effect of low power gallium arsenide laser on healing of venous ulcers. Scand J Reconstr Hand Surg 1991;25:249.
22. Lundeberg T, Malm M: Low-power He-Ne laser treatment of venous leg ulcers. Ann Plast Surg 1991;27:537.
23. Hunter J, Leonard L, Wilson R, et al.: Effects of low energy on wound healing in a porcine model. Lasers Surg Med 1984;3:285.
24. Anneroth G, Hall G, Ryden H, Zetterquist L: The effect of low-energy infra-red laser radiation on wound healing in rats. Br J Oral Maxillofacial Surg 1988;26:12.
25. Smith RJ, Birndorf M, Gluck G, et al.: The effect of low-energy laser on skin-flap survival in the rat and porcine animal models. Plast Reconstr Surg 1992;89:306.
26. Ohta A, Abergel RP, Uitto J: Laser modulation of human immune system: Inhibition of lymphocyte proliferation by a gallium-arsenide laser at low energy. Lasers Surg Med 1987;7:199.
27. Young S, Bolton P, Dyson M, et al.: Macrophage responsiveness to light therapy. Lasers Surg Med 1989;9:497.
28. Amano A, Miyagi K, Azuma T, et al.: Histological studies on the rheumatoid synovial membrane irradiated with a low energy laser. Lasers Surg Med 1994;15:290.
29. Namenyi J, et al.: Effect of laser irradiation and immunosuppressive treatment on survival of mouse skin allotransplants. Acta Chir Acad Sci Hung 1975;16:327.
30. Hendrick DA, Meyers A: Wound healing after laser surgery. Otolaryngol Clin North Am 1995;28:969.

3

ANESTHESIA FOR CUTANEOUS LASER SURGERY

Bill Halmi
Richard H. Epstein
Gary P. Lask

Each passing year brings advances in the field of cutaneous surgery. As new lasers are developed, the spectrum of applications expands. The diversity of cutaneous laser procedures available today demands that laser surgeons be prepared to administer a variety of forms of anesthesia. How best to control intraoperative pain depends on many variables: type of laser, type and site of lesion, size of treatment area, and age of the patient. Various methods for providing analgesia and anesthesia during laser therapy for cutaneous lesions are reviewed. Special attention is paid to safety and to minimizing patient discomfort.

No Analgesia

Adults and some older children can tolerate a variety of laser procedures without analgesia. Treatment of telangiectasias with vascular-specific lasers (e.g., flashlamp-pumped pulsed dye, copper vapor, KTP) and of lentigos and café-au-lait macules with pigment-specific lasers (e.g., Q-switched ruby, Q-switched neodymium:yttrium-aluminum-garnet [Nd:YAG], Q-switched alexandrite) is most often done without analgesia. Similarly, port wine stains in adults and older children can be treated with vascular-specific lasers without anesthesia; although when an area near the eye is treated, topical or local infiltrative anesthesia is usually beneficial. Treatment of port wine stains in children requires special considerations, which are discussed later.

Topical Anesthesia

Cryoanesthesia is one of the oldest forms of topical anesthesia. Cold works on nerves in a similar fashion to local anesthetic agents, blocking pain fibers, then thermal fibers, and finally tactile fibers. Refrigerant sprays such as dichlorotetrafluoroethane (Frigiderm) provide rapid surface anesthesia; however, this effect lasts only a few seconds. This makes them impractical for most laser procedures that require topical anesthesia. Ice packs have the advantage of being inexpensive, readily available, and somewhat longer acting. Application of ice packs can be helpful in treating large port wine stains and tattoos with the Q-switched Nd:YAG and Q-switched alexandrite lasers. Treatment of tattoos with Q-switched laser systems tends to be quite painful. Some patients can tolerate that procedure with no anesthesia or with ice applications, but most prefer local infiltrative anesthesia or eutectic mixture of local anesthetics (EMLA) cream.

EMLA cream is a eutectic mixture of 2.5% lidocaine and 2.5% prilocaine.[1] Since prilocaine produces methemoglobinemia, it is contraindicated for infants younger than one month, because of the reduced activity of neonatal erythrocyte methemoglobin reductase.[2] Proper application is crucial to maximizing the effectiveness of EMLA. The cream must be applied thickly for 60 to 90 minutes. Occlusion can be used when feasible. Reapplication every 15 to 30 minutes to maintain a thick cover is crucial. EMLA can be used successfully to treat port wine stains in children,[3,4] but there is certainly much interpatient and intertreatment variability. The analgesia provided by EMLA is usually nonuniform and variable in intensity. Added to this, the bright flash of the laser, the need to cover the child's eyes, and the child's general anxiety can lead to a disconcerting experience for the patient, the parents, and the physician. In our experience, successful use of EMLA in the treatment of port wine stains has been restricted to adolescents and adults. Only a small number of children younger than 10 years have been able to tolerate their treatments using only EMLA.

Like ice application, EMLA can be helpful in treating tattoos using any of the Q-switched laser systems. EMLA can also be used to provide anesthesia for resurfacing cases using a superpulsed or scanned carbon dioxide (CO_2) laser. With proper application, small regions such as the periorbital or perioral area can be treated. Again, the variable effects of EMLA may necessitate addition of local infiltrative anesthesia or regional blocks for some patients. The efficacy of EMLA can be improved with the addition of an oral sedative (e.g., diazepam) or an oral narcotic (e.g., oxycodone). Iontophoresis of lidocaine has been shown to have efficacy similar to that of EMLA.[5, 6] In addition to being expensive, iontophoresis has the disadvantage of being able to anesthetize only small areas.

Infiltrative Anesthesia

Infiltrative anesthesia is the most common way to anesthetize skin. The anesthetic agent is administered intradermally or subcutaneously at the surgical site. Lidocaine provides rapid onset of anesthesia that lasts 30 to 120 minutes. Because it is an amide anesthetic, it carries far less risk of an allergic reaction than the ester types of anesthetics. These properties make lidocaine the most commonly used anesthetic for routine cutaneous surgical procedures. Lidocaine is a very safe drug, but it is important that recommended dosing guidelines not be exceeded. For adults, this is 4.5 mg/kg; for children, 3 to 4 mg/kg.[7] Adding epinephrine (1:100,000) minimizes systemic absorption and allows more anesthetic to be infiltrated safely. For adults, 7 mg of lidocaine with epinephrine can safely be injected. Techniques to minimize the pain of local anesthetic infiltration include using a 30-gauge needle, slow injection,[8] and buffering the local anesthetic with 8.4% sodium bicarbonate solution at a 1:10 dilution.[9] For procedures that may take a long time, long-acting anesthetic agents such as bupivacaine are preferred.

Nerve Blocks

A peripheral nerve block can be produced by infiltrating local anesthetic along a nerve trunk that contains many nerve fibers.[10] A successful nerve block produces anesthesia along the distribution of that nerve. This has the advantage of anesthetizing large areas of skin with a small amount of anesthetic, which can reduce the risk of anesthetic toxicity and is certainly less painful than locally infiltrating a large area. At times, successful nerve block is difficult to achieve. Often, local infiltration must be added. It is important for the physician to have a good understanding of how to perform nerve blocks, to maximize efficacy and safety.[11, 12]

Oral Sedation

The fearfulness of children and their low threshold for pain make laser treatment very difficult. For pediatric patients who are anxious or unable to cooperate, oral sedatives sometimes facilitate treatment. Infants and small children may be sedated with chloral hydrate (50 to 100 mg/kg), a technique that has been quite successful in allowing completion of magnetic resonance imaging in this age group[13, 14]; however, it should be kept in mind this diagnostic procedure is not painful. Although chloral hydrate may allow the children to be restrained more easily, it provides no analgesia. In our experience, we have not found chloral hydrate to be particularly helpful.

Current standards hold that sedation of pediatric patients be accompanied by cardiorespiratory monitoring (e.g., pulse oximetry). Children should be attended by someone trained in cardiopulmonary resuscitation until they are fully recovered.[15] This person should not be the one who administers the treatment, as it is not possible to monitor the patient adequately and perform the surgery at the same time.

Oral sedation with 0.5 mg/kg midazolam[16] can also make it easier to restrain small children during treatment. The bitter taste of the midazolam must be disguised with a strong, sweet flavor (e.g., chocolate-cherry syrup, simple syrup, cola syrup). Generally, a small volume is used, and the patient should be encouraged to take the entire dose at once. Onset occurs within 15 minutes, and sedation is maximal at about 30 minutes.[15] Although rare, oversedation or serious respiratory complications can be associated with oral midazolam in children. Thus, personnel trained to deal with such problems must be present and appropriate monitoring provided when such sedation is used. Like chloral hydrate, midazolam has no analgesic properties.

Alternative methods of sedative and analgesic delivery include the intramuscular route (e.g., midazolam, ketamine, narcotics), the intranasal route (e.g., ketamine, midazolam), and the rectal route (e.g., methohexital). As drug absorption from these sites can be quite rapid, careful observation and monitoring are necessary when these modes are used. An anesthesiologist should be consulted when such administration is being considered.

Anxious adults may be treated with 5 to 10 mg of oral diazepam or another anxiolytic drug. This can be particularly helpful for CO_2 laser resurfacing that relies on EMLA, local infiltration, or nerve blocks as an anesthetic. A pretreatment dose of oral narcotic analgesic may also be considered, to lessen the discomfort of treatment. An adequate interval (30 to 45 minutes) should be allowed for the medication to take effect. If a narcotic or a sedation is given, it is imperative that someone drive the patient home after the treatment, because full recovery of motor and cognitive function after sedation takes more than 3 hours.[17]

Intravenous Sedation

For laser cases when the stimulus is quite painful (e.g., CO_2 laser for adults, virtually all lasers for children) and the size and site of the lesion preclude comfortably anesthetizing the area by topical or local infiltration alone, intravenous sedation is another possibility. We have generally used fentanyl (a potent synthetic narcotic) and midazolam (a benzodiazepine tranquilizer) for this purpose. It must, however, be kept in mind that these drugs are extremely potent—and potentially lethal when administered by persons inexperienced in their use. A number of deaths associated with use of these or similar medications by medical endoscopists during diagnostic procedures have been reported.[18] We recommend strongly that, when such therapy is contemplated, an anesthesiologist be consulted to provide appropriate monitoring and expertise in administration of the drugs. Administration of such intravenous sedation in a physician's office without the services of an anesthesiologist or anesthetist is strongly discouraged.

General Anesthesia

Pediatric patients may require general anesthesia for treatment of cutaneous vascular lesions, particularly port wine stains. Because of the location of these lesions (e.g., frequently on the face), their size, the need for multiple treatment sessions, and the emotional immaturity of the patients, often there is no alternative to general anesthesia. The extremely small but real risk of general anesthesia must be weighed carefully against the potential harm of having the lesion go untreated until such time as it can be eliminated without general anesthesia. The parents of all of our patients who have opted for general anesthesia after the initial treatment of their children with EMLA much preferred the treatments under anesthesia.

Because of the psychological impact of port wine stains, it has been recommended that they be treated as early as possible.[19] Treatment during infancy is safe,[20] and early treatment is associated with quicker and more complete clearing of lesions.[21] In our practice, generally we have not had to provide general anesthesia for children until age 6 months to a year. Before this age, use of EMLA and immobilization are usually successful. Thus, starting treatment as early as possible may diminish the need to be anesthetized for the treatments or, at least, may decrease the number of anesthetics required.

We recommend that such anesthesia be administered by persons with particular experience and expertise in pediatric anesthesia. Because multiple treatments are usually required, a consistent, individualized anesthetic technique is strongly recommended. The goal is a method that allows the child to awaken quickly with minimal discomfort and to be ready for home discharge in a short time with minimal residual side effects from the anesthetic. Once we establish the technique for a given child, the patient receives the same anesthetic each time unless circumstances indicate the need to change. We have found intraoperative ketorolac, 0.5–1.0 mg/kg into the muscle, to be particularly effective in minimizing the discomfort that some children experience after they awaken from anesthesia. An ice pack applied to the treatment area is usually the only additional treatment required. We have rarely had to administer narcotics for pain control.

Parents are allowed to be present during induction of anesthesia; they leave the room as soon as the child loses consciousness and are not present during the actual laser treatment. The parents are allowed to return when the child is taken to the recovery room; most of the time, the parents are there when the child regains consciousness. The parents' presence has been very useful in helping the children cope with the stress of repeated treatments.

If general anesthesia is provided for laser treatment of cutaneous lesions, special attention must be paid to minimizing the risk of fire. Although the tunable dye laser does not ignite hair in room air at energies in the clinical range, hair can be ignited in the presence of supplemental oxygen or nitrous oxide when struck by the laser.[22] This risk is increased when the patient has dark hair, which absorbs a greater percentage of the laser energy than does light-colored hair. The chance of fire can be minimized by wetting the hair and avoiding spillage of oxygen or nitrous oxide into the laser field. Flammable prep solutions should not be applied to the skin. When mask anesthesia is provided, oxygen frequently leaks around the mask. Thus, we now strongly discourage administering general anesthesia by mask during laser treatment of facial lesions.

Alternatives to mask anesthesia include tracheal intubation and use of a relatively new airway device called a laryngeal mask airway (LMA) (Fig. 3–1). The mask fits inside the patient's mouth, where it forms a low-pressure seal around the larynx. It is placed after anesthesia is induced. Because of the usually brief duration of each laser treatment, our desire to minimize the invasiveness and complexity of the anesthetic, and the fact that properly sized uncuffed pediatric endotracheal tubes often leak oxygen during positive-pressure ventilation, we have chosen to use LMA rather than to intubate our patients. This allows for uninterrupted treatment of facial lesions. As long as the patient breathes spontaneously, the LMA prevents leakage of oxygen from the mouth in more than 95% of cases.[23] We discontinue the anesthetic drugs and remove the LMA at the conclusion of the laser treatment; patients are usually ready to be taken to the recovery room several minutes later. The LMA is readily available and should be familiar to pediatric anesthesiologists.

General anesthesia is also used in some cases of full face resurfacing with the CO_2 laser. Again, the combination of the CO_2 laser beam and flammable gases leads to substantial risk of fire. The LMA is of much benefit for adults as well.

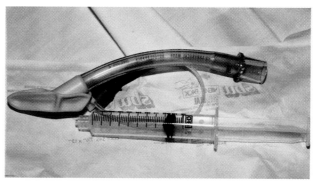

Figure 3–1. Laser treatment of a port wine stain with the laryngeal mask airway (LMA). Being atraumatic, LMA treatment is ideal for laser cases that involve the face. These are performed using general anesthesia.

It is an atraumatic way to maintain an airway that has a very low potential for leaking flammable gases such as oxygen.

Conclusions

In performing any laser procedure, the physician not only must select the most appropriate laser parameters; he or she has to select the most appropriate form of anesthesia. Topical anesthesia using EMLA, ice, or lidocaine delivered by iontophoresis, specific nerve blocks or regional infiltration with local anesthetics, oral sedatives and analgesics, intravenous sedation or analgesia, and general anesthesia may at times be required, depending on the individual needs of the patient. Consultation with an anesthesiologist is recommended to help devise treatment plans for patients who may require more intensive analgesia or sedation than the laser surgeon feels comfortable providing.

REFERENCES

1. Lycka BA: EMLA: A new and effective topical anesthetic. J Dermatol Surg Oncol 1992; 18:859–862.
2. Nilsson A, Engberg G, Henneberg S, et al.: Inverse relationships betweem age-dependent erythrocyte activity of methaemoglobin reductase and prilocaine-induced methaemoglobinaemia during infancy. Br J Anaesth 1990; 64:72–76.
3. Sherwood KA: The use of topical anesthesia in removal of port-wine stains in children. J Pediatr 1993;122:S36–S40.
4. Ashinoff R, Geronemus RG: Effect of the topical anesthetic EMLA on the efficacy of pulsed dye laser treatment of port-wine stains. J Dermatol Surg Oncol 1990; 16:1008–1011.
5. Greenbaum SS, Bernstein EF: Comparison of iontophoresis of lidocaine with a eutectic mixture of lidocaine and prilocaine (ELMA) for topically administered local anesthesia. J Dermatol Surg Oncol 1994; 20:579–583.
6. Bridenstine JB, Olbricht S, Winton GB, et al.: Guidelines for care of local and regional anesthesia in cutaneous surgery. J Am Acad Dermatol 1995; 33:504–509.
7. Maloney JM, Bezzant JL, Stephen RL, Petelenz TJ: Iontophoretic administration of lidocaine anesthesia in office practice. An appraisal. J Dermatol Surg Oncol 1992; 18:937–940.
8. Arndt KA, Burton C, Noe JM: Minimizing the pain of local anesthesia. Plast Reconstr Surg 1983; 72:676–679.
9. Martin AJ: pH-Adjustment and discomfort caused by the intradermal injection of lignocaine. Anaesthesia 1990; 45:975–978.
10. Murphy TM: Somatic blockade of the head and neck. In Cousins MJ, Bridenbaugh PL (eds.): Neural Blockade in Clinical Anesthesia and Management of Pain. Philadelphia: JB Lippincott, 1988.
11. Auletta MJ, Grekin RC: Local Anesthesia for Dermatologic Surgery. New York: Churchill Livingstone, 1991.
12. Carron H, Korbon GA, Rowlingson JC: Regional Anesthesia: Techniques and Clinical Applications. New York: Grune & Stratton, 1984.
13. Greenberg SB, Faerber EN, Aspinall CL, Adams RC: High dose of chloral hydrate for children undergoing MR imaging: Safety and efficacy in relation to age. AJR 1993; 161:639–641.
14. Ronchera CL, Marti-Bonmatí L, Poyatos C, et al.: Administration of oral chloral hydrate to paediatric patients undergoing magnetic resonance imaging. Pharm Weekbl Sci 1992; 14:349–352.
15. Cook BA, Bass JW, Nomizu S, Alexander ME: Sedation of children for technical procedures: Current standard of practice. Clin Pediatr 1992; 31:137–142.
16. McMillan CO, Spahr-Schopfer IA, Sikicj N, et al.: Premedication of children with oral midazolam. Can J Anaesth 1992; 39:545–550.
17. Gale GD: Recovery from methohexitone, halothane and diazepam. Br J Anaesth 1976; 48:691–698.
18. Daneshmend TK, Bell GD, Logan RF: Sedation for upper gastrointestinal endoscopy: Results of a nationwide survey. Gut 1991; 32:12–15.
19. Wagner KD, Wagner RF Jr: The necessity for treatment of childhood port-wine stains. Cutis 1990; 45:317–318.
20. Ashinoff R, Geronemus RG: Flashlamp-pumped pulsed dye laser for port-wine stains in infancy: Earlier versus later treatment. J Am Acad Dermatol 1991; 24:467–472.
21. Goldman MP, Fitzpatrick RE, Ruiz-Esparza J: Treatment of port-wine stains (capillary malformation) with the flash-lamp–pumped pulsed dye laser. J Pediatr 1993; 122:71–77.
22. Epstein RH, Brummett RR Jr, Lask GP: Incendiary potential of the flash-lamp pumped 585-nm tunable dye laser. Anesth Analg 1990; 71:171–175.
23. Epstein RH, Halmi B: Oxygen leakage around the laryngeal mask airway during laser treatment of port-wine stains in children. Anesth Analg 1994; 78:486–489.

4

BENIGN CUTANEOUS LESIONS

Kathleen Behr
Vladislav Chizhevsky
Nicholas J. Lowe
Gary P. Lask

The range of cutaneous lesions amenable to laser therapy is vast and continues to expand as laser technology advances. In this chapter, we focus on benign cutaneous lesions that have been reported to be treated effectively by cutaneous laser systems. For lesions for which the laser system is the treatment of choice, treatment is described in more detail. Other applications that are based on investigational or anecdotal reports are mentioned briefly to make the list as complete as possible, but further investigation may be necessary before determining whether laser is the treatment of choice.

The large category of benign cutaneous lesions can be divided into the following categories: "appendageal" tumors, nonmelanocytic nevi, hyperplasias, cystic lesions, infectious lesions, inflammatory lesions, and ulcerations. Lesions that have been treated by laser therapy in each of these categories are listed in Table 4–1. The largest percentage of these lesions have been treated by the carbon dioxide (CO_2) laser.

Carbon Dioxide Laser

The CO_2 laser has been used to treat a wide variety of benign cutaneous lesions. The physics of laser therapy have been discussed in detail in earlier chapters and will not be repeated here. Briefly, the CO_2 laser emits far infrared radiation at 10,600 nm, and the chromophore of absorption for the CO_2 laser is water. The laser energy is superficially absorbed by tissue water, which limits penetration of the laser to a depth of 0.1 to 0.2 mm with minimal scatter. This superficial penetration explains why benign lesions in the epidermis or superficial dermis are treated most effectively.

Compared with other forms of therapy involving thermal destruction such as cryosurgery and electrodesiccation, in experienced hands the continuous-wave CO_2 laser can produce a more limited area of tissue damage (peripheral damage limited to 50 to 100 μm).[1] The newer CO_2 lasers that produce greater peak powers with shorter pulses allow maximal vaporization with minimal diffusion of energy to adjacent tissues.[2] Many of the lesions that were reported to be amenable to therapy with the older continuous-wave CO_2 laser, with variable results due to side effects such as pigment changes and scarring, may be treated more effectively and with less risk with the higher–peak power, shorter–exposure time CO_2 systems.

The lesions for which the CO_2 laser offers distinct advantages and may be considered the treatment of choice are covered next.

Refractory Warts

In recent years CO_2 laser therapy was the treatment of choice for refractory warts, especially plantar and periungual warts and condyloma. Given recent reports of efficacy of the pulsed dye laser (PDL), this may no longer be the case. For plantar and periungual verrucae that resist electrodesiccation and curettage, cryotherapy, and salicylic acid therapy, 6-month cure rates as high as 80% to 95% have been reported with the CO_2 laser.[3] There have also been reports of lower cure rates with the CO_2 laser and of results no better than those of electrocautery. Obviously, the results are extremely operator dependent with either modality. Other authors who reported comparisons among the continuous-wave CO_2, the superpulsed CO_2, and the ultrapulsed CO_2 lasers found increasing cure rates—68%, 68%, and 90%—with decreased incidence of scarring—54%, 33%, and 7%, respectively—as more precise control of thermal damage was achieved.[4] The limited penetration of ultrapulsed laser increases the treatment time, as more pulses are required.

Therapy begins with paring of dry, hyperkeratotic tissue. Such tissue has low water content and would require higher energy levels to vaporize, which would result in a heat sink with thermal diffusion to surrounding tissue and increased risk of scarring. A margin of 0.5 to 1.0 cm is drawn around the wart, as the papillomavirus can lie latent in this tissue and could produce recurrence (a ring wart) if it is not vaporized.[5] Local anesthesia is usually required with local

Table 4–1. Lesions Amenable to Laser Therapy

Appendageal lesions
  Adenoma sebaceum
  Pearly penile papule
  Trichoepithelioma
  Tricholemmoma
  Syringoma
  Neurofibroma
  Seborrheic keratosis
Nonmelanocytic nevi
  Collagenoma
  Elastoma
  Epidermal nevus
Hyperplasias and hamartomas
  Keloid
  Sebaceous hyperplasia
  Xanthelasma
  Plantar keratoderma
  Chondrodermatitis nodularis chronica helicis
  Pyogenic granuloma
  Lymphangioma circumscriptum
Cystic lesions
  Milia
  Digital mucous cyst
  Apocrine hydrocystoma
Infectious lesions
  Verrucae
Inflammatory lesions
  Hidradenitis
  Hailey-Hailey disease
  Lichen planus
  Lichen sclerosus
  Zoon's balanitis
Ulcerations

infiltration or nerve blocks, depending on the site. The CO_2 laser is then passed over the affected and marked tissue. After one to three passes, a cleavage plane forms at the dermoepidermal junction.[6] This tissue is then removed with scissors, curette, or scalpel. Helpful signs of tissue with residual papillomavirus are opalescent bubbling and residual bleeding points. Healthy tissue tends to show contraction of dermatoglyphs or fingerprint lines with more passes of the laser. It must be remembered that these signs are helpful but not completely reliable. The wart tissue should be wiped with saline-soaked gauze or curette and any residual wart vaporized until there is a uniform appearance to the base of the lesion. The wound is then dressed with antibiotic ointment and Telfa or Duoderm. Wound healing occurs by secondary intention in 3 to 6 weeks.

It is necessary to take precautions when using the CO_2 laser to treat verrucae. Several studies have demonstrated human papillomavirus in the laser plume.[7, 8] These studies raise serious questions about the risk of transmission of the virus to the laser team. Thus, the most important precaution is use of a smoke evacuator with the nozzle held within 1 cm of the treatment site, which removes 99% of plume particulate matter.[9, 10] Surgical masks, gloves, and eye protection further minimize risk of viral particle exposure and spread.

Rhinophyma

Rhinophyma consists of large nodular masses on the nose formed from fibrous tissue, overgrown sebaceous glands, and dilated hair follicles. Treatment with the CO_2 laser affords precise tissue removal and contouring with excellent hemostasis and minimal thermal conduction,[11, 12] all definitive advantages over other established therapies. With dermabrasion, hemostasis and evaluation of desired depth are difficult; sculpting with a scalpel leads to poor visualization secondary to bleeding; and electrosurgical destruction can lead to a large amount of thermal conduction, which can result in significant scarring.[13–22] The older continuous-wave CO_2 laser also carries a definite risk of scarring secondary to heat conduction.[23] This should be decreased with the higher–peak power, shorter–exposure time CO_2 laser systems; however, the small amount of ablation per pass may make these systems impractical for use alone in thick rhinophymas.

Therapy includes anesthesia, with both a topical cream, such as eutectic mixture of local anesthetic (EMLA), and local infiltration with lidocaine. For mild to moderate rhinophyma, the CO_2 laser set on a small spot size is used over the protuberances. This is followed by multiple passes over the entire surface with a large spot size or scanner pattern. For severe rhinophyma the excisional mode may be necessary to remove large protuberances before the entire area is treated with the vaporization mode.[22, 24–28] Continued extrusion of sebum upon squeezing indicates that vaporization has not extended below the sebaceous glands, which could result in scarring.[29] Care is similar to resurfacing for photoaging and includes applications of Crisco or petrolatum for 1 to 2 weeks while reepithelization takes place.

Epidermal Nevi

Effective therapy for epidermal nevi was difficult in the past, before the use of the CO_2 laser.[30–32] If only the epidermal component was treated, as with dermabrasion, lesions often recurred, but when they were treated more aggressively scarring often resulted. Excision left unsightly scars and was often difficult because of the size and configuration of the lesions. With the ultrapulsed CO_2 laser, authors have reported improved results over the continuous-wave CO_2 laser and other methods.[33] They caution that it is still necessary to pay close attention to the level of vaporization, as ablation below the rete ridges is necessary to decrease the chance of recurrence but too deep vaporization is associated with scarring. The higher–peak power, shorter–exposure time CO_2 laser systems offer precision not available with other techniques, but there is still a fine line between resolution of the lesions with excellent results and the side effect of scarring.

Seborrheic Keratoses

Removal of thick and large seborrheic keratoses has been reported to be very successful with the CO_2 laser.[34] In one study using the continuous-wave CO_2 or superpulsed CO_2 laser, all lesions were ablated in one treatment, but 25% of the patients had at least an atrophic scar. When the ultra-pulsed CO_2 laser was used, no scarring or pigment changes were seen, as the thermal damage was more localized to the targeted lesion.[35] These results are encouraging but need further study to verify, as they are very operator dependent. This offers a distinct advantage over cryosurgery, which often leaves hypopigmented scars, especially if thick lesions are treated. Surgical removal with a scalpel or curette is also effective but usually requires injection of local anesthesia. With the newer CO_2 lasers, treatment, as with scalpel or curette, can be performed with topical EMLA if it is applied 1 to 2 hours before the treatment, and multiple lesions can be treated rapidly.

Angiofibromatous and Angiolymphoid Lesions

Such lesions as adenoma sebaceum,[36] angiokeratoma, pyogenic granuloma, and lymphangioma circumscriptum[37-39] are also treated successfully with the argon laser, but owing to their significant fibrous component they are removed more completely with the CO_2 laser. With the less thermally damaging higher–peak power, shorter–exposure time CO_2 laser systems, more selective tissue vaporization should decrease the risk of scarring. For lymphangioma circumscriptum the CO_2 laser is beneficial, as it can seal the lymphatics that often lead to persistent drainage. One should still evaluate the depth of these lesions with other imaging studies before treatment, because aggressive or multiple treatments with the CO_2 laser can still result in scarring. Lesions for which the CO_2 laser is useful and may have a clinical advantage are discussed next.

Benign Dermal Lesions

The CO_2 laser is useful for removing many benign superficial dermal tumors, although many other surgical techniques are also available. Benign dermal tumors reported to have been successfully ablated with the continuous-wave and superpulsed CO_2 lasers include apocrine hidrocystoma, adenoma sebaceum,[40, 41] chondrodermatitis nodularis chronica helicis,[42, 43] collagenoma,[44, 45] elastoma,[44, 45] granuloma faciale,[46] neurofibroma,[47] milia,[44, 45] myxoid cyst,[44, 45] sebaceous hyperplasia, syringoma (Fig. 4–1),[44, 45] trichoepithelioma,[48] tricholemmoma,[51] and xanthelasma.[52, 53] A more recent case report using a higher–peak power and shorter–exposure time CO_2 laser for ablation of xanthelasma showed less scarring and textural change and more complete eradication of the lesions, owing to the enhanced precision of tissue evaporation over the older CO_2 systems.[54] Regardless of which CO_2 laser is used, treatment to a certain depth is necessary to remove lesions, and this can result in pigment loss and textural changes.

Inflammatory Conditions That Respond to Carbon Dioxide Laser Therapy

Several inflammatory conditions including Darier's disease,[55] hidradenitis, Hailey-Hailey disease,[55, 56] lichen planus,[57] lichen sclerosus,[58, 60] and Zoon's balanitis[61] have been treated successfully with the CO_2 laser. Many of these lesions are superficial and are on "intertriginous areas," including the axilla and groin, which gives the CO_2 laser an advantage over other surgical techniques.

Ulcers

European studies have shown that chronic ulcers can be carefully débrided and sterilized by CO_2 and neodymium: yttrium-aluminum-garnet (Nd:YAG) laser systems, which then enhances the healing process.[62, 63]

Pulsed Dye Laser at 585 nm

The PDL is pulsed at 450 μsec with a wavelength of 585 nm, which makes the primary target chromophore hemoglobin.[64] This high energy and short pulse duration impart the capacity to destroy target blood vessels with high specificity and with minimal damage to the epidermis and surrounding structures, which results in a very low incidence of scarring.[65-69] Those lesions considered primarily vascular are discussed in another chapter, and only benign lesions that are not primarily vascular but have a significant vascular component are discussed. This includes verruca vulgaris, verruca plana, keloids, angiofibromas, and acne rosacea.

Verrucae

Verrucae are induced by the human papillomavirus and have an incidence of about 10%.[70] Many methods of destruction have been used successfully to destroy virally infected tissue. Because there are still a number of refractory cases with the current methods, new therapies are continually tested. Tan and coworkers reported successful treatment of recalcitrant verrucae with the PDL.[71] The theory of using the PDL for verrucae involves a characteristic histologic feature of prominent, dilated, and congested blood vessels in the dermal papillae of these lesions.[72] By selectively destroying the vessels supplying

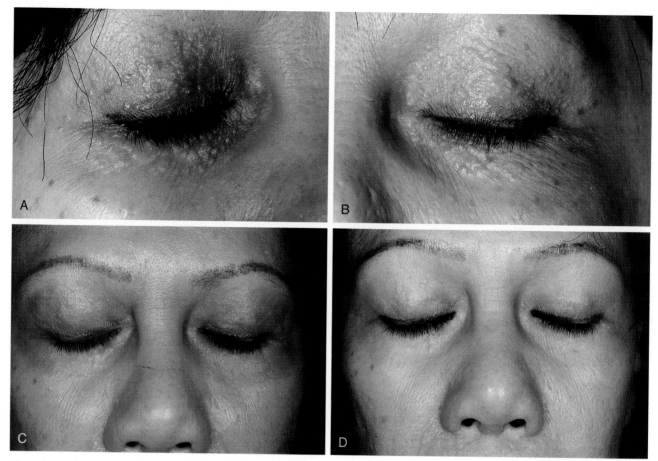

Figure 4–1. Multiple periorbital syringomas. *(A,B)* Pretreatment. *(C)* Twelve weeks after ultrapulsed CO_2 laser therapy (300 mJ, 60 W, density 6): three passes over syringomas, one final pass over syringomas remaining on eyelids. *(D)* Six months after laser treatment.

the virally infected keratinocytes, these rapidly replicating cells are eliminated along with the virus. This would be a specific therapy that minimizes injury to surrounding dermal tissue such as collagen and decreases the reported incidence of scarring associated with the more common nonspecific destructive therapies. Verrucae that are most refractory are those with abundant scar tissue at the base that prevents complete penetration of the laser to the vascular supply. We have found PDL to be effective in the treatment of verrucae.

Treatment includes paring of excess hyperkeratoses with a No. 15 blade, taking special care to avoid frank bleeding on the surface, which would absorb the laser energy and prevent proper penetration. In most cases, topical EMLA is used, but local infiltration may be necessary for digital or plantar lesions owing to their increased sensitivity. Tan and coworkers, who used energies between 6.25 and 7.5 J/cm^2 with a 5-mm spot size, found excellent resolution with 72% total clearance after an average of 1.68 treatments.[71] Bakus and Garden reported lesions to be more resistant, requiring multiple treatments at 7.5 J/cm^2 and noted that those with a scarred base were more refractory.[73] We have used 9 to 10 J/cm^2 with 5-mm spot and multiple impacts, with good results. Larger spot sizes with corresponding energies can be used for large lesions.

Keloids and Hypertrophic Scars

The treatment of keloidal and hypertrophic scars has been reported with both the PDL and argon laser.[74, 75] The target is destruction of the blood vessels, which causes local anoxia in the lesion. The resulting glycolysis produces excess lactic acid, creating low pH, which causes granulocyte lysis and releases enzymes, including collagenase.[76] With increased lysis of collagen, the balance between collagen synthesis and lysis is thought to be altered toward normal in the keloid. Treatment of keloidal and hypertrophic scars is presented in detail in Chapter 15.

Angiofibromas

The earliest sign of angiofibroma associated with tuberous sclerosis is the development of red vascular spots due to an excess of blood vessels in the superficial dermis. Yohn and colleagues have reported treating these early lesions with the PDL to determine whether eliminating the excess vasculature prevents development of the fibrous component seen in more mature angiofibromas.[77] Preliminary results suggest that it requires 2 to 3 treatment sessions to remove the nonfibrous angiofibromas with the PDL, but follow-up will be necessary to determine the long-term results. The benefits include the low risk of scarring from a noninvasive and bloodless therapy.

Acne Rosacea

Acne rosacea is an inflammatory condition often associated with telangiectasia and erythema. The PDL is effective in treating the vascular component of this disease and appears to decrease papular and pustular activity in as many as 59% of the patients treated.[78, 79] Many patients required no further—or less—topical and systemic antibiotic therapy to maintain resolution of the inflammatory component once the telangiectasias were treated.[80, 81]

Argon Laser

The argon laser, with wavelengths of 488 and 514.5 nm, targets hemoglobin and melanin. It is a continuous-wave laser that can be pulsed with a shuttering mechanism. The following benign cutaneous lesions that have either a vascular or pigmented component have been reported to be effectively treated with the argon laser: telangiectasia, rosacea, pyogenic granulomas,[82] angiofibromas, and seborrheic keratoses.[83] The depth of penetration of the argon laser is limited to the upper 1 mm of the dermis, which is one of its limitations.[84] Because it is a continuous laser, the risk of scarring is also a concern.

Neodymium:Yttrium-Aluminum-Garnet Laser

The Nd:YAG has a wavelength of 1064 nm, which is absorbed by proteins of any opaque tissue, darker tissue showing preferential absorption.[85] The laser can be frequency doubled to a 532-nm wavelength. Benign cutaneous lesions treated with the Nd:YAG include keloids and early seborrheic keratoses. Treatment of keloids shows that collagen synthesis by the keloidal fibroblasts is inhibited when exposed to the Nd:YAG laser.[86] Unfortunately, long-term followup has detected similar recurrence rates to those associated with removal of keloids by surgical methods.

Pulsed-Dye Pigmented Laser

The pulsed-dye pigmented laser at a wavelength of 510 nm has been reported to treat flat seborrheic keratoses successfully.[87]

Q-Switched Ruby Laser

The Q-switched ruby laser with a wavelength of 694 nm has also been reported to achieve 75% resolution of seborrheic keratoses.[86]

REFERENCES

1. Schomacker KT, Walsh JT, Flotte TJ, et al.: Thermal damage produced by high irradiance continuous wave CO_2 laser cutting of tissue. Lasers Surg Med 1990; 10:74–84.
2. Hobbs EH, Balin PL, Wheeland RG, et al.: Superpulsed lasers: Minimizing thermal damage with short duration, high irradiance pulses. J Dermatol Surg Oncol 1987; 13:955–964.
3. Street ML, Roenigk RK: Recalcitrant periungual verruca: The role of the carbon dioxide laser vaporization. J Am Acad Dermatol 1990; 23:115–120.
4. Goldman MP, Fitzpatrick RE: Cutaneous Laser Surgery. St. Louis: Mosby–Year Book, 1994:232.
5. Ferenczy A, Mitao M, Nagai N, et al.: Latent papillomavirus and recurring genital warts. N Engl J Med 1985; 313:784–788.
6. Leavitt KM: CO_2 laser surgery for verrucae—a technique. Laser Letter of the International Society of Podiatric Laser Surgery, Winter 1991, issue 23.
7. Garden JM, O'Banion MK, Shelniz LS, et al.: Papillomavirus in the vapor of carbon dioxide laser–treated verrucae. JAMA 1988; 259: 1199–1202.
8. Sawchuck WS, Weber PJ, Lowy DR, et al.: Infectious papillomavirus in the vapor of warts treated with the carbon dioxide laser or electrocoagulation: Detection and protection. J Am Acad Dermatol 1989; 21:41–49.
9. Smith JP, Topmiller JL, Shulman S: Factors affecting emission collection by surgical smoke evacuators. Lasers Surg Med 1990; 10:224.
10. Trevor M: Presence of virus in CO_2 laser plumes raises infection concern. Hosp Infect Control vol 166, 1987.
11. Roenigk RK: CO_2: laser vaporization for treatment of rhinophyma. Mayo Clin Proc 1987; 62:676–680.
12. El-Azhary RA, Roenigk RK, Wang TD: Spectrum of results after treatment of rhinophyma with the carbon dioxide laser. Mayo Clin Proc 1991; 66:899–905.
13. Staindl O: Surgical management of rhinophyma. Acta Otolaryngol 1981; 92:137.
14. Cheney ML, Graves TA, Blair PA: Rhinophyma: A surgical management. J Louisiana State Med Soc 1987; 139:13.
15. Kemble JVH: Correction of deformities of the nose. Practitioner 1980; 224:399.
16. Fulton JE: Modern dermabrasion techniques: A personal appraisal. J Dermatol Surg Oncol 1987; 13:780.
17. Fisher WJ: Rhinophyma: Its surgical treatment. Plast Reconstr Surg 1970; 45:466.
18. Linehan JW, Goode RL, Fajardo LF: Surgery vs. electrosurgery for rhinophyma. Arch Otolaryngol 1970; 91:444.
19. Verde SF, Oliveira ADS, Picoto ADS, et al.: How we treat rhinophyma. J Dermatol Surg Oncol 1980; 6:560.
20. Greenbaum SS, Krull EA, Watnick K: Comparison of CO_2 laser and electrosurgery in the treatment of rhinophyma. J Am Acad Dermatol 1988; 18:363.
21. Eisen RF, Katz AE, Bohigian RK, et al.: Surgical treatment of rhinophyma with the Shaw scalpel. Arch Dermatol 1986; 122:307.
22. Farina R: Rhinophyma: Plastic correction. Plast Reconstr Surg 1950; 6:461.
23. Ali KM, Callari RH, Mobley DL: Resection of rhinophyma with carbon dioxide laser. Laryngoscope 1989; 99:453.
24. Wheeland RG, Bailin PL, Ratz JL: Combined carbon dioxide laser excision and vaporization in the treatment of rhinophyma. J Dermatol Surg Oncol 1987; 13:172.
25. Shapshay SM, Strong MS, Anastasi GW, et al.: Removal of rhinophyma with the carbon dioxide laser. Arch Otolaryngol 1980; 106:257.
26. Hassard AD: Carbon dioxide laser treatment of acne rosacea and rhinophyma: How I do it. J Otolaryngol 1988; 17:336.
27. Haas A, Wheeland RG: Treatment of massive rhinophyma with the carbon dioxide laser. J Dermatol Surg Oncol 1990; 16:645.
28. Greenbaum SS, Krull EA, Watnick K: Comparison of CO_2 laser and electrosurgery in the treatment of rhinophyma. J Am Acad Dermatol 1988; 18:363.
29. El-Azhary RA, Roenigk RK, Wang TD: Spectrum of results after treatment of rhinophyma with the carbon dioxide laser. Mayo Clin Proc 1991; 66:899.
30. Ratz JL, Bailin PL, Lakeland RF: Carbon dioxide laser treatment of epidermal nevi. J Dermatol Surg Oncol 1986; 12:567.

31. Garden JM, Geronemus RG: Dermatologic laser surgery. J Dermatol Surg Oncol 1990; 16:156.
32. Fairhurts MV, Roenigk RK, Brodland DG: Carbon dioxide laser surgery for skin disease. Mayo Clin Proc 1992; 67:49–58.
33. Goldman MP, Fitzpatrick RE: Cutaneous Laser Surgery. St. Louis: Mosby–Year Book, 1994:246.
34. Fitzpatrick RE, Goldman MP, Ruiz-Esparza J: Clinical advantage of the CO_2 laser superpulsed mode: Treatment of verruca vulgaris, seborrheic keratoses, lentigines and actinic cheilitis. J Dermatol Surg Oncol 1994; 20:449–456.
35. Goldman MP, Fitzpatrick RE: Cutaneous Laser Surgery. St. Louis: Mosby–Year Book, 1994; 230.
36. Wheeland RG, Bailin PL, Kantor GR, et al.: Treatment of adenoma sebaceum with carbon dioxide laser vaporization. J Dermatol Surg Oncol 1985; 11:861–864.
37. Eliezri YD, Skylar JA: Lymphangioma circumscriptum: Review and evaluation of carbon dioxide laser vaporization. J Dermatol Surg Oncol 1988; 14:357.
38. Bailin PL, Kanter GR, Wheeland RG: Carbon dioxide laser vaporization in lymphangioma circumscriptum. J Am Acad Dermatol 1986; 14:257.
39. Arndt KA, Noe JM, Rosen S (eds): Cutaneous Laser Therapy: Principles and Methods. New York: John Wiley & Sons, 1983.
40. Wheeland RG, Bailin PL, Kantor GR, et al.: Treatment of adenoma sebaceum with carbon dioxide laser vaporization. J Dermatol Surg Oncol 1985; 11:861.
41. Bellack GS, Shapshay SM: Management of facial angiofibromas in tuberous sclerosis: Use of the carbon dioxide laser. Otolaryngol Head Neck Surg 1986; 94:37.
42. Karam F, Bauman T: Carbon dioxide treatment of chondrodermatitis nodularis helicis. Ear Nose Throat J 1988; 67:757.
43. Taylor MB: Chondrodermatitis nodularis helicis: Successful treatment with the carbon dioxide laser. J Dermatol Surg Oncol 1991; 17:862.
44. Bailin PL, Ratz JL: Use of the CO_2 laser in dermatologic surgery. In Ratz JL (ed): Lasers in Cutaneous Medicine and Surgery. Chicago: Year Book, 1985; 73–104.
45. Ratz JL: Laser Therapy Update. Boston: GK Hall, 1984; 244–251.
46. Wheeland RG, Ashley JR, Smith DA, et al.: Carbon dioxide laser treatment of granuloma faciale. J Dermatol Surg Oncol 1984; 10:730.
47. Roenigk RK, Ratz JL: CO_2 laser treatment of cutaneous neurofibromas. J Dermatol Surg Oncol 1987; 13:187.
48. Groot DW, Johnson PA: Lasers and advanced dermatologic instrumentation. Austral J Dermatol 1987; 28:77.
49. Apfelberg DB, Maser MR, Lash H, et al.: Superpulse CO_2 laser treatment of facial syringomata. Lasers Surg Med 1987; 7:533.
50. Wheeland RG, Bailin PL, Reynolds OD, et al.: Carbon dioxide laser vaporization of multiple facial syringomas. J Dermatol Surg Oncol 1986; 12:225.
51. Wheeland RG, McGillis ST: Cowden's disease—treatment of cutaneous lesions using carbon dioxide laser vaporization: A comparison of conventional and superpulsed techniques. J Dermatol Surg Oncol 1989; 15:1055.
52. Gladstone GJ, Beckman H, Elson LM: CO_2 laser excision of xanthelasma lesions. Arch Ophthalmol 1985; 103:440–442.
53. Apfelberg DB, Maser MR, Lash H, et al.: Treatment of xanthelasma palpebrarum with carbon dioxide laser. J Dermatol Surg Oncol 1987; 13:149–151.
54. Alster TS, West TB: Ultrapulse CO_2 laser ablation of xanthelasma. J Am Acad Dermatol 1996; 34:848–849.
55. McElroy JA, Mehregan DA, Roenigk RK: Carbon dioxide laser vaporization of recalcitrant symptomatic plaques of Hailey-Hailey disease and Darier's disease. J Am Acad Dermatol 1990; 23:893–897.
56. Don PC, Carney PS, Lynch WS, et al.: Carbon dioxide laser abrasion: A new approach to management of familial benign chronic pemphigus (Hailey-Hailey disease). J Dermatol Surg Oncol 1987; 13:1187.
57. Bain L, Geronemus R: The association of lichen planus of the penis with squamous cell carcinoma in situ and verrucous squamous cell carcinoma. J Dermatol Surg Oncol 1989; 15:413.
58. Ratz JL: Carbon dioxide laser treatment of balanitis xerotica obliterans. J Am Acad Dermatol 1984; 10:925.
59. Rosenberg SK, et al.: Continuous wave CO_2 treatment of balanitis xerotica obliterans. Urology 1982; 19:539.
60. Greenbaum S, Glogau R, Stegman S, et al.: Carbon dioxide laser treatment of erythroplasia of Queyrat. J Dermatol Surg Oncol 1989; 15:747.
61. Baldwin H, Geronemus R: Carbon dioxide laser vaporization of Zoon's balanitis: A case report. J Dermatol Surg Oncol 1989; 15:491.
62. Mester E, et al.: Effect of laser rays on wound healing. Am J Surg 1971; 122:532.
63. Mester E, Syende B, Spiry T, Scher A: Stimulation of wound healing by laser rays. Acta Chir Acad Sci Hung 1972; 13:315.
64. Tan OT, Murray S, Kurban AK: Action spectrum of vascular specific injury using pulsed irradiation. J Invest Dermatol 1989; 92:868.
65. Glassberg E, et al.: The flashlamp pumped 577 nm tunable dye laser: Clinical efficacy and in vitro studies. J Dermatol Surg Oncol 1988; 14:1200.
66. Anderson RR, Parish JA: Microvasculature can be selectively damaged using dye lasers: A basic therapy and experimental evidence in human skin. Lasers Surg Med 1981; 1:263.
67. Garden JM, Polla LL, Tan OT: The treatment of port-wine stains by the pulsed dye laser: Analysis of pulse duration and long-term therapy. Arch Dermatol 1988; 124:889.
68. Glassberg E, Lask GP, Tan EM, Vitto J: Cellular effects of the pulsed tunable dye laser at 577 nanometers on human endothelial cells, fibroblasts and erythrocytes: An in vitro study. Lasers Surg Med 1988; 8:567.
69. Polla LL, Tan OT, Garden JM, Parrish JA: Tunable pulsed dye laser for the treatment of benign vascular ectasias. Dermatologica 1987; 174:11.
70. Rowson KEK, Maghy BWJ: Human papova-(wart) virus. Bacteriol Rev 1967; 31:100.
71. Tan OT, Hurwitz RM, Stafford TJ: Pulsed dye laser treatment of recalcitrant verrucae: A preliminary report. Lasers Surg Med 1993; 13:127.
72. Lever WF, Schaumberg-Lever G: Diseases caused by viruses. In Histopathology of the Skin. Philadelphia: JB Lippincott, 1983; 371.
73. Bakus AD, Garden JM: Pulsed dye laser treatment of plantar verrucae. Lasers Surg Med 1993; Suppl 5:59.
74. Ginsbach G, Kohnel W: The treatment of hypertrophic scars and keloids by argon laser: Clinical data and morphological findings. ASPRS-EF-ASMS Plastic-Surgical Forum 1978; 1:61.
75. Henderson DL, Cromwell TA, Mes LG: Argon and carbon dioxide laser treatment of hypertrophic and keloidal scars. Lasers Surg Med 1984; 3:271.
76. Peacock BE Jr, van Winkle W Jr: Surgery and Wound Repair. Philadelphia: WB Saunders, 1970.
77. Yohn J: The treatment of skin disorders associated with tuberous sclerosis. NTSA Parent & Clinical Brochure. Perspective 1995; Spring/Summer: 16.
78. Apfelberg DB (ed): Atlas of Cutaneous Surgery. New York: Raven, 1992. Cases 7.6, 7.7, 7.22, 7.30.
79. Waner M, Dinehart S: Lasers in facial plastic and reconstructive surgery. In Davis RK (ed): Lasers in Otolaryngology: Head and Neck Surgery. Philadelphia: WB Saunders, 1989.
80. Lowe NJ, Behr KL, Fitzpatrick R, et al.: Flashlamp pumped dye laser for rosacea-associated telangiectasia and erythema. J Dermatol Surg Oncol 1991; 17:522.
81. Tan OT, Kurban AK: Noncongenital benign cutaneous vascular lesions: Pulse dye laser treatment. In Tan OT (ed): Management and Treatment of Benign Cutaneous Vascular Lesions. Philadelphia: Lea & Febiger, 1992.
82. Arndt KA: Argon laser therapy of small cutaneous vascular lesions. Arch Dermatol 1982; 118:220.
83. Pasyk KA: Case 5.49: Seborrheic keratosis. In Apfelberg DB (ed): Atlas of Cutaneous Laser Surgery. New York: Raven Press, 1992.
84. Garden JM, Geronemus RG: Dermatologic laser surgery. J Dermatol Surg Oncol 1990; 16:156.
85. Hanke CW: Lasers in dermatology. Indiana Med J 1990; 83:394.
86. Ohtsuka H, et al.: Ruby laser treatment of pigmented skin lesions. Jpn J Plast Reconstr Surg 1991; 44:615.

5

VASCULAR LESIONS

Bernard I. Raskin
Vladislav Chizhevsky
Gary P. Lask
Nicholas J. Lowe

Types of Vascular Lesions

This chapter reviews treatment of telangiectasias of the face and body, vascular birthmarks, and vascular lesions amenable to laser therapy. Leg veins are addressed in Chapter 6.

Telangiectasias: Definition and Causes

Telangiectasia is clinically defined as a visible, permanently dilated cutaneous blood vessel.[1] Facial telangiectasias are the most common entity in the authors' experience. Telangiectasias and vascular proliferations are best divided into those of intrinsic and of extrinsic causes (Table 5–1).[2] Telangiectasias are seen in approximately 50% of healthy children and 15% of normal adults[3, 4]; however, in the authors' opinion, adult telangiectasias are far more frequent in areas of high exposure to ultraviolet (UV) light.

Clinically, telangiectasias are considered to be vessels with diameters from 0.1 to 1 mm.[5] The terms that describe these vessels on examination are *single* or *multiple, linear, arborizing, discrete, confluent, macular, papular, nodular,* and *red, blue,* or *purple.* The wiry red vessels are derived from arterioles, whereas blue vessels are from venules. There may be a papular or nodular component to the vessel. Over time, red telangiectasias sometimes become bluer.[5] Spider telangiectasias have red vessels radiating from a central arteriolar punctum and blanch when pressure is applied centrally.[6]

Development is multifactorial.[7–11] It may be based on the underlying anatomic circumstance, such as wound closure under tension; on direct physical damage; or on biochemical stimulation such as estrogen or corticosteroid excess. Treatment decisions are based on the history, physical features, vessel size, and diagnosis.

Congenital Vascular Malformations: Port Wine Stains and Capillary Hemangiomas

Among the congenital and neonatal vascular proliferations, the two most responsive to laser are port wine stains and capillary hemangiomas. Large vascular malformations are beyond the purview of this chapter. Port wine stain is most common. This capillary malformation is seen in 0.3% of the population, most often on the face.[12] At birth these are blanchable pink, red, or purple macular patches that may darken and show a papulonodular surface and underlying tissue hypertrophy. These are composed of thin-walled ectatic vessels in the superficial dermis.[13] Port wine stains can be associated with congenital syndromes, including Sturge-Weber, Klippel-Trenaunay-Weber, and Cobb syndromes. They may also overlie arteriovenous malformations. Port wine stains can improve spontaneously, although this is extremely rare.[14]

The "salmon patch"[2] is a macular stain that is paler pink and blanches. It is noted at birth or shortly thereafter, and usually is located medially on the eyelids or glabella or on the nuchal regions. On the neck they have been called "stork bites." These very light pink patches can be seen in as many as one third of all neonates. No histologic abnormalities are demonstrated. Facial lesions usually vanish within the first year of life; nuchal lesions persist in 30% to 40% of cases.

Capillary hemangiomas are present at birth or shortly thereafter. They enlarge by proliferation during the first several months and regress spontaneously, but often not completely, over 5 to 10 years. They are composed of aggregates of plump, proliferating endothelial cells and are different from port wine stains.[13] The incidence varies according to sex, race, and gestational age. Girls are two to three times more likely to be affected than boys. Premature newborns may have a higher incidence than term infants. Hemangiomas are most often noted on the head, neck, and

Table 5–1. Intrinsic and Extrinsic Causes of Telangiectasis

Intrinsic causes
    Genetic disorders
        Bloom's syndrome
        Rothmund-Thomson syndrome
        Goltz's syndrome
        Benign hereditary telangiectasias
        Rendu-Osler-Weber syndrome (benign hereditary hemorrhagic
          telangiectasias)
    Collagen vascular diseases
        Systemic lupus erythematosus
        Progressive systemic sclerosis
    Other systemic conditions
        Liver disease
        Internal malignancy
        Discoid lupus
        Telangiectasia muscularis eruptiva perstans (mastocytosis)
        Cushing's disease and other elevated corticosteroid states
        Pregnancy
Extrinsic causes
    Drugs
        Systemic estrogen
        Topical steroids (excessive local application)
    Environmental
        Overexposure to the sun (photoaging)
        Actinic dermatitis (sunny climates)
    Direct trauma
    Surgery
        Wound closure under tension
        Rhinoplasty
        Sclerotherapy
    Therapeutic radiation

trunk. The pathogenesis of hemangiomas is not understood. One theory suggests that inappropriate release of angiogenic factors results in neovascularization and subsequent capillary proliferation.

Nontelangiectasia Vascular Lesions

Other entities that are vascular[15] include venous lakes, nevus araneus, Kaposi's sarcoma, pyogenic granulomas, lymphangioma circumscriptum, angiokeratomas, and cherry angiomas. Spider angiomas are both a vascular lesion and a telangiectasia.

Medical Indications for Treatment

Indications for treatment are multiple. Many telangiectasias have a papular component that bleeds easily from minor trauma.[16] Treatment of telangiectasias may be part of the reconstruction toward normal after trauma, surgery, or irradiation. Therapy may be part of the total medical care required for an underlying disease such as collagen disease, rosacea, or Cushing's or liver disease. Clusters of vessels (as in rosacea) contribute to flushing reactions that may lead to additional vascular dilatation or inflammatory states.[17, 18] Certainly, neonatal and rapidly evolving childhood vascular proliferations have clear medical indications for treatment. Residual congenital vascular nevi may develop a resistant

papular component in adult years, so treatment of residual lesions should be considered at an early stage.

Nontelangiectatic vascular conditions such as pyogenic granulomas and traumatized hemangiomas require treatment to prevent bleeding, further growth, and potentially significant scarring if the lesions become infected. Other lesions subject to potential trauma such as venous lakes deserve treatment at an asymptomatic stage.

Nonlaser Treatment Modalities

Therapy of the underlying systemic condition or cause is mandatory to prevent (when possible) continued development of vessels. Thus, medical workup and evaluation of the patient's overall clinical status is necessary. For photoaging, sun protection and sunscreens are indicated. If the cause is excessive application of topical steroids, the steroids must be reduced or discontinued. Pregnancy-induced vessels resolve or shrink significantly over the first few months after delivery, so conservative care may be appropriate. In children, isolated telangiectasias sometimes resolve but often persist.[19] In general, however, telangiectasias do not resolve spontaneously and usually require therapy. Port wine stains only rarely improve spontaneously.[14]

Treatment decisions about capillary hemangiomas of early childhood are based on the lesion, history, size, and site. Systemic steroids or surgery may be indicated. Many do resolve spontaneously[2] or improve over several years with no treatment, but a scar, residual lesion, or skin atrophy may result. Systemic corticosteroids have been shown to produce regression of growing lesions and are the first line of treatment for potentially harmful hemangiomas; however, many months' therapy is often necessary,[20] and severe complications can result (e.g., arrested linear growth, hypertension, adrenal insufficiency). Embolization can be useful for visceral hemangiomas, but the risks associated with it, including thrombosis, inadvertent embolization of normal vessels, extensive necrosis and sloughing of skin, and loss of vision, must be considered.[20, 21] Interferon alpha has been used successfully to treat internal and cutaneous hemangiomas that are refractory to other forms of therapy, and with minimal side effects. More studies are still required. Current recommendations are for early laser treatment of macular lesions (see section on Pulsed-Dye Laser [PDL]).

Kaposi's sarcoma is often treated with radiation. The lesions can also be treated by other modalities. Nontelangiectasia vascular lesions such as venous lakes, pyogenic granulomas, and angiokeratomas, among others, generally do not resolve spontaneously and virtually always require treatment. In addition to lasers other surgical modalities may be effective.

The usual nonlaser method for treating fine and medium-sized facial telangiectasias or telangiectasias on other body regions (excepting lower leg spider vessels) has been low-amperage electrodesiccation.[16] While this may be very successful, generation of heat results in superficial necrosis. Results are not consistently effective, and there is substantial risk of scarring.[22]

Sclerotherapy is utilized infrequently on the face because of the risk of scarring and the theoretical risks of sclerosant effects on adjacent vital organs.[16] Since most telangiectasias are arteriolar in origin, they lie close to an artery and this increases the risk of necrosis. When sclerosing solutions are injected into high-flow systems, complete local destruction does not occur. Instead, there is patchy, necrotic endothelial cell damage that forms microemboli and sludge that can lodge in vessels downstream. Also, vasospasm may occur. Regardless, Goldman[16] reported on 300 patients treated with modified solutions, with minimal morbidity. Another study[23] demonstrated that supplemental modified microsclerotherapy increased the effectiveness of copper vapor laser with minimal morbidity for facial lesions.

Over the past several years laser technology has allowed for effective and relatively safe treatment of port wine stains, early capillary hemangiomas, cutaneous telangiectasias, and other vascular lesions.

Lasers for Vascular Lesions: Theory, Definition of Terms, Absorption Spectra, and Basics of Pulsed and Continuous-Wave Systems

Laser (*light amplification by stimulated emission of radiation*) light is monochromatic, coherent, and collimated.[15, 24–26] Continuous-wave (CW) lasers emit energy as long as the foot pedal is depressed. Pseudocontinuous-wave units use a manual shuttering system to try to make the laser more like a pulsed beam. Another adaptation CW lasers employ is a scanning device to make the laser move over the skin rapidly, so that the skin "sees" the laser for only a short time.

Pulsed lasers have extremely short pulses and prolonged intervals between pulses. Long-pulsed lasers work best on larger structures such as telangiectasias, whereas short-pulsed systems such as the Q-switched neodymium:yttrium-aluminum-garnet (Nd:YAG) target smaller structures such as melanin. Lasers deliver light energy to the skin. The measurement utilized is the amount of energy delivered per unit of area, a measure referred to as *fluence*. Obviously, if more energy is delivered per unit of area, the destructive forces are greater. The greater the energy delivered per unit of area, the higher the fluence. Energy fluence is expressed in joules per square centimeter.[26] For a given fluence, the machine setting (measured in joules) required for a 3-mm spot size is different than for a 5- or 7-mm spot size, because the concept is *energy per unit area*. Energy fluence is used principally with pulsed lasers.

Irradiance[26, 27] is the rate of energy delivery, and this is the measurement most often utilized with CW systems, as the amount of energy delivered with a continuous wave varies with the time that the wave is on the area of skin. Irradiance thus describes the intensity of delivery. It is expressed in watts per square centimeter.

The theory of selective photothermolysis describes the effect of the laser. In this concept, first espoused in 1980 by Anderson and Parrish,[15] selective heating is achieved by preferential laser light absorption and heat production in the target chromophore when the pulse duration is shorter than the thermal relaxation time of the target.

The molecule that absorbs the specific laser wavelength is known as a *chromophore*.[27] In lasers designed for vascular lesions, the chromophore is oxyhemoglobin, which absorbs best with yellow light at either 577 or 585 nm. Selective photothermolysis uses a combination of selective absorption and thermal energy confinement to damage only specific microscopic structures, in this case blood vessels. Thus, a small amount of energy entirely absorbed by a chromophore can produce substantial heating of that chromophore. Alternatively,[15] large amounts of laser energy can be delivered through nonabsorbing substances, including skin, without causing damage if no chromophore is available for absorbing laser light and converting it into heat.

The laser light turns to heat upon impact with the correct chromophore. Heat diffusion to other structures is guided by the *thermal relaxation time*,[27] the time required to lose 50% of the heat generated by the absorbed light energy. If the pulse is shorter than the thermal relaxation time of the target (chromophore), then the majority of the absorbed energy is retained by the target structure and nonspecific thermal damage in adjacent tissue is minimized. The chromophore becomes extremely hot. The size of the target determines the thermal relaxation time for that chromophore: small objects cool faster than large ones. So, for example, the thermal relaxation time of venules (which are fairly large) in a port wine stain[15] is a few thousandths of a second, as compared with that of melanosomes (which are quite small)—on the order of nanoseconds (tenths of a millionth of a second). Thus, the pulse duration required for a blood vessel is different from that needed for a smaller target such as melanin pigment.

Thermal relaxation time helps to explain why CW lasers have the potential to produce relatively widespread heat injury. For example, argon ion laser exposures might be tens of milliseconds, which allows heat to diffuse 100 μm or more[15] and that is greater than the distance between blood vessels. Thus, the entire superficial dermis might be heated even though the wavelength of 488 nm is quite specific for hemoglobin. In theory, then, a pulse system designed to take advantage of a specific chromophore and its thermal relaxation time produces a less adverse reaction than a CW system that is inherently less specific for thermal relaxation time, even though both lasers are set at the same wavelength.

Pulse duration is extremely important, and considerable clinical variability occurred with the initial pulsed systems[28, 29] until empiric studies demonstrated that pulses of several hundred microseconds were needed along with the proper fluences. It was also determined that selective laser microvascular damage[15, 27] involves both photocoagulation and mechanical injury, thrombosis and complement fixation, a necrotizing vasculitis, and neovascularization without scarring.

The absorbing chromophore is the hemoglobin and oxyhemoglobin molecule,[24] and the wavelength utilized for these lasers is between 488 and 600 nm. Melanin also absorbs to some extent in this region, more at the lower wavelengths and less at 577 to 600 nm. So, depigmentation can be a problem, principally with the CW lasers, which are at 532 nm and less. Optimal absorption for oxyhemoglobin is in the 577- to 600-nm range, whereas melanin absorbs less in these wavelengths. Most CW systems are in the 532-nm range and lower; thus, those all have higher potential for pigmentation alteration problems.

The PDL at 585-nm wavelength (yellow) with 450-μsec pulse has been optimized for oxyhemoglobin absorption and small vessel (40- to 100-μm) thermal relaxation time. These parameters, however, may not work as well for vessels larger than 100 μm in diameter. Different laser parameters are needed, for example, on lower extremity spider telangiectasias, as the initial standard PDL system (450 μsec) was ineffective. Thus, in some cases CW lasers may have been more effective than the 450-μsec PDL, even when the wavelength or thermal relaxation time is not matched exactly. With the newer longer-pulse systems (1.5 msec at 595 to 600 nm), these larger-caliber vessels can be treated.

Laser Safety

The main safety issue discussed in this section is eye safety for both patient and operating personnel. The specific Occupational Safety and Health Administration (OSHA) designated eye protection for each specific laser must be worn by all operating personnel. Knowledge of and adherence to standard OSHA safety guidelines for eye protection are mandatory. Near-total functional vision loss can occur in an eye exposed to a very small amount of laser energy, like the amount in reflected light.

Fire safety precautions should be observed per OSHA, including wet drapes, wetting hair, and a functioning fire extinguisher nearby. When oxygen is used for conscious sedation or general anesthesia, the incendiary potential of the laser is substantially increased because of the oxygen-rich environment. There have been reports of scalp and eyebrow hair ignition[30] in this circumstance with the flashlamp-pumped pulsed-dye laser (FLPDL). Dark, thick hair is most prone to ignition.

The issue of patient protection was recently addressed[31] for wavelengths produced by vascular lasers when a number of available shields were tested. Few are specifically designed for laser use. In this study, four plastic shields, a metal shield, and two types of tanning goggles were evaluated. The temperature rise at the surface of the shields was

not more than 0.2°C; however, white light penetrated several of the shields at significant levels, but yellow light transmittance occurred only through the green-colored shield. All except green, therefore, were safe from transmission of the 585-nm light. The conclusion of the study is that the ideal patient laser eye shield does not exist.

Another study reviewed laser safety of eye shields for all laser spectrums.[32] The shields tested were the standard white eye external eye protector used in tanning salons, Storz blue plastic corneal shields, Danker black and Danker red corneal shields, Stefanovsky metallic corneal protectors, and Cox stainless corneal protectors. The Storz makes no mention of laser use in product literature, and the Dankers indicate they are not intended for laser use. All shields showed minimal damage if any with the FLPDL, but light leakage was as much as 10%. There was 7% leakage in the eye shields supplied with the flashlamp dye laser (FLDL). These authors recommended Stefanovsky metal shields. The thin Cox shields were deemed to carry a risk of heat conduction and higher risk of reflection. The overall risk of reflection from metal shields back toward the operator was not addressed in this study.

The same study performed with the argon laser demonstrated burn-through in the plastic shields.[32] The temperature rise in the Cox shield was over 100°C, whereas with the Stefanovsky it increased up to 30°C. The overall recommendation was Stefanovsky corneal shields for all laser modalities. Again, the investigators opined that the ideal shields have yet to be developed.

Laser Therapy: Pulsed Versus Continuous-Wave Lasers and a List of Available Sources

A variety of lasers are available for vascular lesions and telangiectasias (Table 5–2). CW units utilize wavelengths from 488 to 578 nm. The target chromophore is oxyhemoglobin, although some melanin absorption also occurs, principally at shorter wavelengths. Penetration is approximately 1 mm and is greatest at longer wavelengths.

The pulsed laser, the FLPDL, was developed specifically for vascular lesions. Originally, machines were set at 577 nm, later at 585 nm, and most recently at 595 to 600 nm. At 577 nm, penetration was 0.5 mm, but at 585 nm,

Table 5–2. Lasers for Vascular Lesions

LASER	WAVELENGTH (nm)	COLOR	TYPE
Argon	488–514	Blue-green	CW
Argon dye	577–630	Yellow-red	CW
KTP	532	Green	Pulse train
Q-switched Nd:YAG	532	Green	20-nsec pulse
Krypton	568	Yellow	CW
Copper vapor	578	Yellow	Pulse train
PDL	585	Yellow	450 μsec pulse
PDL	585, 590, 595, 600	Yellow	1.5 msec pulse

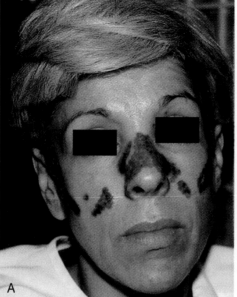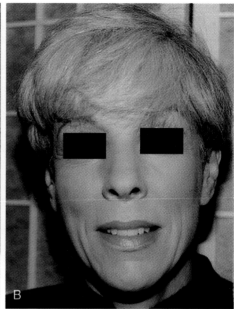

Figure 5–1. Temporary purpura caused by pulsed dye laser used to treat facial telangiectasias. *(A)* After treatment with the Candela flash lamp pulsed dye laser (FLPDL) at 6 J/cm², 5-mm spot size. *(B)* Purpura can be camouflaged with corrective cosmetics such as Dermablend.

penetration increased to 1.2 mm. Also, melanin absorbs less, so irregular pigmentation is reduced. Initially, the pulse duration was 450 µsec. This is considerably shorter than the 1- to 5-msec thermal relaxation time of superficial blood vessels.[33] The laser pulse ends before heat is diffused, thus limiting damage to the target only. The newer system has wavelengths of 585, 590, 595, and 600 nm and a pulse width of 1.5 msec. The longer wavelength allows deeper penetration, and the longer pulse width allows treatment of larger-caliber vessels.

The pulsed laser is more desirable for treating vascular lesions, as the primary target is oxyhemoglobin and the pulse duration prevents heat diffusion, thus limiting the laser energy to the target tissue. However, pulsed laser machines are more expensive and larger and require more maintenance. CW units do not cause purpura. All PDLs cause temporary purpura, lasting from 5 to 14 days (Fig. 5–1).

Laser Treatment, Techniques, Vessel Size, and Anatomic Considerations

The spectrums outlined from 480 through 600 nm are blue-green to yellow-red and are absorbed by red, brown, and black pigments. The port wine stains best treated with CW lasers are the mature, more deeply pigmented blue-purple lesions, especially those with an irregular cobblestone or textured surface.[25] The 450-µsec PDL technique is more effective for macular lesions. The current standard of care is PDL for childhood vascular lesions. Only a few published articles have addressed the use of other lasers in children.[25]

For CW lasers, anesthesia usually is needed to treat port wine stains. The laser is used almost as an airbrush over the vessel, and the end point is slight whitening or opalescence.

More severe local changes must be avoided, lest scars or discoloration develops. Intervals between treatments may be as short as 1 month, but if depigmentation or significant epidermal changes supervene, the interval might be as long as several months. Fading may continue for 1 year. Some 60% to 70% of port wine stains heal well; scars occur in 5%. The upper lip and sides of the nose are at greatest risk for scar formation.[34]

For small vascular lesions, CW lasers (argon, krypton, copper vapor, copper bromide, argon-pumped tunable dye, potassium titanyl phosphate [KTP]) are often very effective. For small vascular lesions a handpiece is used that is approximately the diameter of the vessel, usually 0.1 mm. The beam is slowly traced over the vessel at a rate sufficient to cause disappearance of the vessel or blanching but not so slowly as to induce obvious thermal necrosis or significant epidermal changes. With 0.1-mm spot size, magnification loupes are often helpful. At this level, patients feel heat and burning but rarely much pain. Local anesthesia may be used, most often without epinephrine, or eutectic mixture of local anesthesia (EMLA) may be effective.

In general, large lesions require larger spot sizes or robotic scanners[22] for effective management. Lesions on the extremities are most difficult to clear and require repeat treatment. Lesions on thin skin like that of lips, neck, and eyelids are most safely treated with PDL, which produces minimal thermal injury.[24] Longer wavelengths may penetrate deeper into the skin; thus, yellow light may be needed for deeper lesions. Vessels larger than 100 µm respond less well to 0.5-µsec PDL and often require conjunctive CW or long-pulsed yellow light laser.[22] Vessels with long flow rates respond less well to PDL[22] and require long-pulsed yellow or green light for best results.

PDL treatment may or may not require local anesthesia. Infants and young children need sedation or general anesthesia. Energy densities vary depending on the wavelength, pulse width, and spot size and are delivered in individual pulses or with very slightly overlapping pulses to ensure blending. Purpura occurs immediately and lasts as long as 2 weeks. Improvement occurs over 4 to 8 weeks, and repeat treatments at 6- to 8-week intervals typically are required.

Skin types 1 and 2 can be treated[25] with either green or yellow light lasers. Types 3 and 4 are best treated with yellow light to reduce melanin absorption. Types 5 and 6 are more prone to crusting and pigmentary changes with reduced response.

Continuous-Wave Lasers

A variety of CW lasers are available that have wavelengths from 488 to 578 nm, the target being oxyhemoglobin. Longer wavelengths of 577 nm and above have the deepest penetration, and the greatest selectivity of oxyhemoglobin over melanin.

Facial telangiectasias are the most common application, as the diameters of most telangiectasias vary from 100 to 200 μm.[22] The PDL is matched to the thermal relaxation time of a median vessel size of 50 to 100 μm (the size typically seen in port wine stains). The larger vessels of many facial telangiectasias are thus often treated appropriately with the CW modality. With the longer-pulsed (1.5 msec) laser, larger vessels can now be treated with PDLs; however, the PDL is also exceptionally effective for facial telangiectasias.[30] Next we discuss the specifics of various CW lasers available today.

ARGON LASER

This was the first vascular-specific laser introduced, so for several years it was the standard of care. It has six different wavelengths from 488 to 514 nm, with 80% of emissions at 488 and 514 nm. The medium is argon gas.[24] Currently, it is used on large vessels. Typical penetration is 1 mm. Usually, little or no anesthesia is needed, and the laser is delivered through fiberoptic cable using 50 msec to 0.3 sec pulses with energy levels of 0.8 to 2.9 W at spot sizes of 0.1 to 1 mm.[35]

Minimal crusting follows treatment, which resolves in 5 to 10 days. Scarring can occur. Pigment alteration is also seen. A limiting factor is the penetration depth of 1 mm. This makes it effective principally for superficial papillary dermal lesions. On darker skin, melanin absorption decreases oxyhemoglobin absorption and increases the risk of pigment changes, which can be permanent. Skin texture changes can also occur: studies have shown that both vascular and nonvascular structures are damaged, partially because argon laser light is scattered by the skin and not precisely absorbed by hemoglobin. The result is coagulative necrosis of the epidermis and dermis.[23, 34] Skin texture changes have been shown to occur in 5% to 38% of patients, and permanent hypopigmentation is more than 20%.[24, 36]

The PDL is considered the standard of care for port wine stains[24, 37]; however some considered the argon to be the treatment of choice[24] for hypertrophic port wine stains or nodular areas within them. The laser result depends on fibrosis around the vessel wall; so, evaluation of full response may require 4 to 12 months. Another effective application is low-flow hemangiomas[37] that are venous in origin, such as venous lakes of the lip and mucosal venous malformations.

Facial telangiectasias can also be treated. The recommended beam diameter is 0.5 to 1.0 mm and the pulse duration less than 0.1 sec.[22] Contraindications are port wine stains located on the upper lip and jaw and any lesions on persons younger than 17 years, owing to the increased risk of scarring. Lesions on the lower extremities are a relative contraindication.[24]

ARGON-PUMPED TUNABLE DYE LASER (APTDL)

The APTDL uses a shuttering mechanism to alter its CW properties into 30-msec pulses.[38] Using various organic dyes,[24] a range of 50 to 1200 nm is covered, and this output is filtered by a prism to allow a chosen setting from blue to near infrared. As currently adapted, it is used at 577 or 585 nm transmitted through a fiberoptic cable. While power output is low, the small spot size yields high energy density. Facial telangiectasias are treated with the tracing technique outlined earlier in this chapter for continuous-wave lasers. Settings are 100-μm spot size with pulses of 0.05 to 0.1 sec, power settings 0.1 to 0.4 W, and wavelengths of 577 or 585 nm.[39] Because of an extremely small spot size, power densities are 1000 to 2000 W/cm^2. Blanching is observed with treatment, and erythema and edema subsequently.[24]

Results superior to those of standard argon laser are reported,[39, 40] and results are comparable to those of PDL.[39] The narrow spot size is well-suited to treating telangiectasias, and the 577-nm wavelength is theoretically an advantage over the standard argon.

In general, benign vascular lesions of 30 to 300 μm should be amenable to this laser at 577 nm. Success has been reported for port wine stains, facial telangiectasias, hemangiomas, angiofibromas, and vascular rhinophymas.[39–41]

The technique involves performing a test first and evaluating the result at 4 to 6 weeks. The procedure is performed by tracing the vessel, either in a continuous pass or with a series of pulses. The end point is clinical disappearance or blanching of the vessel without epidermal charring or contraction. Vessels turn brown a few days after treatment and disappear within 5 to 10 days. Occasionally epidermal blistering occurs. One problem with this technique is that it is very slow. Adverse sequelae have been minimal.[42]

A robotic scanner (Hexascan) aids in treating small, diffuse lesions. Comparable results have occurred with the Hexascan using 585 nm (yellow) and 532 nm (green) at similar fluences.[43–45] In smaller vessels, recommended pulse width is 30 to 100 msec with fluences of 18 to

$20 J/cm^2.[22]$ Larger vessels use the same pulse width, with fluences of 22 to 30 J/cm^2. This laser may be used for vessels from 30 to 300 μm.[22]

POTASSIUM TITANYL PHOSPHATE 532 NANOMETER LASER

This CW system[22] is pulsed with a mechanical shuttering system. The 532-nm wavelength is obtained by frequency doubling an Nd:YAG crystal (1064 nm), and this results in a system similar to the argon laser's. Recently, the KTP lasers have become more widely used due to lower-cost, more portable units. The availability of larger spot sizes and wider pulse durations is effective for vessels larger than those that are otherwise treated with a PDL. The advent of cooling heads decreases the risk of epidermal damage and the sequelae of scarring and pigmentation abnormalities. Typical settings for facial telangiectasias are 2 mm spot size at 10 to 15 J at 15 to 25 msec. However, settings vary with each manufacturer. The treatment technique is that described earlier in the chapter, with the airbrush movement over the vessel. With the Hexascan, for large confluent telangiectasias, the energy used is 10 to 18 J/cm^2 with the shortest pulse possible.[46]

COPPER VAPOR LASER

Light is emitted at 578 nm from a gas medium of copper vapor.[24] Results are comparable to those of the APTDL.[47] The system has 30- to 50-nsec pulses at a rate of 6000 to 15,000 per second, so effectively it is a CW laser system. The large number of pulses results in heating beyond the thermal relaxation time; however, a mechanical shuttering system produces 200-msec exposure intervals every 400 msec and the heating is more in keeping with the thermal relaxation time. Thus, the risk of scarring is lessened, as 200 msec results in 3000 pulses, which is sufficient to cause precise vascular destruction.[27] Recommended settings are 150-μm handpiece, 450 to 500 mW, 0.2-sec shutter intervals.[48, 49]

Treatment creates a fine eschar that heals within 2 weeks. Transient posttreatment hyperpigmentation has been noted in 10%; other scarring is unusual.[49–51] Walker and colleagues[52] demonstrated selective damage to port wine stain vessels without involvement of avascular structures. Histologically, there is necrosis of the endothelial cells without vessel rupture, and the mechanism of action is considered to be erythrocyte coagulation and vessel vasoconstriction (in contrast to PDL).[27] These lasers are considered appropriate for nodular port wine stains, larger telangiectasias, venous malformations, raised vascular lesions, and pyogenic granulomas.[27] It has been shown that copper vapor laser treatment of port wine stains is not as selective on brown skin as on fair skin because of epidermal melanin.[53] Again, the clinical end point[24] is blanching or whitening of the vascular lesions, similar to that with argon lasers. The handpiece may be hand directed, and a computer-controlled scanning device is available. Epidermal disruption and posttreatment weeping are common.

KRYPTON LASER

The krypton laser, a CW system using a shuttering mechanism, emits yellow at 568 to 577 nm. It can also be set to green at 520 to 530 nm. Treatment is performed with the 100-μm collimated or a 1-mm noncollimated handpiece. The settings are 0.4 to 0.6 W with 0.2-sec pulse or CW with the 100-μm handpiece; or 0.7 to 0.9 W with 0.2-sec pulse while using the 1-mm handpiece.[22] The airbrush technique along the vessel is utilized, as described earlier in the chapter for CW lasers. There is a paucity of clinical data on this laser for evaluating long-term efficacy.[54]

COPPER BROMIDE LASER

This quasipulsed system emits at 511 and 578 nm, the latter for vascular lesions. The spot size is 0.7 mm, with pulses as short as 7 msec.[22] The copper bromide laser has been demonstrated to be effective in treating telangiectasias, spiders, and vascular nevi with only rare minor skin atrophy when larger vessels are treated.[55] To understand why multiple CW systems enter the market, one can use the example of this laser. The limitations of other yellow light lasers in common use are two: with argon and standard copper vapor, the output power is low, so sufficient energy density for vessel ablation is produced only with relatively long pulses (50 msec or longer) and very small spot sizes. Until recently, the PDL systems did not permit the prolonged pulse needed for treating vessels 80 μm in diameter or larger. The copper bromide laser to some extent overcomes these limitations with its substantial output of 2 W and exposure times of 10 to 50 msec. In theory, these parameters achieve the selective destruction of vessels in the size range of most telangiectasias of the face and neck. There is a paucity of studies on this laser, and the one cited evaluated only 23 patients.

Pulsed Lasers

The literature refers to the *flashlamp dye laser* (FLDL), *flashlamp-pumped pulsed-dye laser* (FLPDL), or *pulsed dye laser* (PDL). The initial 450-μsec FLPDL was designed expressly for vascular lesions, principally for port wine stain–sized vessels in the 40-μm range (Figs. 5–2, 5–3). Although initially it was established at 577 nm, which correlates with oxyhemoglobin absorption, it was found that deeper penetration occurred at 585 nm.[56] The pulse duration of 450 μsec is less than the 1- to 5-msec thermal relaxation time of skin vessels.[57] The medium is liquid rhodamine-based organic dye.[24]

This laser was specifically designed for port wine stains. Initial studies were at 577 nm, but this penetrated only

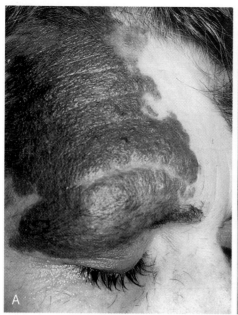
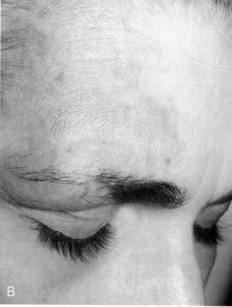

Figure 5–2. Extensive port wine hemangioma in a 54-year-old patient. *(A)* Before treatment, patient underwent surgical repair of upper-lid ptosis caused by the hemangioma. *(B)* Appearance after treatments with FLPDL at 6, 6.5, 7, 7.5, and 8 J/cm^2.

0.5 mm. Increasing to 585 nm changed the penetration depth to 1.2 mm; plus, less light is absorbed by melanin at 585 nm, maximizing absorption by oxyhemoglobin.[56]

In port wine stains, histology demonstrates[56] agglutination of erythrocytes and vessel wall degeneration extending to 1.2 mm. Microvascular rupture and hemorrhage are relatively minimal. Vascular damage is minimal, and so is perivascular thermal tissue damage (in contrast to CW lasers).[27] After about a week, fine granulation tissue replaces the vessels. After 1 month there is normal-looking epidermis and dermis, with normal adnexa, no fibrosis, and fine capillaries.[58–61] This histologic picture confirms the theoretical advantage of PDL over CW lasers for port wine stains. Thus, the PDL is considered the standard of care for port wine stains (Fig. 5–4).[62, 63] Clinically, purpura lasts 7 to 14 days, and partial to complete vessel clearing takes 1 to 2 months. Because of the slow vessel resolution, a minimum

interval of at least 1 month is recommended between treatments.

Understanding the use of the PDL requires appreciation of the specificities of laser-tissue interaction. Absorption is varied by changing the spot size of the beam.[32] Currently, there are 2-, 3-, 5-, 7-, and 10-mm handpieces. Reducing the spot size changes the effective energy[32] delivered, and thus a change in output is necessary to produce an equivalent result when a smaller beam size is utilized. Melanin can also interfere with absorption, and energy delivery is greater in less heavily pigmented skin.[16]

Thus, it is the authors' recommendation that physicians consider test sites when deciding how best to handle any particular telangiectasias or vascular lesions. Clinical response to test pulses can be used to decide on the proper settings. The correct setting should produce purpura without excessive edema, blistering, crusting, or other epidermal

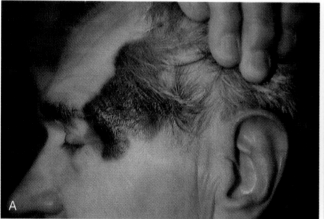
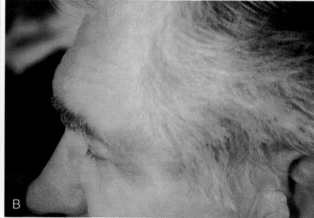

Figure 5–3. Elevated "purple" port wine hemangioma before treatment *(A)* and *(B)* after six treatment sessions with FLPDL at 6, 6.5, 7, 7.5, 8, and 9 J/cm^2 and 5-mm spot size.

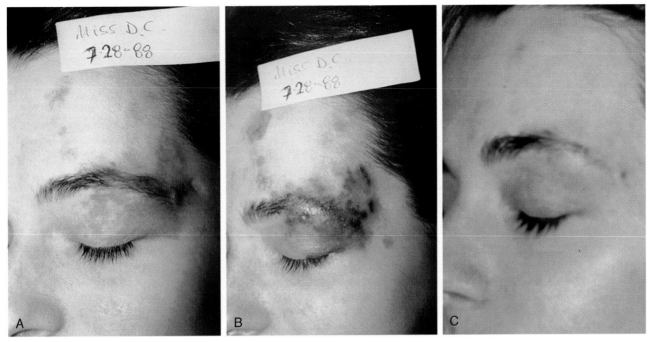

Figure 5–4. Port wine stain. *(A)* Flat pink stain preoperatively. *(B)* Purpura immediately following treatment with Candela FLPDL. *(C)* Six months after two Candela FLPDL treatments at 6 and 6.5 J/cm², 5-mm spot size.

changes. It may be appropriate to wait 4 to 8 weeks after testing a small area to judge the clinical response.

Recent research has indicated interlaser variability[64]— among machines from one manufacturer and among manufacturers. Currently, two companies in the United States sell PDLs: Candela and Cynosure. One study demonstrated spot size variations of 4% to 35% between machines, even from the same manufacturer when the size of the spot was measured. This resulted in varied fluences. Also, the Cynosure uses a top-hat beam configuration, whereas the Candela uses a gaussian curve. Thus, care must be exercised when moving from machine to machine whether they are from one or different manufacturers.

Clinical Technique. Technique is fairly straightforward with PDLs.[24] This is in contrast to the CW systems, whose results are more technique and operator dependent. There is a fixed-distance handpiece with a green aiming light. The system is operated either by hand or foot switch. Eye protection is necessary as even reflected light can cause damage. The patient needs to wear eye protection also. Care must be taken to avoid laser beam exposure to plastic tubing, endotracheal tubes, and other combustible materials. Similarly, hair should be moistened if it is in the field.

The lowest effective energy should be employed. Often, several test sites are chosen at the first session and different energies are employed. The sites are then observed for 4 to 6 weeks, and the results of those test sites dictate the energies chosen for treatment. In general, for children, for pink lesions, or for the thin skin of the neck and eyelids, lower energies are chosen. Darker or purplish lesions, adult

skin other than thin-skinned areas, and raised lesions require higher energy.

Pulses can be placed adjacent to one another or with 10% overlap.[24] Greater overlap results in more nonspecific damage and increased risk of scarring or discoloration. The reticular bridging pattern that results in treating larger areas is eliminated by treating the interspaces between the pulses at another session in 6 to 8 weeks. The immediate clinical response—blue or gray purpura—develops within 30 seconds of a pulse. In general, isolated facial telangiectasias respond with only one treatment, whereas port wine stains require several sessions.

Clinically, the PDL causes stinging with each pulse, similar to the sensation of a snapped rubber band. Some patients in the authors' experience find this quite uncomfortable; others do not much mind. Pretreatment with EMLA is effective, but the vasoconstriction it causes often makes it difficult to see the vessels clearly while wearing protective goggles. The transient purpura is very noticeable to patients, especially on the face, and considerable pretreatment counseling is necessary. Wound care is minimal, as epidermal integrity is usually preserved. Crusting or vesiculation develops in fewer than 4%.[35] Postoperatively, patients typically compare the pain to that of a sunburn.

Contraindications. Contraindications to treatment are few. The primary problem is heavily pigmented skin.[24, 65, 66] For skin types I to IV on untanned skin, melanin absorption[30] generally is not significant enough to cause problems. In more heavily pigmented skin, the melanin impedes absorption by deeper vascular structures, so risks are increased. There are no age restrictions, and the literature reports treatment as early as the 6th day of life.[66] Vascular lesions of questionable origin should be biopsied first. Lesions scarred by previous treatment with other modalities may appear more atrophic and hypopigmented after PDL. In general, one can site test any lesion first to avoid problems later.

Complications. In a study of 500 patients,[67] both children and adults, treated for port wine stain, telangiectasia, or hemangioma, there were no hypertrophic scars. Persistent atrophic scars occurred in fewer than 0.1%. Permanent hyperpigmentation occurred in 1%, and transient hypopigmentation developed in 2.6%. Transient dermatitis was noted in fewer than 1% after multiple treatments with PDL. These authors conclude that the PDL solves many of the problems associated with CW lasers.

Other authors have seen hyperpigmentation rates as high as 10% to 15%,[30] usually in darker-pigmented persons or with higher energy levels. In general, most hyperpigmentation gradually diminishes over a few months.[30] Hypopigmentation occurred in fewer than 5% in another study,[68, 69] and, again, usually resolved over a few months. Permanent hypopigmentation can be vascular—a laser-induced nevus anemicus. Small, depressed areas sometimes seen after treatment in small children generally resolve after several months. Infections are rare, as the epidermis usually is not violated.

Retinal damage can occur (see section on Laser Safety). Superficial burns have resulted from ignition of hair, and care must be taken when using general anesthesia as oxygen concentrations are high.[24] The overall incidence of scarring[30] is less than 1% for port wine stain with this modality, as compared with 5% or greater with the argon laser.

PORT WINE STAINS

The laser was designed primarily for port wine stains. Studies have shown 50% to 75% lightening within two or three treatments[70] and, in many cases, 30% to 40% show complete resolution.[24, 71, 72] In early lesions, 50% clearing may be achieved with one treatment.[73] Lighter, pinker port wine stains respond better than more mature, nodular or darker ones. Typically, younger children need fewer treatments than adults. Sometimes, however, children need more treatments because of growth of residual vessels.[74] Treatment can start at any time from several days after birth,[66] although waiting about a month is common.[75]

The recommendation is to first test energy levels at various levels.[30] The energy varies with spot size, pulse width, and wavelength. Test sites are observed for up to 8 weeks. Children's lesions, macular pink vascular spots, and eyelid and neck skin typically require less energy. The darker or elevated or adult lesions often need higher energy levels. Care should be taken with higher energy levels in olive or darker skin, lest prolonged hyperpigmentation result.

The majority of lightening[37] usually occurs by 2 months after a session, although in some patients lightening continues for several months. A significant number of port wine stains do not achieve significant lightening, even after multiple additional treatments.[76] This problem seems to be associated with hypertrophic or nodular changes, extensive areas of involvement, and certain sites, including[77] the central areas of the face such as the medial aspect of the cheek, upper lip, and nose; the temporal distribution of the second branch of the trigeminal nerve; and the limbs. Fortunately, the selective vascular injury allows multiple treatment sessions with low risk.[27] Patients' assessment of outcomes in PDL treatment of port wine stains correlates well with the clinical results.[78]

After multiple treatments, there may be no further fading, and this may be the end point, although[30] some physicians have found that, after waiting 6 months to a year, further treatments can again be effective. If there is a substantial nodular component, as in adult lesions, trying a CW modality may be considered.

Port wine stains do not recur after FLDL treatment; however, any residual lesion can vary in intensity over time. The PDL is the treatment of choice for port wine stains.[62, 63] Many also consider it the treatment of choice for various vascular lesions.[62, 63] This concept is expanded in the next paragraph and in the summary section at the conclusion of the chapter.

TELANGIECTASIAS

PDL is effective for other telangiectasias and vascular lesions. Parameters are determined by location and morphology. Spider telangiectasias clear after one treatment in 93% of adults and 70% of children, with 5-mm spot, 450-μsec pulse width, and fluence of 6 to 7.5 J/cm^2.[22] Higher fluences should not be used at the first session but would be used at subsequent sessions on adults, older children, or refractory vessels. Some lesions are smaller than the spot size, and in that case one pulse directed at the central punctum is effective. Clinically, purpura should be present immediately and the vessel should no longer blanch with pressure. Radiating vessels are treated with not more than 10% overlap. While a smaller spot may produce less adjacent tissue purpura, fluence must be adequate for the vessel, as occasionally fluence of 8.5 to 10 J/cm^2 is needed.[35]

Facial telangiectasias respond well but may require more than one treatment (Figs. 5–5, 5–6). Linear telangiectasias such as those around the nasal alae show texture changes less often with PDL than with CW systems. Some 91% showed good to excellent response after one treatment for facial telangiectasias.[68] Fluences above 7 J/cm^2 may be needed.[68, 79] Larger blue vessels respond less well owing to a larger ratio of deoxygenated hemoglobin and prolonged thermal relaxation times.[68] With a 5-mm spot, keeping fluence at 6.5 J/cm^2 or lower minimizes risk of hyperpigmentation.[30]

With 5-mm spot size, parameters are the same as for port

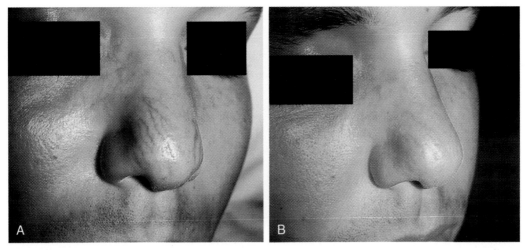

Figure 5–5. Nasal telangiectasias. *(A)* Pretreatment, and *(B)* after three treatments with Candela FLPDL at 9, 10, and 10 J/cm^2, 3-mm spot size.

wine stain—5.5 to 7.6 J/cm^2 in most cases.[30] To minimize purpura when treating small vessels, a 2- or 3-mm spot size may be chosen. To maintain the same fluence, energy levels need to be increased to achieve the same results. With a 3-mm spot size, energy levels must be in the 7- to 7.5-J/cm^2 range, and more than 8 J/cm^2 with a 2-mm spot size.

LEG VEIN SPIDER TELANGIECTASIAS

With the FLDL, results on leg veins have been inconsistent at best, with persistent postinflammatory pigmentation; however, after sclerotherapy matted vessels have responded.[80] Recently, another FLPDL with parameters designed for leg veins has been introduced in the market. It is discussed elsewhere in this book.

DIFFUSE FACIAL TELANGIECTASIAS

Rosacea, actinic damage, and chronic steroid use are often associated with diffuse facial telangiectasias. PDL can be quite effective. Rosacea is an inflammatory disease, usually of the face. It affects both sexes, most often between ages 30

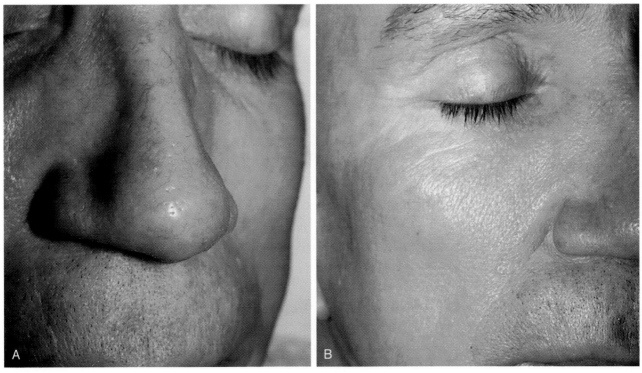

Figure 5–6. Nasal telangiectasias. *(A)* Before treatment and *(B)* after one treatment with Candela FLPDL at 10 J/cm^2, 2-mm spot size.

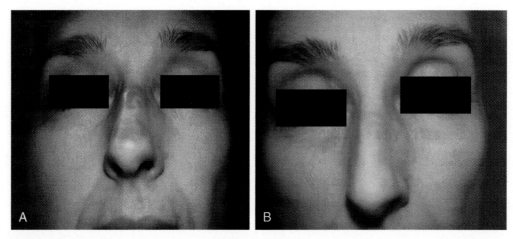

Figure 5–7. *(A)* Rosacea of the nose shows persistent erythema despite treatment with oral minocycline and metronidazole gel. *(B)* After one treatment with the Candela FLPDL at 6 J/cm², 5-mm spot size.

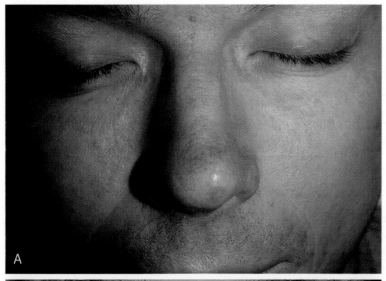

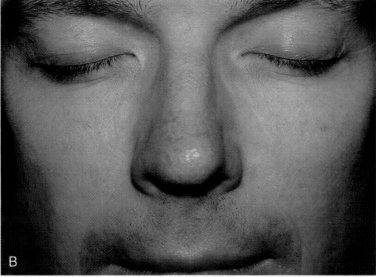

Figure 5–8. *(A)* Diffuse erythema and telangiectasias in a patient with partially controlled rosacea. *(B)* Appearance after one treatment with the Candela FLPDL at 6.5 J/cm², 5-mm spot size.

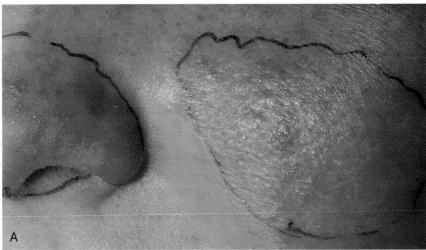

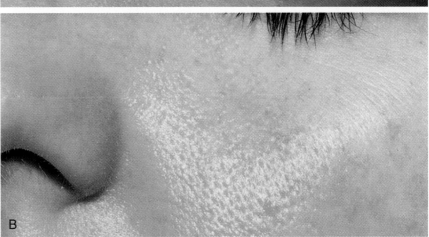

Figure 5–9. *(A)* Severe facial erythema improved with oral minocycline and metronidazole gel. *(B)* After three treatments with the Candela FLPDL at 6, 6.5, and 6.5 J/cm², 5-mm spot size.

and 50 years, and is prone to relapsing papulation and pustulation.[81–83] In addition, almost all patients have telangiectasias of the face, particularly the nose and cheeks.[83, 84] Patients frequently experience skin flushing, which has been suggested to be an important component of the pathogenesis of rosacea papules and pustules.[81, 82, 85]

Successful forms of therapy for rosacea papules and pustules include topical[86–88] and systemic antibiotics,[87, 89] isotretinoin,[82, 90–92] and systemic[82, 86] and topical metronidazole.[81, 89, 93] Usually, however, these agents are not effective at reducing the telangiectasia and flushing observed in most rosacea patients (Fig. 5–7).

FLPL tuned at 585 nm with a 450-μsec pulse width and a 5-mm spot-size handpiece[94] was used to treat patients with rosacea and associated persistent telangiectasia (Figs. 5–8 and 5–9). Some transient adverse cutaneous reactions were reported,[94, 95] including purpuric responses with purplish gray discoloration, crusting and mild scabbing, and mild crusting and peeling. No permanent pigmentation changes or scarring resulted from FLPDL treatment. Clinical observations[81, 94] suggest that ablation of the superficial dermal vasculature using the FLPDL may be a useful adjunct in the management of facial rosacea by reducing flushing induced by vasodilatation and the pustular papular inflammatory component.[96] Genetic syndromes such as Bloom's,

Rothmund-Thomson, and Goltz's syndrome respond well also.[97, 98] In these cases, the recommendation is 5- to 7-mm spot sizes with fluences of 6 to 7.5 J/cm².[96] Some authors recommend overlap of 10% to 33%, whereas some feel this leads to increased risk of scarring.[22] Multiple treatments are needed when there are extensive confluent vessels.

EXTRAFACIAL TELANGIECTASIAS

Results with extrafacial lesions are more variable. Poikiloderma of Civatte,[99] a sun-induced reticulated hyperpigmented and vascular process on the neck and chest, responds effectively at fluences of 6.5 to 7 J/cm² and requires about four treatment sessions.[99] The neck and chest are more susceptible to atrophic scarring, so a test with low-energy fluence is recommended. Lask indicates that the neck and chest are particularly prone to scar and recommends lower fluences, such as 6 J/cm², and avoiding extensive overlap.[30] It is also noted[30] that poikiloderma of Civatte may cover large areas, and an unnatural demarcation of untreated areas can occur, leading to patient dissatisfaction. Thus, the need for multiple sessions should be resolved with the patient before treatment of large areas is initiated. Essential telangiectasias—multiple dilated netlike vessels on the extremities[22]—also respond effectively to this modality.

CAPILLARY HEMANGIOMAS

Certain capillary (strawberry) hemangiomas are also effectively treated. In particular, early macular lesions in the first few weeks of life can be aborted with minimal or no sequelae.[62, 100–103] Low fluences are recommended[30] to begin (6 to 6.5 J/cm², 5-mm spot), and treatment is repeated at 2- to 4-week intervals to impede further growth.

Treatment is terminated when the lesion has resolved or when no further growth is anticipated. No cases of scarring have been reported, and the cosmetic results have been superior to those obtained when lesions were left to resolve. Thus, these lesions should be treated within the first few weeks of life when they are small and macular.

Once the lesion has matured and thickened, the response is much less dramatic. If the lesion is deeper than 1.2 mm, the laser light cannot penetrate to be effective; however, this can be partially overcome by compressing with a glass slide before lasering. Telangiectatic sequelae of resolved[24] hemangiomas respond well. Cavernous or mixed hemangiomas cannot be treated, because the vascular channels are too large for this laser light.

OTHER VASCULAR LESIONS

Venous lakes, small cherry hemangiomas, and small angiokeratomas also respond, although vascular compression may be necessary before treatment. In general, if the vascular lesion is composed of small vessels it should respond to PDL.[68] Telangiectasia macularis eruptiva perstans responds, but results are temporary.[104] *Treatment parameters[105] for various lesions are noted in Table 5–2, which is specific for the Cynosure laser. Each manufacturer's recommendations differ.*

Carbon Dioxide Laser

The CO_2 laser is no longer considered appropriate for telangiectasias, owing to the risk of scar; however, this laser may be effective for ablation of lesions such as angiokeratomas, larger hemangiomas, pyogenic granulomas, and similar lesions. The energies chosen should be the lowest sufficient to ablate the lesion. The CO_2 laser may be useful for debulking large capillary or cavernous hemangiomas.[24] The newer resurfacing lasers (Ultrapulse 5000C, Sharplan Silktouch, and others) have not been studied specifically for vascular lesions. It is the authors' opinion that superficial vascularity is significantly diminished after facial resurfacing in many patients.

Nd:YAG Laser

This laser, when set on 1064 as a continuous (non–Q-switched) wave, can function as a deeper penetrating laser to ablate larger lesions, as outlined above for the CO_2 laser.

Some degree of fibrosis and scarring is inevitable.[106] Penetration is 4- to 6-mm with coagulation of vessels up to 4 mm in diameter. A glass slide can be used to compress larger vessels. Multiple treatments may be necessary. At the frequency-doubled rate of 532, which is accomplished by using KTP crystal, the laser becomes the KTP system and vascular lesions can be treated[106] (see section of this chapter on KTP).

Summary: Which Laser for Which Problem?

CW or PDL often can be used for the same vascular problems. Various CW lasers have been effective in treating facial telangiectasias with minimal problems and excellent results. Comparison studies between CW and PDL[22] have often produced equivocal results. Discomfort may be less pronounced with CW lasers, but this could be due to the small spot size. Used correctly, there is no purpura with the CW systems, whereas the limiting factor with the PDL is often the purpura. On the other hand, studies have demonstrated an extremely low risk of adverse results with the PDL overall,[67] and technique with the unit is straightforward and less operator dependent.

The PDL was designed specifically for port wine stain–sized vessels and is considered the standard of care.[62, 63] The technique with the PDL is very straightforward, as previously noted, the primary issue being choosing the proper energy setting. Even choosing the energy setting is minimized by simply performing several small tests at various settings at the first visit and then waiting 6 weeks. On the other hand, CW lasers are far more technique and operator dependent. Many authors, therefore, consider the PDL to be the standard of care for most vascular lesions.[62, 63] For larger vessels, CW lasers may be more efficacious based on the pulse duration needed. Many lasers are available to treat vascular lesions, but no single one is appropriate in all instances, although for most clinical lesions, the FLPDL would be the initial choice.

REFERENCES

1. Waldorf HA, Lask GP, Geronemus RG: Laser treatment of telangiectasia. In Alster TS, Apfelberg DB (eds): Cosmetic Laser Surgery. New York: Wiley-Liss, 1996;93–109.
2. Sanchez JL, Ackerman AB: Vascular proliferations of skin and subcutaneous fat. In Fitzpatrick TB, Eisen AZ, Wolff K, et al. (eds): Dermatology in General Medicine. New York: McGraw-Hill, 1993; 1209–1237.
3. Bean WB: Vascular Spiders and Related Lesions of the Skin. Springfield: Charles C. Thomas, 1958.
4. Alderson MR: Spider naevi—Their incidence in healthy school children. Arch Dis Child 1963; 38:286–288.
5. Goldman MP, Bennet RG: Treatment of telangiectasia: A review. J Am Acad Dermatol 1987; 17:167–182.
6. Mullikan JB, Young AE: Vascular Birthmarks, Hemangiomas and Malformations. Philadelphia: WB Saunders, 1988.
7. Moy JA: Cutaneous manifestations of drug abuse. In Fitzpatrick TB, Eisen AZ, Wolff K, et al. (eds): Dermatology in General Medicine. New York: McGraw-Hill, 1993; 1807–1812.

8. Freinkel RK: Cutaneous manifestations of endocrine diseases. In Fitzpatrick TB, Eisen AZ, Wolff K, et al. (eds): Dermatology in General Medicine. New York: McGraw-Hill, 1993;2113–2131.

9. Stoughton RB, Corness RC: Corticosteroids. In Fitzpatrick TB, Eisen AZ, Wolff K, et al. (eds): Dermatology in General Medicine. New York: McGraw-Hill, 1993;2846.

10. Kligman AM, Kligman LH: Photoaging. In Fitzpatrick TB, Eisen AZ, Wolff K, et al. (eds): Dermatology in General Medicine. New York: McGraw-Hill, 1993;2972–2979.

11. Goslen JB: Wound healing for the dermatologic surgeon. J Dermatol Surg Oncol 1988; 14:959–972.

12. Geronemus RG, Ashinoff R: The medical necessity of evaluation and treatment of portwine stain. J Dermatol Surg Oncol 1991;17:76–79.

13. Cooper P: Vascular tumors. In Farmner ER, Hood AF (eds): Pathology of the Skin. Norwalk: Appleton & Lange, 1990;816.

14. Wilson B, Brewer PC: Spontaneous improvement of a port wine stain. Cutis 1995; 56:93–95.

15. Anderson RR, Levins PC, Grevelink JM: In Fitzpatrick TB, Eisen AZ, Wolff K, et al. (eds): Dermatology in General Medicine. New York: McGraw-Hill, 1993;1755–1766.

16. Goldman MP, Weiss RA, Brody JH, et al.: Treatment of facial telangiectasia with sclerotherapy, laser surgery, and/or electrodesiccation: A review. J Dermatol Surg Oncol 1993;19:889–906.

17. Marks R. Concepts in the pathogenesis of rosacea. Br J Dermatol 1968;80:170–177.

18. Wilkin JK: Flushing reactions. In Rook AJ, Maibach HI (eds): Recent Advances in Dermatology, No. 6. New York: Churchill-Livingstone, 1983;157–187.

19. Geronemus R: Treatment of spider telangiectasias in children using the flashlamp-pumped pulsed dye laser. Pediatr Dermatol 1991; 8:61–63.

20. Dermuth RJ, Miller SH, Keller F: Complication of embolization treatment for problem cavernous hemangioma. Ann Plast Surg 1984; 13:135–177.

21. Esterly NB: Cutaneous hemangiomas, vascular stains, and associated syndrome. Curr Probl Pediatr 1987;17:1–69.

22. Waldorf HA, Lask GP, Geronemus RG: Laser treatment of telangiectasias. In Alster TS, Apfelberg DB (eds): Cosmetic Laser Surgery. New York: Wiley-Liss, 1996;93–109.

23. Thibault KP: Copper vapor laser and microsclerotherapy of facial telangiectases: Patient questionnaire. J Dermatol Surg Oncol, 1994; 20:48–54.

24. Glassberg E, Walker K, Lask G: Lasers in dermatology. In Lask GP, Moy RL (eds): Principles and Techniques of Cutaneous Surgery. New York: McGraw-Hill, 1996; 445–468.

25. Dover JS: Course Syllabus: Lasers in Dermatology. Course 108, American Academy of Dermatology Annual Meeting, 1996.

26. Ratz JL: Laser physics. Clin Dermatol 1995;13:11–20.

27. Spicer MS, Goldberg DJ: Lasers in dermatology. J Am Acad Dermatol 1996;34:1:1–25.

28. Morelli JG, et al: Tunable dye laser (577 nm) treatment of port wine stains. Lasers Surg Med 1986; 6:94.

29. Garden JM, et al.: Effect of dye laser pulse duration on selective cutaneous vascular injury. J Invest Dermatol 1986;87:653.

30. Lask GP, Glassberg E: 585-nm Pulsed dye laser for the treatment of cutaneous lesions. Clin Dermatol 1995;13:63–67.

31. Russell SW, Dinehart SM, et al.: Efficacy of corneal eye shields in protecting patients' eyes from laser irradiation. Dermatol Surg 1996; 22:613–616.

32. Ries WR, Clymer MA, Reinisch L: Laser safety features of eye shields. Lasers Surg Med 1996;18:309–315.

33. Garden JM, Tan OT, Kerschmann R, et al.: Effect of dye laser pulse duration on selective cutaneous vascular injury. J Invest Dermatol 1986;87:653–657.

34. Geronemus RG: Argon laser for the treatment of cutaneous lesions. Clin Dermatol 1995;13:55–58.

35. Goldman MP, Fitzpatrick RE: Treatment of cutaneous vascular lesions. In Goldman MP, Fitzpatrick RE (eds): Cutaneous Laser Surgery: The Art and Science of Selective Photothermolysis. St Louis: Mosby–Year Book, 1994; 19–105.

36. Ratz JL, et al.: Post-treatment complications of the argon laser. Arch Dermatol 1985; 121:714.

37. Garden JM, Geronemus RG: Dermatologic laser surgery. J Dermatol Surg Oncol 1990; 16:156.

38. Key DJ: Argon-pumped tunable dye laser for the treatment of cutaneous lesions. Clin Dermatol 1995;13:59–61.

39. Orenstein A, Nelson JS: Treatment of facial vascular lesions with a 100-micron spot 577-nm pulsed continuous wave dye laser. Ann Plast Surg 1989; 23:310–316.

40. Scheibner A, Wheeland RG: Argon-pumped tunable dye laser therapy for facial port wine stain hemangiomas in adults: A new technique using small spot size and minimal power. J Dermatol Surg Oncol 1989; 15:277.

41. Scheibner A, Wheeland RG: Use of argon-pumped tunable dye laser for port wine stain in children. J Dermatol Surg Oncol 1991; 17:735.

42. Hanke CW: Lasers in dermatology. Indiana Med 1990; 83:393–402.

43. Mordon S, Beacco C, et al.: Relation between skin surface temperature and minimal blanching during argon, Nd:YAG, and CW dye 585 laser therapy of portwine stain. Laser Surg Med 1993;13:124–126.

44. Apfelberg DB, Smoller B: Preliminary analysis of histological results of Hexascan device with continuous tunable dye laser at 514 (argon) and 577 (yellow). Laser Surg Med 1993;13:106–112.

45. McDaniel DH: Cutaneous vascular disorders: Advances in laser treatments. Cutis 1990;45:339–359.

46. Keller GS: Use of the KTP laser in cosmetic surgery. Am J Cosmetic Surg 1992;9:177–180.

47. Schliftman AB, Brauner G: The comparative tissue effects of copper vapor laser (578 nm) on vascular lesions. Laser Surg Med 1988;8:188.

48. Waner M, Dinehart S, et al.: A comparison of copper vapor and flashlamp-pumped dye lasers in treatment of facial telangiectasia. J Dermatol Surg Oncol 1993;19:992–998.

49. Dinehart S, Waner M, Flock S: The copper vapor laser for treatment of cutaneous vascular and pigmented lesions. J Dermatol Surg Oncol 1993;19:370–375.

50. Key MJ, Waner M: Selective destruction of facial telangiectasia using a copper vapor laser. Arch Otolaryngol Head Neck Surg 1992;118:509–513.

51. Pickering JW, Walker EB, Butler P, et al: Copper vapour laser treatment of port-wine stains and other vascular malformations. Br J Plast Surg 1990;43:273–282.

52. Walker EP, Butler PH, Pickering JW, et al.: Histology of portwine stains after copper vapour laser treatment. Br J Dermatol 1989; 121:217.

53. Chung JH, Koh WS: Histological responses of port wine stains in brown skin after 578 nm copper vapor laser treatment. Lasers Surg Med 1996; 18:358–366.

54. Wheeland RG: Treatment of port wine stains for the 1990s. J Dermatol Surg Oncol 1993;19:348–356.

55. McCoy S, Hanna M: An evaluation of the copper bromide laser for treating telangiectasia. Dermatol Surg 1996;22:551–557.

56. Tan OT, Murray S, Kurban AK: Action spectrum of vascular specific injury using pulsed irradiation. J Invest Dermatol 1989;92:868–871.

57. Garden JM, Tan OT, Kerschmann R, et al.: Effect of dye laser pulse duration on selective cutaneous vascular injury. J Invest Dermatol 1986;87:653–657.

58. Glassberg E, Lask GP, Tan EML, Uitto J: Cellular effects of the pulsed tunable dye laser at 577 nm on human endothelial cells, fibroblasts and erythrocytes. An in vitro study. Lasers Surg Med 1988;8:567–572.

59. Glassberg E, Lask GP, Tan EML, Uitto J: The flashlamp pumped 577 nm tunable dye laser: Clinical efficacy and in vitro studies. J Dermatol Surg Oncol 1988;14:1200–1208.

60. Anderson RR, Parish JA: Microvasculature can be selectively damaged using dye lasers: A basic theory and experimental evidence in human skin. Lasers Surg Med 1981;1:263–276.

61. Garden JM, Polla LL, Tan OT: The treatment of portwine stains by the pulsed dye laser: Analysis of pulse duration and long term therapy. Arch Dermatol 1988;124:889–896.

62. Geronemus RG: Pulsed dye laser treatment of vascular lesions in children. J Dermatol Surg Oncol 1993;19:303–310.

63. Day TW, Pardue CC, Dinwiddie C: Pulsed dye laser therapy for port wine stains in children. J Tenn Med Assoc 1991;84:173–175.

64. Brooke AJ, Arndt AK: Are all 585 nm pulsed dye lasers equivalent? J Am Acad Dermatol 1996;34:1000–1004.

65. Glassberg E, Lask GP, Tan EM, et al.: The flash-lamp pumped 577-nm pulsed tunable dye laser: Clinical efficacy and in vitro studies. J Dermatol Surg Oncol 1988;14:1200–1208.

66. Glassberg E, Lask GP, Rabinowitz LG, et al.: Capillary hemangiomas: Case study of a novel laser treatment and a review of therapeutic options. J Dermatol Surg Oncol 1989; 15:1214–1223.

67. Levine VJ, Geronemus RG: Adverse effects associated with the 577 and 585 nanometer pulsed dye laser in the treatment of cutaneous vascular lesions: A study of 500 patients. J Am Acad Dermatol 1995;32:613–617.

68. Gonzalez E, Gange RW, Momatz KT: Treatment of telangiectases and other benign vascular lesions with the 577 nm pulsed dye laser. J Am Acad Dermatol 1992;27:220–226.

69. Reyes BA, Geronemus R: Treatment of port wine stains during childhood with the flashlamp pumped pulsed dye laser. J Am Acad Dermatol 1990;23:1142–1148.

70. Tan OT, Carney M, Margolis R, et al.: Histologic responses of port wine stains treated by argon, carbon dioxide and tunable dye lasers. Arch Dermatol 1986;122:1016–1022.

71. Tan OT, Sherwood K, Gilchrest BA: Treatment of children with port wine stains using the flashlamp pumped tunable dye laser. N Engl J Med 1989;320:416–421.

72. Reyes BA, Geronemus RG: Treatment of port wine stains during childhood with the flashlamp pumped dye laser. J Am Acad Dermatol 1990;22:136–137.

73. Goldman MP, Fitzpatrick RE, Ruiz-Esparza J: Treatment of port wine stains (capillary malformation) with the flashlamp pumped pulsed dye laser. J Pediatr 1993;122:71–77.

74. Alster TS, Wilson F: Treatment of port wine stains with the flashlamp pumped pulsed dye laser: Extended clinical experience in children and adults. Ann Plast Surg 1994;32:478–484.

75. Lask GP: Personal communication.

76. Kauver AN, Geronemus RG: Repetitive pulsed dye laser treatments improve persistent port wine stains. Dermatol Surg 1995;21:515–521.

77. Renfro L, Geronemus RG: Anatomical differences of port wine stains in response to treatment with the pulsed dye laser. Arch Dermatol 1993;129:182–188.

78. Tan E, Vinciullo C: Pulsed dye laser treatment of port-wine stains, a patient questionnaire. Dermatol Surg 1996;22:119–122.

79. Fitzpatrick RE, Goldman MP: Treatment of facial telangiectasia with the flashlamp pumped dye laser. Lasers Surg Med 1991;3(Suppl):70.

80. Goldman MP, Fitzpatrick RE: Pulsed dye laser treatment of leg telangiectasia with and without simultaneous sclerotherapy. J Dermatol Surg Oncol 1990;16:338–344.

81. Decauchy F, Beauvais L, Meunier L, et al.: Rosacea. Rev Prat 1993;43(18):2344–2348.

82. Jansen T, Plewig G, Kligman AM: Diagnosis and treatment of rosacea fulminans. Dermatology 1994;188(4):251–254.

83. Marks R: Rosacea in Acne and Related Disorders. London: Martin Dunitz, 1989;293–299.

84. Borrie P: The state of the blood vessels of the face in rosacea. Br J Dermatol 1955;67:5.

85. Wilkin JK: Oral thermal-induced flushing in erythematotelangiectatic rosacea. J Invest Dermatol 1981;76:15–18.

86. Chu T: Treatment of rosacea. Practitioner 1993;237:941–945.

87. Wilkin JK, DeWitt S: Treatment of rosacea: Topical clindamycin versus oral tetracycline. Int J Dermatol 1993;32(1):65–67.

88. Pierard-Franchimont C, Arrese JE, Pierard GE: Pharma-clinics. How I treat rosacea. Rev Med Liege 1996;51(6):393–395.

89. Thiboutot DM: Acne rosacea. Am Fam Physician 1994;50(8):1691.

90. Ertl GA, Levine N, Kligman AM: A comparison of the efficacy of topical tretinoin and low-dose oral isotretinoin in rosacea. Arch Dermatol 1994;130(3):319–324.

91. Gajardo J: Severe rosacea treated with oral isotretinoin. Rev Med Child 1994;122(2):177–179.

92. Jansen T, Plewig G: The oral treatment of rosacea with isotretinoin. Dtsch Med Wochenschr 1995;120(50):1745–1747.

93. Signore RJ: A pilot study of 5 percent permethrin cream versus 0.75 percent metronidazole gel in acne rosacea. Cutis 1995;56(3):177–179.

94. Lowe NJ, Behr KL, Fitzpatrick R, et al.: Flash lamp pumped dye laser for rosacea-associated telangiectasia and erythema. J Dermatol Surg Oncol 1991;17:522–525.

95. Landthaler M: Argon laser in rosacea. Hautarzt 1993;44(5):328.

96. Lowe NJ, Behr KL, Fitzpatrick R, et al.: Flashlamp pumped dye laser for rosacea associated telangiectasias and erythema. J Dermatol Surg Oncol 1991;17:522–525.

97. Potozkin JR, Geronemus RG: Treatment of poikilodermatous component of the Rothmund-Thomson syndrome with the flashlamp pumped pulsed dye laser.: A case report. Pediatr Dermatol 1991;8:162–165.

98. Alster TS, Wilson F: Treatment of focal dermal hypoplasia (Goltz syndrome) with the 585 nm flashlamp pumped pulsed dye laser. Arch Dermatol 1995;131:143–144.

99. Wheeland RG, Applebaum J: Flashlamp pumped pulsed dye laser therapy for poikiloderma of Civatte. J Dermatol Surg Oncol 1990;16:12–16.

100. Waner M, et al.: Laser photocoagulation of superficial proliferating hemangiomas. J Dermatol Surg Oncol 1994;20:43–46.

101. Glassberg E, Lask GP, Rabinowitz LG, Tunnessen WW: Capillary hemangiomas: Case study of a novel laser treatment and a review of therapeutic options. J Dermatol Surg Oncol 1989;15:1214–1223.

102. Ashinoff R, Geronemus R: Capillary hemangiomas and treatment with flashlamp pumped dye laser. Arch Dermatol 1991;127:202–205.

103. Garden JM, Bakus AD, Paller AS: Treatment of cutaneous hemangiomas by the flashlamp pumped pulsed dye laser: Prospective analysis. J Pediatr 1992;120:555–560.

104. Ellis DB: Treatment of telangiectasia macularis eruptiva perstans with the 585 nm flashlamp pumped dye laser. Dermatol Surg 1996;22:33–37.

105. Cynosure Peer Reference Manual for the Photogenica 5 Laser. Cynosure Clinical Service Dept., Chelmsford, MA, 1995.

106. Lask GP, Glassberg E: Neodymium:yttrium-aluminum-garnet laser for the treatment of cutaneous lesions. Clin Dermatol 1995;13:81–86.

6

TELANGIECTASIAS OF THE LEGS

Patrick K. Lee
Gary P. Lask

Abnormal leg veins occur in 29% to 41% of women and 6% to 15% of men in the United States.[1] Genetic predisposition, hyperestrogenemia, jobs that demand prolonged standing, and obesity are all major etiologic factors.[2] Localized trauma can also contribute, as can any condition that causes the hemodynamic changes seen when the valves of the major superficial veins become incompetent and fail to function properly.[3]

Abnormalities of the leg veins can be roughly divided into two categories: varicosities of the greater and lesser saphenous veins, which are connected to the deep venous system, and superficial telangiectasias, which have negligible deeper connections. The former can often be a medical as well as cosmetic concern: inflammation can lead to symptoms of cramping and tenderness and the pruritus of stasis dermatitis.[4] Conventional treatments have included support hose, surgery, aggressive sclerotherapy,[4] and, more recently, ambulatory phlebectomy,[5] and have had a great deal of success. Superficial telangiectasias of the leg are primarily a cosmetic concern, and cosmesis is what most often prompts patients to seek treatment.[6]

Sclerotherapy

The most common method of treating leg telangiectasias is sclerotherapy,[6] and it is the gold standard against which all other therapies are measured. Its effectiveness is well-documented and has been reliable and predictable for more than two decades.[5] The most widely used, and only FDA-approved, sclerosants in the United States are hypertonic (23.4%) saline and sodium tetradecyl sulfate (Sotradecol); however, only sodium tetradecyl sulfate is FDA approved as a sclerosant; hypertonic saline being approved as an abortifacient.[7] Although highly effective on small vessels, hypertonic saline causes pain on administration and has ulcerogenic potential.[7] Sotradecol works well on small and large vessels, but its drawbacks include hypersensitivity reactions.[7] Polidocanol (Aethoxysclerol) is another sclerosant awaiting FDA approval that is very effective and relatively painless and has little, if any, ulcerogenic potential. Rare allergic hypersensitivity reactions have been reported.[8, 9]

One of the most frequent side effects of sclerotherapy is postsclerosis pigmentation, which has been estimated to occur in 30% or more of patients. It is induced by extravasation of erythrocytes through the damaged or destroyed vessel and is more likely to occur if the sclerosant is too strong.[10] Often, the therapy is merely watchful waiting for resolution.

Another common side effect of sclerotherapy is telangiectatic matting, which has been estimated to occur in 5% to 40% of patients. The trauma of the sclerosants and the injections themselves can contribute to the development of these veins, and they may occur immediately or several months after one or more treatments. Often, the vessels can resolve partially without treatment or become responsive to future treatments after an interval of 3 months to 2 years.[11]

Laser Therapy

Because of the side effects of sclerotherapy described above, alternative therapies for superficial telangiectasias of the leg, such as laser therapy, have been sought. In the past, continuous-wave (CW) laser systems, such as carbon dioxide (CO_2) and argon lasers, were tested for their effect on leg veins[12]; however, there were a number of adverse sequelae, including scarring, hypo- and hyperpigmentation, pain, and recurrence in treated vessels. These complications far outweighed the side effects of sclerotherapy.[6]

When the pulsed-dye laser (PDL) proved effective for cutaneous vascular lesions, the treatment of leg veins seemed to be a natural application, but results were disappointing because of inconsistent responses and persistent postinflammatory hyperpigmentation.[13] These poor results may have been due to deeper localization of leg telangiectasias, the larger diameter, or the presence of connections with the deep venous system, which resulted in rapid recanalization of the coagulated vessel.[14] In addition, PDL treatment of leg veins, combined with sclerotherapy, offered no greater resolution than treatment by sclerotherapy alone.[6]

The investigation of alternative therapies such as lasers must be viewed in the context of sclerotherapy complications. Many patients, even those treated successfully with sclerotherapy, had a large number of veins that did not improve with injections. They often inquire as to whether another treatment modality is available for those unresponsive veins. Moreover, often these very same patients have developed telangiectatic matting as a result of sclerotherapy and are not reassured when the only forms of treatment offered for these vessels are "tincture of time" and further sclerotherapy. Some patients have vessels of very small caliber that make sclerotherapy extremely difficult, if not impossible.

Another group who would benefit from an alternative such as laser treatment are patients with telangiectasias of the ankles and feet. Often, it is only an aggressive sclerotherapist who is willing to inject such veins, because of the risk of ulcers. Such patients could benefit much from effective laser treatment. Finally, there are patients who fear injections of any kind. Laser can be a relatively noninvasive treatment-modality for those who desire no injections yet seek improvement of their superficial leg veins.

Laser Systems

As of this writing, there are six systems that are advocated for the treatment of leg veins:

ScleroPLUS The PDL resulted in excessive postinflammatory hyperpigmentation after treatment of superficial leg telangiectasias. The hyperpigmentation was hemosiderin deposited as a result of mechanical shock and cavitation of blood vessels by the laser.[14] This effect was thought to be secondary to the short pulse duration (450 µsec) of the laser; this brief energy exposure time would contribute to rupturing the vessel. The ScleroPLUS (Candela) was developed to address this concern. With a longer pulse duration (1500 µsec), the ScleroPLUS attempts slower, more temporally uniform heating of the chromophore (the hemoglobin of red blood cells). In addition, the exposure wavelengths are 585, 590, 595, and 600 nm, which are longer than the PDL's wavelength of 585 nm. The intention is that longer wavelengths produce deeper penetration of the beam and, therefore, more complete heating of the blood vessel target. Kienle and Hibst[16] recently demonstrated that wavelengths close to 600 nm may be necessary for optimal treatment of leg veins. At these longer wavelengths, melanin is also less of a competing chromophore. Finally, with the longer pulse duration, higher fluences can be achieved—in the range of 1 to 30 J/cm², as opposed to the traditional 6 to 10 J/cm² of the PDL.[13] Garden and coworkers[15] have shown that a pulse duration of 1500 µsec at 585 nm can be effective for superficial leg veins at fluences of 7 to 10 J/cm²; therefore, higher fluences will be necessary at 590 through 600 nm because of decreased absorption by the hemoglobin chromophore. The ScleroPLUS also utilizes a 2-mm by 7-mm elliptical spot size so that vessels can be traced out, minimizing energy exposure to uninvolved skin and thus decreasing the risk of complications. The ScleroPLUS is recommended for vessels up to 1 mm in diameter (Figs.

6–1, 6–2). Clinical treatment usually consists of one pass over a leg vein with the resultant effect being a delayed purpura, conforming to the shape of the vessel. Many studies have proven the ScleroPLUS laser's effectiveness. Using 595 nm for one treatment, Hsia and coworkers[17] reported >50% clearance by 6 weeks in 11 out of 26 patients (42.3%) using 15 J/cm² and 6 out of 13 patients (45.2%) using 18 J/cm²; by 5 months, >50% clearance was noted in 18 out of 34 patients (53.0%) using 15 J/cm², and 11 out of 17 patients (64.7%) using 18 J/cm². Reichert[18] reported complete resolution of leg vessels <0.5 mm in diameter after one or two treatments at 590 nm and 8 J/cm²; for vessels between 0.5 and 1.0 mm, 80% clearance was achieved with up to four separate treatments at 595 and 600 nm with fluences between 16 and 22 J/cm². Bernstein and coworkers[19] demonstrated >75% clearance of leg veins in ten patients after three treatments at 595 nm and 15 to 20 J/cm². Although its success rate is far below that of sclerotherapy, the ScleroPLUS is safe, with the most common side effects being transient hyper- and hypopigmentation, and no scarring has been reported.[17–19] Previous studies had shown that cooling of the epidermis could increase the effectiveness of laser treatment of leg veins,[20] and findings are similar for the ScleroPLUS.[17, 19, 20] There are now available several different devices which can cool the epidermis while a laser

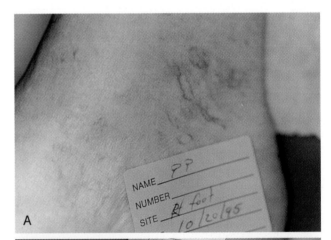

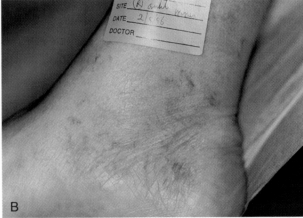

Figure 6–1. Superficial ankle veins *(A)* before treatment, and *(B)* after treatment with the ScleroPLUS (595-nm wavelength, 20 J/cm², 2-mm × 7-mm spot size).

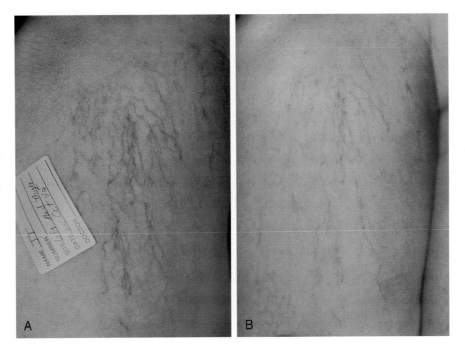

Figure 6–2. Superficial veins of the medial thigh *(A)* before treatment and *(B)* after treatment with the ScleroPLUS (595-nm wavelength, 15 and 20 J/cm², 2-mm × 7-mm spot size).

is in use, and they can increase the ScleroPLUS laser's efficacy as well as possibly reduce its side effects.[17–20] In the authors' experience, treatment has been effective but unpredictable. Many patients achieve significant improvement after one treatment; others have minimal improvement after several treatments. Areas that seem to respond best are vessels above the knee that are smaller than 1 mm in diameter. Complications have been rare, consisting of superficial scabbing, transient hypo- and hyperpigmentation (Fig. 6–3); there has been no scarring.

Orion/Aura Laser Laserscope has developed a variation of the CW, frequency-doubled Nd:YAG or potassium titanyl phosphate (KTP) laser called the Orion/Aura Laser. This laser utilizes what is called StarPulsing technology, which is basically pulsing the laser's beam at high frequencies, making it "quasicontinuous-wave". This system emits at 532 nm, still well within the hemoglobin absorbance range; however, at this wavelength melanin is theoretically a much more competitive chromophore. The fluences available range from 1 to 999 J/cm², and the pulse widths are

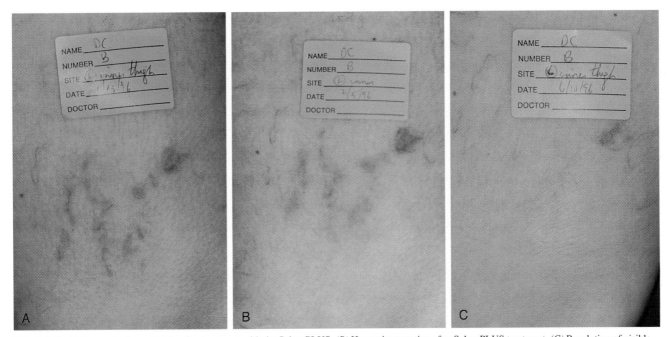

Figure 6–3. *(A)* Leg veins immediately after treatment with the ScleroPLUS. *(B)* Hyperpigmentation after ScleroPLUS treatment. *(C)* Resolution of visible leg veins and postinflammatory hyperpigmentation 6 months after ScleroPLUS treatment.

adjustable from 1 to 50 msec. The handpieces are available with 1- and 2-mm spot sizes, and the recommended parameters for treating leg veins are 24 to 30 J/cm^2 with a pulse width of 15 msec at 5 to 10 pulses per second, and 14 to 20 J/cm^2 with a pulse width of 10 to 15 msec at 1 to 3 pulses per second, respectively. As with the ScleroPLUS, the small spot sizes decrease the chance of exposing uninvolved skin to the laser beam and so avoid any related complications. The longer pulse widths allow greater fluences to be applied to the target vessels. One pass over a particular leg vein is the standard approach, with the clinical endpoint being vessel blanching. In the authors' experience, vessels of 0.5 mm or smaller are most likely to respond; larger vessels may exhibit significant scabbing (Fig. 6–4), which might increase the chance for skin texture changes. Also, because of the 532-nm wavelength, the risk of hypopigmentation from melanin competition is a significant risk.

Versapulse VPW Coherent Medical Corporation has developed a device similar to the Orion/Aura laser. The Versapulse is also a frequency-doubled Nd:YAG laser emitting at the 532 nm wavelength and has selectable pulse widths of 2, 5, 7, and 10 msec. Spot sizes from 2 through 10 mm are available coupled with pulse frequencies of 1–6 Hz. Pulse energies up to 38 J/cm^2 can be achieved using a 2 mm spot size. In addition, the device has the capability of cooling the skin during the treatment, with a novel sapphire "chill tip," which can be cooled to a temperature as low as 4°C by means of circulating chilled water. Adrian[21] treated patients with fluences between 9.5 and 16 J/cm^2 at pulse frequencies of 2–4 Hz; spot sizes ranged between 3 and 4 mm, with a chill tip temperature of 5.5°C. The clinical endpoint was either vessel disappearance or persistent intervascular coagulation, which usually required multiple passes. He reported 83% of patients with clearances >50% after two treatments, and patients graded as 75%–100% clearance increased from 18% after one treatment to 63% after a second treatment. Adverse effects mentioned included mild to moderate epidermal crusting,

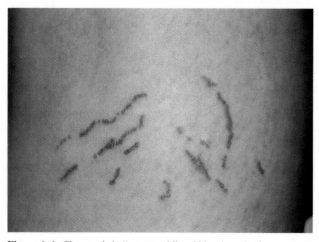

Figure 6–4. Characteristic "cat-scratch" scabbing 1 week after treatment with the Orion/Aura laser.

erosions, and occasional blister formation, which was often related to poor contact between epidermis and chill tip. Incidence of hyperpigmentation was reported as 36% and hypopigmentation as 12%; both were transient. No scarring was reported. A distinct advantage discussed about this laser was the absence of posttreatment purpura, normally seen with pulsed-dye lasers.

Veinlase This Nd:YAG laser is available from HGM and represents technology similar to that of the Aura and Versapulse lasers. The Veinlase has "quasi-continuous wave" pulsing at 532 nm and also at 1064 nm. This laser's "Captured-Pulsing" is a form of rapid pulsing of the beam, allowing fluences of up to 100 J/cm^2 with a 2 mm spot. Spot sizes of .6 mm to 4 mm are available with pulse widths adjustable from 8 to 50 msec. The 532 nm is recommended for leg veins up to 1.5 mm in diameter, and the 1064 nm for vessels up to 3 mm in diameter.

PhotoDerm The PhotoDerm VL system is not a laser, but is a noncoherent, intense pulsed light source developed to treat a variety of benign cutaneous lesions, including leg veins.[22] The device uses a flashlamp as a light (i.e., thermal) source to generate energy. The energy is directed into the skin and used to heat the vessels, to coagulate them. By its inherent design for energy application, the PhotoDerm is reportedly able to transfer heat so that it dissipates within the vessel's thermal relaxation time, thus conforming to the principle of selective photothermolysis. Because of the varying calibers and depths of leg veins, the PhotoDerm was developed with a great range of parameters. Since it is not a laser, it does not emit light at a specific wavelength; rather, it uses a series of "cutoff" filters. A cutoff filter cuts out the spectrum of light emitted by the flashlamp below the particular wavelength (e.g., a 550-nm cutoff filter allows transmission of the light spectrum from 550 nm to approximately 900 nm[22]). In the clinical treatment of leg veins, cutoff filters at 515, 550, 570, and 590 nm are available, fluences reach from 25 to 70 J/cm^2, and pulse durations range from 3 to 14 msec.[22] The spot size is 8 mm by 35 mm, and the PhotoDerm is recommended for leg veins up to 3 mm in diameter. The success of this system has been controversial. Goldman and Eckhouse[22] reported 94% of patients had clearances >50% after up to five treatments with few side effects, and Schroeter and Neumann[23] described that 73.6% of patients had immediate clearing, with 84.3% of patients having clearing after 1 month, again with few side effects reported. However, Green[24] reported only 9.5% of patients had complete or almost complete clinical clearing, with 56% showing no change. In addition, adverse effects were frequent and significant: hyperpigmentation in 50% of patients, hypopigmentation in 20%, epidermal desquamation in 42%, and scarring and textural change in 21%.[24] The correct parameters for leg vein treatment with the PhotoDerm and its predictability and reliability have been greatly debated[24–27] and still do not have a consensus.

Vasculight This system, also available from ESC, is a 1064 nm Nd:YAG laser with variable pulse durations for treatment of reticular veins. One theoretical advantage of this system, as opposed to previous laser and light source systems for leg veins, is that at 1064 nm, melanin is only absorbed at high fluences, so the incidence of pigment alteration, which occurred often with previous systems, should be markedly diminished. The Vasculight system has a spot size of 6 mm, fluences up to 150 J/cm^2, and pulse duration variabilities ranging from 2 to 20 msec, with single, double, and triple pulsing capabilities. At present, the parameters for the treatment of reticular veins are 120–140 J/cm^2, with 14–16 msec pulse duration, at a single pulse, using one pass.[28, 29] Sadick and coworkers[28] reported that an average of 2.5 treatments produced 100% clearing in 8 out of 10 patients. Other investigators have claimed good response using multiple passes over the same vein in one treatment session.[30] Further investigation is necessary for refinement of the parameters.

Conclusion

Documented effective treatment of superficial leg telangiectasias has been available for a number of years; however, the contribution of laser technology has so far been frustrating. Now, although they will never replace current leg vein treatments, a number of laser modalities show promise as alternative or complementary therapy for leg telangiectasias. Future clinical studies will define their role in the leg vein therapy armamentarium.

REFERENCES

 1. Engel A, Johnson ML, Haynes SG: Health effects of sunlight exposure in the United States: Results from the first national health and nutrition examination survey: 1971–1974. Arch Dermatol 1988;124:72–79.
 2. Sadick NS: Predisposing factors of varicose and telangiectatic leg veins. J Dermatol Surg Oncol 1992;18(10):883–886.
 3. Lofgren KA: Varicose veins: Their symptoms, complications, and management. Postgrad Med 1979;65(6):131–139.
 4. Fitzpatrick TB, Eisen AZ, Wolff K, et al. (eds): Dermatology in General Medicine. New York: McGraw-Hill, 1993;2095–2096.
 5. Weiss MA, Weiss RA: Sclerotherapy in the U.S. Dermatol Surg 1995; 21:393–396.
 6. Goldman MP, Fitzpatrick RE: Pulsed-dye laser treatment of leg telangiectasia: With and without simultaneous sclerotherapy. J Dermatol Surg Oncol 1990;16:338–344.
 7. Sadick NS: Advances in sclerosing solutions. Cosmetic Dermatol 1996;9(3):9–13.
 8. Conrad P, Malouf GM, Stacey MC: The Australian polidocanol (Aethoxysklerol) study—results at 2 years. Dermatol Surg 1995; 21:334–336.
 9. Conrad P, Malouf GM, Stacey MC: The Australian polidocanol (Aethoxysklerol) study—results at 1 year. Phlebology 1994;9:17–20.
10. Goldman MP, Kaplan RP, Duffy DM: Postsclerotherapy hyperpigmentation: A histologic evaluation. J Dermatol Surg Oncol 1987;13: 547–550.
11. Duffy DM: Understanding sclerotherapy. In Lask GP, Moy RL (eds): Principles and Techniques of Cutaneous Surgery. New York: McGraw-Hill, 1996:411–412.
12. Apfelberg DB, Maser MR, Lash H, et al.: Use of the argon and carbon dioxide lasers for treatment of superficial venous varicosities of the lower extremity. Lasers Surg Med 1984;4:221–231.
13. Lask GP, Glassberg E: 585-nm Pulsed dye laser for the treatment of cutaneous lesions. Clin Dermatol 1995;13(1):63–67.
14. Polla LL, Tan OT, Garden JM, et al.: Tunable pulsed dye laser for the treatment of benign cutaneous vascular ectasia. Dermatologica 1987; 174:11–17.
15. Garden JM, Kauvar ANB, Bakus AD, et al.: Pulsed dye laser treatment of superficial leg veins. Lasers Surg Med 1995; Supplement 7, Abstracts:57–58.
16. Kienle A, Hibst R: Optimal parameters for laser treatment of leg telangiectasia. Lasers Surg Med 1997; 20:346–353.
17. Hsia J, Lowery J, Zelickson B: Treatment of leg telangiectasia using a long-pulse dye laser at 595 nm. Lasers Surg Med 1997; 20:1–5.
18. Reichert D: Evaluation of the long-pulse dye laser for the treatment of leg telangiectasias. Dermatol Surg 1998; 24:737–740.
19. Bernstein EF, Lee J, Lowery J, et al: Treatment of spider veins with the 595 nm pulsed-dye laser. J Am Acad Dermatol 1998; 39:746–750.
20. Hohenleutner U, Walter T, Matthias W, et al.: Leg telangiectasia treatment with a 1.5 ms pulsed dye laser, ice cube cooling of the skin and 595 vs. 600 nm: preliminary results. Lasers Surg Med 1998; 23:72–78.
21. Adrian RM: Treatment of leg telangiectasias using a long-pulse frequency-doubled Neodymium:YAG laser at 532 nm. Dermatol Surg 1998; 24:19–23.
22. Goldman MP, Eckhouse S: Photothermal sclerosis of leg veins. Dermatol Surg 1996; 22:323–330.
23. Schroeter CA, Neumann HAM: An intense light source: the Photoderm VL-Flashlamp as a new treatment possibility for vascular skin lesions. Dermatol Surg 1998; 24:743–748.
24. Green D: Photothermal removal of telangiectases of the lower extremities with the PhotodermVL. J Am Acad Dermatol 1998; 38: 61–68.
25. Green D: Letter to the editor: Photothermal sclerosis of leg veins. Dermatol Surg 1997; 23:303–304.
26. Weiss RA: Reply to letter. Dermatol Surg 1997; 23:304–305.
27. Green D: Pitfalls in the evaluation of ablative therapy for telangiectases. Dermatol Surg 1998; 24:1143–1146.
28. Sadick NS, Weiss R, Goldman M: The utilization of a new Nd:YAG pulsed laser (1.064 microns wavelength) for the treatment of varicose veins. Lasers Surg Med 1999; Supplement 11:21.
29. Weiss RA: Initial results with a new synchronized pulsed 1064 nm laser for larger leg telangiectasias. Lasers Surg Med 1999; Supplement 11:21.
30. Bush RG, Hammond K: Multiple same site same session applications of Vasculight. Lasers Surg Med 1999; Supplement 11:65.

7

TATTOOS

Edward Glassberg
Gary P. Lask
Nicholas J. Lowe
Vladislav Chizhevsky

Decorative and ceremonial tattooing are ancient practices that date back thousands of years. Evidence exists of tattooing as early as the Bronze Age and on Egyptian mummies.[1–3] The practice has become quite sophisticated and continues to be widespread. Teenagers and young adults, in particular, have repopularized it. Some tattoos serve principally for cultural identity; others are purely decorative. Years after acquiring a tattoo (sometimes sooner), many people have regrets or no longer wish to have their skin marked in this way and seek to have the tattoo removed. It is estimated that 50% or more of persons in the United States who acquire tattoos eventually regret it and wish to have them removed.[4, 5]

Tattoos may be strictly amateur in design and application or more elaborate, usually more colorful, and professional in design and application. Some tattoos are placed for medical purposes, as to delineate radiation fields, and still others may be acquired by trauma or by exposure to various metals used in dentistry (''amalgam tattoo''). In this chapter we focus primarily on professional and amateur skin tattoos.

The natural history of a tattoo has been studied and is somewhat predictable. The ink particles generally reside in dermal fibroblasts and often around blood vessels. Approximately 2 months after application, there is some degree of fibrosis in the area. The particles remain fairly stable indefinitely.[6] Professional tattoo ink tends to reside predominantly in the upper, or papillary, dermis, whereas amateur tattoos are highly variable and the tattoo ink may reside in the papillary or reticular dermis and occasionally as deep as subcutaneous tissue.[7, 8] The size of tattoo ink particles has been measured at an average 4.42 μm $\pm$ 0.72 μm.[9] This size becomes important in laser treatment of tattoos, as it relates to the thermal relaxation time of particles of this size—approximately 30 ns to 1 ms.[10] Amateur tattoos do seem to be more variable in ink granule size, shape, and sites than professional tattoos, whereas the depth and density of tattoo ink varies much in both types.[11]

Both amateur and professional tattoos, which are principally black ink, generally contain carbon-based pigments, although iron oxide pigments can also create black tattoo ink. Professional tattoos, with their ever increasing array of colors, generally use many different metal ions in the various pigments: red ink may contain mercury, cadmium, or iron; yellow ink generally contains cadmium or ochre; black ink usually contains carbon or iron oxide; blue ink generally contains cobalt; green ink, chromium; white inks, usually titanium.[12, 13] These pigments, because of their granule size, composition, absorption, and reflectance properties, are amenable to fairly specific destruction by several laser modalities.

In this chapter, multiple methods, past and present, for removing tattoos are reviewed; however, the focus of the chapter is the most efficacious and safest methods of treatment, revolving around various laser systems, including the Q-switched ruby laser (QSRL), the Q-switched alexandrite laser, the 510-nm flashlamp-pumped pulsed dye pigment laser (FLPDL), and the Q-switched neodymium: yttrium-aluminum-garnet (QS-Nd:YAG) laser.

Methods of Tattoo Removal, Old and New

Many approaches have been developed over the years for removing tattoos. These have met with various degrees of success, and historically most have been fraught with the risk of scarring or permanent pigment changes. Attempts at removal have been documented as early as ancient Greece, approximately 1400 years ago.[14] The method was salabrasion, which has met with some success and is still in use. Methods previously and currently used to treat tattoos can be divided into mechanical forms such as dermabrasion and salabrasion; excisional therapy using full-thickness or tangential excisions; chemical methods using forms of acids such as trichloroacetic acid (TCA) or caustic chemicals such as phenol; cryotherapy; and thermal methods, which include electrodesiccation and cautery, the infrared coagulator, continuous-wave (CW) lasers such as the ruby, carbon dioxide (CO_2), and argon. The latest modality, which overlaps partly with thermal treatments but involves more specific destruction of pigmentation, is laser systems developed on the principle of selective photo-thermolysis.

Mechanical Destruction

Salabrasion (abrasion with a salt preparation) has been around for at least 1400 years.[14] A more modern variation on this sort of mechanical destruction involves the use of dermabrasion with either a diamond fraise or a wire brush. More recently, a series of shallow dermabrasions has been recommended, to minimize scarring and pigment changes.[15] Variations on this treatment have also involved the use of caustic chemicals to promote loss of pigment in wound exudate.[16] Although this method can be effective, there is a reasonably high risk of scarring, or at least moderate texture changes, as well as hypopigmentation, which may persist, and the possibility of hyperpigmentation.

Excision

Small, very limited tattoos can be excised successfully (depending on their site and size), leaving a very subtle or barely noticeable scar. Staged excisions may be necessary for larger tattoos, and tissue expansion can be used as well to minimize stretch-back. With this method, some scarring is inevitable, but it may be cosmetically quite acceptable and preferable to the original tattoo.[17, 18] A more recent variation of excisional therapy for tattoos reported by O'Donnell and colleagues in 1995 involves thin tangential excision of tattoos using a Brown dermatome set to 0.2 mm in depth plus application of gentian violet to the wound area for 5 days. These authors reported that four of five patients had no "significant" scarring 3 months after this procedure. One patient did have significant scarring, and another had what was described as *relatively insignificant* scarring. Three of the five patients had slight residual pigment. Two others had significant amounts of pigment left. This method, though less traumatic and extensive than full-thickness excision, still carries relatively high risk for scarring.[19]

Chemical Destruction

In one form or another, chemical ablation has been around for more than 100 years[20] and has used tannic acid or silver nitrate, and more recently phenol or TCA.[21, 22] Both of these methods have been associated with significant scarring and pigment changes, but they can be relatively successful.

Cryotherapy

Cryotherapy has been reported to be successful; however, results are very unpredictable, and significant scarring is a risk.[23] It is not currently recommended, owing to its unpredictability and high risk for scarring.

Thermal Destruction

Thermal destruction of tattoos can be performed with electrodesiccation or electrocautery under local anesthesia, but scarring is very common. For very small lesions, this may be an acceptable modality, but it generally results in scarring or pigment changes. The infrared coagulator is a noncoherent light source[24] in the infrared range at approximately 900 to 960 nm. It was developed in 1979 and has been used fairly extensively for tattoo removal. The method is fairly effective; however, it results in nonspecific tissue destruction and frequent scarring.

Other sources of thermal destruction of tattoos involve one of the earliest applications of lasers to medical therapy. In particular, the CW ruby laser at 694 nm was first used on tattoos in the mid-1960s.[25] In addition, an early version of the QSRL was also used on tattoos and was described in articles published in 1967 and 1968.[8, 26] These early findings were largely dismissed or ignored until the advent of the modern QSRLs in the last decade. The CW Nd:YAG laser has also been used for thermal destruction of tattoos,[27] with moderate success but frequent scarring. Much more widely used for thermal destruction of tattoos are the CW argon and CW CO_2 lasers. The use of the argon laser for tattoo removal was reported in 1979 to achieve relatively complete removal and "acceptable" cosmesis in 29% to 33% of cases.[28, 29] The destruction by this laser is relatively nonspecific. Hypertrophic scars and incomplete removal have also resulted.[11] The CW CO_2 laser was also reported for tattoo treatments, beginning in 1978.[30, 31] The laser vaporized the tissue overlying and involving the tattoo, resulting in fairly extensive dermal damage and nonspecific tissue necrosis. Atrophic and hypertrophic scarring have been relatively common with this treatment, as have permanent pigment changes.[11]

Selective Photothermolysis

The use of high-energy, rapidly pulsed, or Q-switched lasers to specifically destroy or fragment tattoo ink particles has revolutionized the treatment of tattoos and allowed complete or partial removal of tattoos with minimal risk of scarring. The Q-switched and pulsed systems are described next and are discussed in detail with regard to their relative efficacy for tattoos of various types and colors.

Current Lasers for Tattoo Removal

The parameters and wavelengths of the lasers discussed in this section are based primarily on the theory of selective photothermolysis as propounded by Parrish and Anderson,[32, 33] which uses very brief high-energy pulses at selected wavelengths to damage specific chromophore or tissue targets while sparing the surrounding tissue. The Q-switched and pulsed lasers described here all use pulses of high energy in the nanosecond range, which are, generally speaking, shorter than the thermal relaxation time of the target tissue. This allows the full impact of the energy of the laser pulse to be absorbed by the chromophore and offers minimal opportunity for thermal conduction, which would result in nonspecific peripheral thermal destruction. Rapid mechanical expansion or shock waves from the rapidly absorbed energy results in breakup or destruction of the pigment or target chromophore (Fig. 7–1). The advantages and disadvantages of the various wavelengths and pulse durations are discussed.

Q-Switched Ruby Laser

The technique of Q switching was first reported by Goldman and coworkers in 1965,[34] and as early as 1967 and 1968[8, 26] was used for dermal pigmentation. Reid and associates, as early as 1983, reported excellent results using the QSRL on tattoos, and they recently reported an extensive 9-year experience.[35, 36] Since that time, multiple reports have described the efficacy of the QSRL and tattoo removal.

The term *Q-switched* refers to a change in the quality of the optical resonating structures of the laser so that light is emitted in very brief high-energy pulses, usually in the range of nanoseconds.[37] The mechanism of tattoo dye pigment destruction involves rapid absorption of energy with vaporization or rapid thermal expansion and the concomitant shock wave effect and destruction of the pigment. The pigment can be absorbed by phagocytic cells and eliminated by exudation through breaks in the epidermis or possibly through thermally mediated chemical changes, which may alter the optical properties of the tattoo pigment, resulting in clinical lightening.[11, 38]

INDICATIONS

The QSRL, with a wavelength of 694 nm and pulse width of 20 to 40 nsec, has been shown effective in the eradication of professional, amateur, traumatic, medical, and chemical tattoos of the skin and mucosa. Blue and black pigments appear to respond best to the QSRL wavelength, and the response of many types of green tattoo pigment is good.[39]

Erasing other colors has been less successful. Red is generally fairly resistant to QSRL.

In 1990, Taylor and colleagues[7] reported treating 35 amateur and 22 professional tattoos. After three or four treatments, 74% of the amateur and 22% of the professional tattoos were 75% to 100% cleared. The incidence of scarring was minimal. Another report of 101 amateur and 62 professional tattoos from 1990 had very similar results. It showed superior response with amateur tattoos.[40] Reid and associates, in Scotland, reported fairly comparable results in a cumulative 9-year experience with 418 patients. Ashinoff and Geronemus[41] reported a series of traumatic and medical tattoos that were also treated successfully without scarring or permanent pigment changes. The QSRL was also successful on an amalgam tattoo of the gingiva—at least in lightening the lesion.[42] Another very large series by Levins' group in 1991[43] reported on 200 tattoos treated with the QSRL. Superior response was cited for black, blue, green, and brown pigments. It should be noted that the QSRL is also absorbed fairly avidly by melanin; thus, overlying pigmentation of the patient may play a role in efficacy. Posttreatment hypopigmentation is fairly common though usually transient.[44, 45]

TREATMENT METHODS AND EFFICACY

As with all medical lasers, proper safety and precautions must be taken before and during treatment. Appropriate goggles or eye protection for the operator, all personnel in the room, and the patient is critical to avoiding retinal damage. Ignition of combustible material, including gauze on the field, the patient's hair or skin, and other equipment, anesthesia tubing, and oxygen-delivery systems, must be appropriately guarded from the beam and from sparks. The QSRL is a high-voltage machine, and care must be taken to avoid electrical shock and contact of water with the machine. Virtually all of the Q-switched lasers have the potential to aerosolize tissue and splatter viable debris; thus, masks, eye shields, and splatter shields or clear biologic dressings should be employed to avoid or contain tissue splatter. Although the latter technique of biologic dressing may reduce energy by 10%, it is an effective method of containing potentially infectious material.[43]

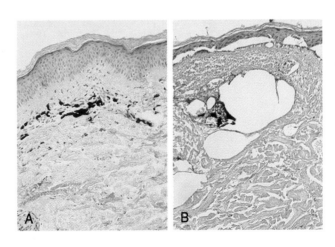

Figure 7–1. Amateur blue-black tattoo. *(A)* Skin biopsy before laser treatment. *(B)* Skin biopsy after two treatment sessions with Q-switched ruby laser (694-nm wavelength, 28-nsec pulse, 10 J/cm², 5-mm spot size).

Tattoos can be erased with or without anesthesia. Pain varies with the energy level and the individual patient's tolerance. Some can be treated without anesthesia, but some require or request either topical anesthesia such as eutectic mixture of local anesthetics (EMLA) or infiltration with lidocaine or another local anesthetic. Particular care must be taken with disinfecting agents, particularly alcohol, to avoid potential ignition.

Typical spot sizes for ruby lasers range from 3 to 8 mm with energy levels of 4 to 10 J/cm^2. Clinically, uniform whitening of the area, which appears almost immediately, is the usual end point. The tissue whitening is usually transient and may resolve after 10 to 20 minutes. There may be some moderate purpura or pinpoint bleeding at higher energy levels. Some erythema and edema also appear. Often, during the first 2 weeks after laser treatment, a scale crust forms that may exude pigment granules. The patient may also experience vesiculation at the treatment site. Postoperative wound care may consist of cleansing of the wound and topical antibiotic or bland ointments, plus sun protection once the epidermis is again intact. In general, multiple treatment sessions are necessary, ranging from approximately two to ten sessions or more at 4- to 8-week intervals.

In general, amateur tattoos respond somewhat more quickly than professional tattoos (Figs. 7–2, 7–3). Kilmer and associates reported good clearing of tattoos with the QSRL at 6 to 8 J/cm^2 and an average of four to six treatments for amateur tattoos and six to ten treatments for professional tattoos.[45] Other reports have documented good to excellent clearing of amateur tattoos in four to six sessions at 4 to 10 J/cm^2 and of professional tattoos in six to twelve sessions at fluences of 8 to 10 J/cm^2. Treatment frequency was every 3 to 4 weeks.[43] The most responsive colors were blue-black, black, green, and brown. Lowe and

colleagues reported average energy densities of 10 J/cm^2 treated at 6- to 8-week intervals for an average of five treatments (Figs. 7–4, 7–5). Under this regimen, 22 of 28 patients experienced better than 75% clearing.[46] Similar responses have been reported by many authors.[11, 41, 47]

COMPLICATIONS AND CONTRAINDICATIONS

The incidence of complications with the use of the QSRL appears to be quite low overall and is related to energy level, the patient's skin color, and the overall number of treatments. Early reports have shown scarring to be quite rare at or below 4 J/cm^2, but a few cases of scarring have been reported. One case (out of 57 patients) of localized scarring of approximately 2 cm^2 in a professional tattoo treated at 7 J/cm^2 has been reported.[35, 36, 40] More recently, a large study reported transient texture changes, which were fairly common early on but resolved within a couple of months. Fewer than 5% were permanent. This same study showed true hypertrophic scarring in approximately 0.5% of cases.[43] The most common reported complication or side effect of the QSRL is transient—possibly prolonged or possibly permanent—confetti-like hypopigmentation at the treatment site. In an early study, 39% of patients treated with 4 J/cm^2 or less and 46% treated with more than 5 J/cm^2 demonstrated this side effect 1 month after treatment.[7] Often, the hypopigmentation normalizes in 4 to 12 months, although one report showed that as many as 40% of patients had some degree of hypopigmentation after 1 year. Another study reported a high incidence of transient hypopigmentation (more than 50% of patients) lasting 2 to 6 months. In some cases, it was permanent.[43, 45] One very limited study on five dark-skinned patients (Fitzpatrick types V and VI) did report complete depigmentation with the QSRL at one test site on one patient.[48] Hyperpigmentation appears to be

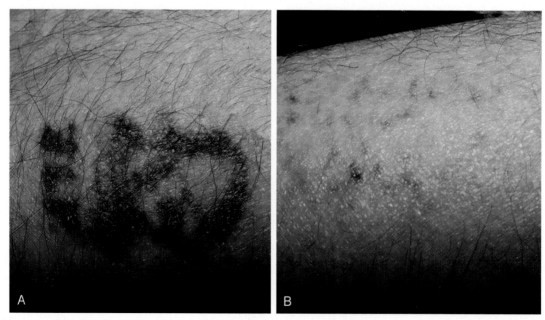

Figure 7–2. A 30-year-old amateur tattoo on the forearm *(A)* before treatment and *(B)* after two treatments using Q-switched ruby laser (694-nm wavelength, 28-nsec pulse, 10 J/cm^2, 5-mm spot size).

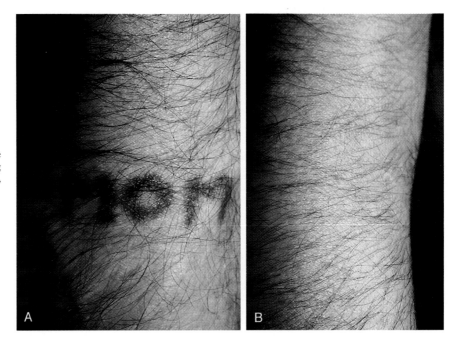

Figure 7–3. A 20-year-old tattoo *(A)* before treatment and *(B)* after two treatments using Q-switched ruby laser (694-nm wavelength, 28-nsec pulse, 10 J/cm², 5-mm spot size).

very uncommon—and usually transient—in perhaps 2% to 3% of patients. The frequency is somewhat increased in very dark-skinned patients.[7, 35]

Of particular note is the phenomenon sometimes observed in cosmetic tattoos of pigment darkening upon laser treatment. The QSRL, the QS-Nd:YAG and alexandrite lasers, and in particular, the 510-nm PDPL, can all make cheek rouge or lip tattooing turn black. Also, white and flesh-colored pigments can turn dark after treatment. This may or may not be amenable to further lasering to treat the black pigment.[11] Thus, it would be prudent to test small areas of any cosmetic tattoo, particularly lip liner or rouge and flesh- or white-colored tattoos before treating large areas. The darkening is usually quite immediate. Further laser treatment of the resulting black pigment has been successful in some cases.

It is assumed that darker-skinned patients such as Fitzpatrick types V and VI may be more prone to hypertrophic scarring, keloids, and pigment changes. One very limited initial study showed that tattoos can be treated successfully in these patients with minimal side effects. Grevelink and

associates published a study in 1996 of five dark-skinned patients treated on the face, neck, and chest with the QS-Nd:YAG laser and reported no significant scarring. In this study the QSRL was abandoned early on because of some depigmentation at test sites. Thus, very dark skin is a relative contraindication to treating patients with the QSRL. The authors of this study recommend using the QS-Nd:YAG for tattoo removal in darker-skinned patients, which showed fewer side effects.[48]

QS-ND:YAG LASER

The Nd:YAG laser has been in use in dermatology for more than 10 years, initially as a cutting and vaporizing tool and later for treating vascular lesions. Recently, when the Q switching technique was applied to the Nd:YAG laser, it was found to be useful in the treatment of tattoos and melanotic pigmentation. The QS-Nd:YAG laser emits principally 1064 nm with a pulse width of approximately 10 nsec and can be pulsed at 1 to 10 Hz. The beam size is 1.5 to 4 mm in current models. The laser can be frequency-

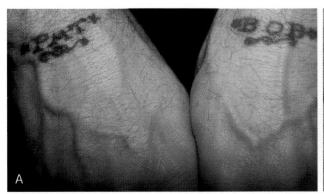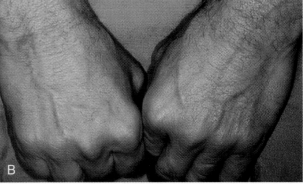

Figure 7–4. A professional tattoo *(A)* before treatment and *(B)* after three treatments using Q-switched ruby laser (694-nm wavelength, 28-nsec pulse, 10 J/cm², 5-mm spot size).

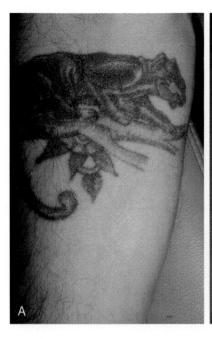
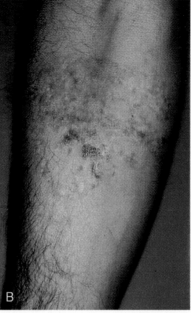

Figure 7–5. A professional tattoo *(A)* before treatment. *(B)* Some dye persists after six treatments using Q-switched ruby laser (694-nm wavelength, 28-nsec pulse, 10 J/cm², 5-mm spot size).

doubled to a wavelength of 532 nm, which is effective for more superficial melanin pigment or red tattoo ink (Fig. 7–6). The QS-Nd:YAG laser is similar in many ways to the QSRL, with some exceptions in efficacy. Both make use of the principle of selective photothermolysis in destroying pigment. Mechanisms of action of destruction of tattoo ink appear to be similar to those of the QSRL, including fragmentation of particles, changes in optical property, possible lymphocyte or phagocyte removal, and transepidermal removal of pigment.[49]

Indications. The QS-Nd:YAG laser is most useful on black or blue-black tattoos (Fig. 7–7), as well as red, orange, and purple pigments when frequency-doubled to 532 nm.[35, 49] In an early study of 28 patients with blue-black tattoos whose response to the QSRL was poor, better than

50% lightening was noted after a single treatment with the QS-Nd:YAG laser.[50] In overall terms, the QS-Nd:YAG appears to be comparably effective to the QSRL for blue-black tattoos. Fewer sessions may be needed with ruby laser treatment; however, there is also more hypopigmentation than with the QS-Nd:YAG.[51] Green tattoo pigment appears to be very resistant to the QS-Nd:YAG laser in general.[49] For darker-skinned patients, the QS-Nd:YAG appears to be superior to the QSRL, as one limited study demonstrated.[48]

Treatment Methods and Efficacy. In one study of black and blue-black tattoos at energy levels of 6 to 12 J/cm² with a 2-mm spot size, better than 75% clearing was seen in 77% of tattoos. No hypopigmentation was noted in this study, and no scarring was reported.[50] General response was poor at 1064 nm to green, yellow, white, and red pigments;

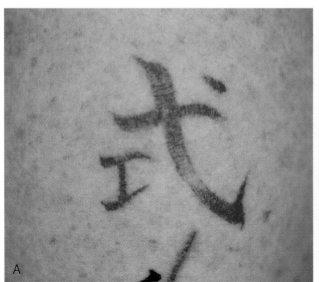
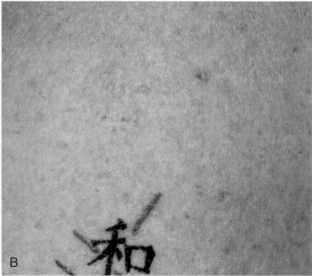

Figure 7–6. A red tattoo on the right arm *(A)*. *(B)* After four treatments with Q-switched Nd:YAG laser (5 J/cm², 2-mm spot size, 532-nm wavelength).

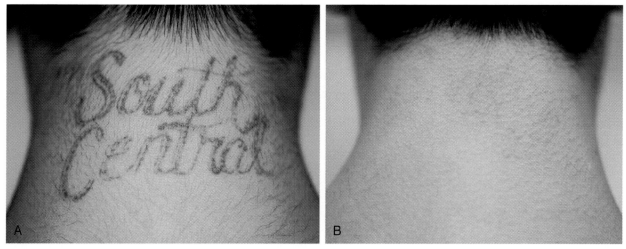

Figure 7–7. A blue-black tattoo of the posterior neck *(A)*. *(B)* After seven treatments with Q-switched Nd:YAG laser (12 J/cm², 2-mm spot size, 1064-nm wavelength).

however, at 532 nm, response was approximately 75% with red ink and good with purple and orange pigment.[11] Other studies have reported similar response rates using 8 to 12 J/cm² at 1 to 10 Hz and 1064 nm and treating at 4 to 5 J/cm², 2-mm spot size, at 532 nm on red pigment. In treating patients with this laser, the normal safety precautions outlined above for eye protection and spark ignition should be observed. Eye protection is particularly important because the laser beam emitted is not in the visible wavelength but near infrared. Thus, the normal protective reflexes are absent. The laser has an articulated arm mechanism and no aiming beam. Spot size varies from 1.5 to 4 mm with the most common spot size being about 3 mm. As with the QSRL, whitening of the tissue occurs immediately upon treatment, sometimes accompanied by some tissue splatter, particularly with smaller spot sizes. A clear plastic cylinder is often used to contain the splatter and help aim the beam, or a clear dressing such as Vigilon or Second Skin is important to contain splatter. At 1064 nm, there is significantly less melanin absorption than with the QSRL, and, consequently, less hypopigmentation.[51] General parameters for energy levels are around 10 to 12 J/cm² using the 2-mm spot size, and around 6 J/cm² using the 3-mm spot. These power settings vary with the amount of pigment and the density of the tattoo. As tattoo pigment is cleared, higher energy levels may be needed to get an adequate clinical response. The rapidity of the beam can be set anywhere from 1 to 10 Hz. The 532-nm beam can also be set at 1.5 to 4 mm with energy levels usually in the range of 2 to 6 J/cm² for treating red, orange, or purple pigments. Postoperative care is similar to that for any partial-thickness or epidermal wound, and the areas can be treated again at 4- to 8-week intervals.[45, 49]

Complications and Contraindications. Much like the QSRL, complications and side effects of the QS-Nd:YAG laser are generally minor and relatively uncommon. White, red, or flesh-colored cosmetic tattooing can turn black, particularly when treated with the 532-nm wavelength.[52] These tend to be titanium or iron-based pigments, which may be undergoing a form of oxidation resulting in changes in optical properties.[11] Extreme care must be taken when treating these types of tattoos. Many otherwise red, noncosmetic tattoos respond extremely well to the 532-nm wavelength. Pretreatment spot testing is indicated.

With the QS-Nd:YAG laser, some transient hyperpigmentation can be seen, particularly using the 532-nm wavelength, which is absorbed more avidly by melanin in the epidermis. Transient hypopigmentation is less common than with the QSRL. Scarring is quite rare, although it is possible at the highest fluences.[49] No cases of true depigmentation have been reported at this point, even in patients of Fitzpatrick types V and VI skin. Limited studies with the Nd:YAG laser have shown excellent response of black tattoos; only one in five patients showed persistent hypopigmentation and none had evidence of scarring or lasting texture changes. Further and larger studies of darker-pigmented patients are needed before accurate complication risks can be determined and recommendations made.

Q-SWITCHED ALEXANDRITE LASER

The QS alexandrite laser, with wavelength output from 750 to 760 nm and a pulse width of 50 to 100 nsec is similar in efficacy and indications to the QSRL.[53–55] The initial, relatively long pulse width of 100 nsec did, however, result in a lower peak power at any given fluence as compared with the QSRL and the QS-Nd:YAG lasers.[56] The decreased peak power clinically resulted in less tissue splatter and less clinical bleeding and purpura.[57] In addition, at the higher wavelength of 755 nm, somewhat less melanin is absorbed than with the ruby laser, resulting in less clinical hypopigmentation. The newer, shorter pulse width of 50 nsec results in a clinical profile more comparable to the QSRL, and fewer treatments are required for tattoo clearance. Proposed mechanisms of tattoo pigment removal are virtually the same as with the other Q-switched lasers, including pyrolytic chemical changes, possible phagocytosis, transepidermal elimination, and changes in dermal light-scattering coefficients.[58]

Indications. The QS alexandrite laser has been most successful in clearing black, blue-black, and green tattoo pigments, and some red pigments.[56] No difference between blue-black and green pigment removal was reported in one recent study.[57] Both amateur and professional tattoos respond extremely well to this laser, but newer, more recent, tattoos require somewhat more treatments.

Treatment Methods and Efficacy. Many recent reports have documented the efficacy of the QS alexandrite laser in treating blue-black and green tattoos. One study indicated that approximately five sessions or treatments are needed to clear approximately 75% of these tattoos, and an average 6.4 sessions to clear 90% of tattoos.[59] The average energy used was 8 J/cm^2 at treatment intervals of 4 to 8 weeks. The spot size is usually 3 mm; wavelength, 755 nm; and pulse width, 100 nsec. The clinical response is quite similar to that of the QSRL and the QS-Nd:YAG lasers: immediate whitening and some edema. Purpura and bleeding points may be seen at higher energy levels; however, they tend to be less significant with the alexandrite than with other Q-switched lasers. In 1995, Alster and colleagues reported treatment of 24 multicolored professional tattoos and 18 blue-black amateur tattoos with the QS alexandrite laser at 2-month intervals until all lesions were completely cleared. The 510-nm pulsed dye pigment laser was used for red pigment. Energies ranged from 4.75 to 8.0 J/cm^2 with whitening of the lasered area used as a clinical threshold, and energy decreased if bleeding occurred. Professional tattoos cleared in an average of 8.5 treatments; amateur tattoos, in an average of 4.6 treatments. Another study also reported excellent clinical results with professional and amateur tattoos in skin types I to III using fluences of 4 to 8 J/cm^2. Better than 95% clearing was achieved in 20 of 23 tattoos— all of 8 amateur ones and 12 of 15 professional tattoos. The average number of treatments for amateur tattoos was 7.8, whereas professional required 9.7 treatments on average.[60] Stafford and coworkers treated 22 professional and amateur blue-black tattoos and reported an average of 11.6 treatments for professional and 10.3 treatments for amateur tattoos to complete clearing.[61] Treatments ranged from 6.5 to 8.5 J/cm^2 at 4- to 6-week treatment intervals.

Complications and Contraindications. Complications of the QS alexandrite laser are very similar to those of other Q-switched lasers. Transient hypopigmentation has been reported in as many as 50% of patients, ranging in duration from 1 to 12 months.[11, 60] Alster and colleagues reported much less frequent, but also transient, hypopigmentation that resolved within approximately 3 months.[57] Transient hyperpigmentation was reported in 1 of 23 cases in one study, and this cleared in 4 months. The patient had

Fitzpatrick III–type skin.[60] Some transient texture changes have also been noted in approximately 12% of patients.[60] Even though several authors report no persistent scarring or texture changes, there are reports of two patients with focal areas of scarring after significant excoriation.[60] In general, minimal pain is reported with treatment; use of anesthesia is rare, and with normal wound care no infections were reported.[57]

With the alexandrite laser, as with all other Q-switched lasers, transient, brief flashes of light have been observed in treated areas which may represent formation of a plasma state.[61] The threshold for formation of plasma may be somewhat higher with the alexandrite laser. It has been estimated to be approximately 7.5 J/cm^2 in untreated tattoos and 9.0 J/cm^2 in older, faded, or previously treated tattoos. This higher threshold of plasma formation may be attributable to the lower peak power and more prolonged pulse width (100 nsec) as compared with other Q-switched lasers. This higher threshold and decreased plasma formation in general may contribute to lessen tissue splatter and punctate bleeding and purpura.[11, 61]

PULSED-DYE PIGMENT LASER

The FLPDL at 510 nm wavelength was designed principally for epidermal pigment, particularly melanin, which absorbs energy avidly at this wavelength.[61] The laser was found to be effective for red tattoo pigment, with efficacy very similar to that of the 532-nm frequency-doubled QS-Nd:YAG laser. The PDPL can sometimes be found housed in a single modified unit with the alexandrite laser for comprehensive treatment of pigmented lesions to treat red tattoo dye in conjunction with the alexandrite laser, which effectively treats blue-black and green pigments.

Indications. The PDPL has a pulse width of 300 nsec and a typical spot size of 3 to 5 mm. It is particularly effective for red tattoo pigment, which may be resistant to higher-wavelength lasers (694 to 1064 nm).[61]

Treatment Methods and Efficacy. Relatively little has been published on the PDPL. The limited available reports show excellent efficacy in treating red tattoo dye at fluences of 2 to 4 J/cm^2.[62, 63] One report indicated an excellent response in three to seven treatments at 1-month intervals without scarring or lasting hypopigmentation. Red, orange, purple, and yellow pigments were found to be responsive to treatment with this laser.[11, 64] The typical clinical response also involves whitening of the treatment area, with or without purpura. Crusting or vesiculation can occur at higher fluences with significant absorption by epidermal melanin.[62, 65] Pain appears to be minimal to moderate, and anesthesia is not usually necessary with this modality.

Complications and Contraindications. Hyperpigmentation or hypopigmentation can occur with the PDPL, although it is usually transient.[38] The incidence of scarring is extremely low, but localized atrophic areas can result with higher fluences, especially at sites below the neck. Sub-threshold energy levels or excessive energy can result in hyperpigmentation.[65] As mentioned previously, when treating red, white, or flesh-colored pigment with any laser, care must be taken to avoid darkening of the pigment in certain dyes.[11]

Conclusions and Summary

Clearly, the advent of Q-switched and flashlamp-pumped lasers has revolutionized the treatment of tattoos while minimizing long-term complications and risks. The systems described here can produce excellent clearing of tattoos with minimal risk of complication when used prudently. No single laser system can treat all tattoo pigments and colors; however, all of the Q-switched systems are excellent at clearing blue and black tattoos. The ideal laser system might combine the properties of the alexandrite or ruby laser with the Nd:YAG laser with frequency-doubling capacity, or the 510-nm PDPL. This would cover the most common tattoo pigments—blue, black, red, green—plus the less common colors. While the QSRL may clear some tattoos more rapidly than other systems, it carries a higher risk of hypopigmentation, particularly in darker-pigmented patients. The Nd:YAG laser is least likely to cause lasting hypopigmentation, owing to its relatively long wavelength. It is the laser of choice for darker-pigmented skin. The alexandrite laser at 100 nsec, perhaps because of its longer pulse width, may result in less tissue splatter and spread of viable tissue. Thus, each laser has its advantages and drawbacks.

Ideally, one would have access to multiple lasers and base the treatment of various tattoos and tattoo pigments on the wavelengths of the treating laser, the pulse width, and the patient's overlying pigmentation.[50, 66] The opening of various laser centers at private and university facilities should make it possible to obtain the best of all possible results with access to all of the appropriate laser systems. It is important to remember, and to make our patients aware, that not all lesions can be completely cleared, even with multiple treatments; however, most lesions are amenable to significant, if not complete, clearing with the laser systems now available.

REFERENCES

1. Scutt R, Gotch C: Art, Sex and Symbol: The Mystery of Tattooing. Cranbury, NJ: AS Barnes, 1974.
2. Grumet GW: Psychodynamic implications of tattoos. Am J Orthopsychiat 1983;53:482.
3. Ebensten H: Pierced Hearts and True Love. London: Derek Verschoyle, 1953.
4. Pers M, von Herbst T: The demand for removal of tattoos: A plea for regulations against tattooing of minors. Acta Chir Scand 1996; 131:201.
5. Goldstein N: Psychological implications of tattoos. J Dermatol Surg Oncol 1979;5:883.
6. Mann R, Klingmuller G: Electron-microscope investigation of tattoos in rabbit skin. Arch Dermatol Res 1981;271:367.
7. Taylor CR, et al.: Treatment of tattoos by Q-switched ruby laser. A dose-response study. Arch Dermatol 1990;126:383.
8. Laub DR, et al.: Preliminary histopathological observation of Q-switched ruby laser radiation on dermal tattoo pigment in man. J Surg Res 1968;8:220–224.
9. Lea PJ, Pawlowski A: Human tattoo: Electron microscopic assessment of epidermis, epidermal-dermal junction and dermis. Int J Dermatol 1987;26:453–458.
10. Anderson RR, Parrish JA: The optics of human skin. J Invest Dermatol 1981;77:13–19.
11. Goldman MP, Fitzpatrick RE: Cutaneous Laser Surgery. St. Louis: Mosby–Year Book, 1994.
12. Rostenberg A, Brown RA, Caro MR: Discussion of tattoo reactions with report of a case showing a reaction to a green color. Arch Dermatol Syph 1950;62:540.
13. Everett MA: Tattoos: Abnormalities of pigmentation. In Clinical Dermatology, vol 2, units 11–21. Hagerstown, Md: Harper & Row, 1980.
14. Scutt RWB: The chemical removal of tattoos. Br J Plast Surg 1972; 25:189.
15. Clabaugh W: Removal of tattoos by superficial dermabrasion, Arch Dermatol 1968;98:515.
16. Goldstein N, Penoff J, Price N, et al.: Techniques of removal of tattoos. J Dermatol Surg Oncol 1979;5:901.
17. Bunke HJ, Conway H: Surgery of decorative and traumatic tattoos. Plast Reconstr Surg 1957;20:67.
18. Goldstein N: Tattoo removal. Dermatol Clin 1987;5:349.
19. O'Donnell BP, et al.: Thin tangential excision of tattoos. Dermatol Surg 1995;21:601.
20. Variot G: Nouveau procede de destruction des tatouages. Compte Rendu Soc Biologie (Paris) 1888;8:836.
21. Piggot TA, Norris RW: The treatment of tattoos with trichloroacetic acid: Experience with 670 patients. Br J Plast Surg 1988;41:112.
22. Lindsay DG: Tattoos. Dermatol Clin 1989;7:147.
23. Colver GB, Dawber RPR: The removal of digital tattoos. Int J Dermatol 1985;24:567.
24. Colver GB, Jones RL, Cherry GW, et al.: Precise dermal damages with an infrared coagulator. Br J Dermatol 1986;114:603.
25. Bailey BN: Treatment of tattoos. Plast Reconstr Surg 1976;40:361.
26. Yules RB, et al.: The effect of Q-switched ruby laser radiation on dermal tattoo pigment in man. Arch Surg 1967;95:179.
27. Goldman L, et al.: Laser treatment of tattoos: A preliminary survey of three years' clinical experience. JAMA 1967;201:841.
28. Apfelberg DB, Maser MR, Lash H: Argon laser treatment of decorative tattoos. Br J Plast Surg 1979;32:141.
29. Apfelberg DB, Rivers J, Maser MR, et al.: Update on laser usage in treatment of decorative tattoos. Lasers Surg Med 1982;2:169.
30. Brady SC, Blokmanis A, Jewett L: Tattoo removal with the carbon dioxide laser. Ann Plast Surg 1978;2:482.
31. McBurney EI: Carbon dioxide laser treatment of dermatologic lesions. South Med J 1978;71:795.
32. Anderson RR, Parrish JA: Selective photothermolysis: Precise microsurgery by selective absorption of pulsed irradiation. Science 1983; 220:524.
33. Anderson RR, Parrish JA: Microvasculature can be selectively damaged using dye lasers: A basic theory and experimental evidence in human skin. Lasers Surg Med 1981;1:263.
34. Goldman L, et al.: Radiation from a Q-switched ruby laser. J Invest Dermatol 1965;44:69.
35. Reid WH, et al.: Q-switched ruby laser treatment of tattoos: A nine year experience. Br J Plast Surg 1990;43:663.
36. Reid WH, et al.: Q-switched ruby laser treatment of black tattoos. Br J Plast Surg 1983;36:455.
37. Lipow M: Laser Physics Made Simple. Chicago: Year Book, 1986.
38. Glassberg E, et al.: Lasers in dermatology. In Lask GP, Moy RL (eds): Principles and Techniques of Cutaneous Surgery. New York: McGraw-Hill, 1996.
39. Lowe NJ, et al.: Q-switched ruby laser: Further observations on treatment of professional tattoos. J Dermatol Surg 1994;20(5):307.
40. Scheibner A, et al.: A superior method of tattoo removal using the Q-switched ruby laser. J Dermatol Surg Oncol 1990;16:1091.
41. Ashinoff R, Geronemus RG: Rapid response of traumatic tattoos to treatment with the Q-switched ruby laser (abstract). Lasers Surg Med 1992;(Suppl 4):71.

42. Ashinoff R, Tanenbaum D: Treatment of amalgam tattoo with the Q-switched ruby laser. Cutis 1994;54:269.

43. Levins PC, et al.: Q-switched ruby laser treatment of tattoos. Lasers Surg Med 1991;11(Suppl 3):255.

44. Levins PC, Anderson RR: Q-switched ruby laser for the treatment of pigmented lesions and tattoos. Clin Dermatol 1995;13:75.

45. Kilmer SL, Anderson RR: Clinical use of the Q-switched ruby and the Q-switched Nd:YAG (1064 nm and 532 nm) lasers for treatment of tattoos. J Dermatol Surg Oncol 1993;19:330.

46. Lowe NJ, et al.: Q-switched ruby treatment of professional tattoos. Lasers Surg Med 1993;5(Suppl):54.

47. Geronemus RG, Ashinoff R: Use of the Q-switched ruby laser to treat tattoos and benign pigmented lesions of the skin. Lasers Surg Med 1991;3(Suppl):64.

48. Grevelink JM, et al.: Laser treatment of tattoos in darkly pigmented patients: Efficacy and side effects. J Am Acad Dermatol 1996;34:653.

49. Glassberg E, Lask GP: Neodymium:yttrium-aluminum-garnet laser. Clin Dermatol 1995;13:81.

50. Kilmer SL, Lee M, Grevelink JM, et al.: The Q-switched Nd:YAG laser (1064 nm) effectively treats tattoos: A controlled dose-response study. Arch Dermatol 1993;129:971–978.

51. DeCoste SD, Anderson RR: Comparison of Q-switched ruby and Q-switched Nd:YAG laser treatment of tattoos (abstract). Lasers Surg Med 1991;Suppl 3:64.

52. Anderson RR, Geronemus R, Kilmer SL, et al.: Cosmetic tattoo ink darkening: A complication of Q-switched and pulsed laser treatment. Arch Dermatol 1993;8:1010.

53. Brauner GJ, Schliftman AB: Treatment of pigmented lesions of the skin with alexandrite laser (abstract). Lasers Surg Med 1992;Suppl 4:72.

54. Fitzpatrick RE, et al.: The alexandrite laser for tattoos: A preliminary report (abstract). Lasers Surg Med 1992;Suppl 4:72.

55. Tan OT, Lizek R: Alexandrite (760 nm) laser treatment of tattoos (abstract). Lasers Surg Med 1992;Suppl 4:72.

56. Stafford TJ, Tan OT: 510-nm Pulsed-dye laser and alexandrite crystal laser. Clin Dermatol 1995;13:69.

57. Alster TS: Q-switched alexandrite laser treatment (755 nm) of professional and amateur tattoos. J Am Acad Dermatol 1995;33:69.

58. Dozier, et al.: The Q-switched alexandrite laser's effects on tattoos in guinea pigs and harvested human skin. Dermatol Surg 1995;21:237.

59. Fitzpatrick RE, Goldman MP, Ruiz-Esparza J: The use of the alexandrite laser (755 nm, 100 microsec) for tattoo pigment removal in an animal model. J Am Acad Dermatol 1993;28:745.

60. Fitzpatrick RF, Goldman MP: Tattoo removal using the alexandrite laser. Arch Dermatol 1994;130:1508.

61. Stafford TJ, et al.: Role of the alexandrite laser for removal of tattoos. Lasers Surg Med 1995;17:31.

62. Ruiz-Esparza J, et al.: Selective melanothermolysis: A histologic study of the Candela 510 nm pulsed-dye laser for pigmented lesions (abstract). Lasers Surg Med 1992;Suppl 4:73.

63. Brauner GJ, Schliftman AB: Treatment of pigmented lesions with the flash-lamp pumped PLDL ("brown spot") laser (abstract). Lasers Surg Med 1992;Suppl 4:73.

64. Grekin RC, Shelton RM, Geisse JK, et al.: 510 nm Pigmented lesion dye laser: Its characteristics and clinical uses. J Dermatol Surg Oncol 1993;19:380.

65. Fitzpatrick RE, et al.: Treatment of benign pigmented lesions with the Candela 510 nm pulsed laser (abstract). Lasers Surg Med 1992;Suppl 4:73.

66. McMeekin TO, Goodwin DP: A comparison of the alexandrite laser (755 nm) with the Q-switched ruby laser (694 nm) in the treatment of tattoos. Lasers Surg Med 1993;Suppl 5:43.

8

BENIGN PIGMENTED LESIONS

David Sawcer
Joshua Wieder
Peter Burrows

Vladislav Chizhevsky
Nicholas J. Lowe
Gary P. Lask

Benign pigmented lesions are extremely common. It is estimated that such lesions in the U.S. population today number well in excess of 10 billion.[1] Only a tiny fraction are treated each year, but because of the numbers involved they still represent great expenditures of time and effort. The most common reason for requesting treatment is that the lesions are physically undesirable or emotionally disabling. Occasionally there is concern that they might be malignant.[1]

Patients with a wide variety of benign pigmented lesions that require treatment consult physicians. For convenience, these lesions may be divided into three groups, according to the site of the pigment within them. *Epidermal lesions,* commonly encountered, include benign melanocytic lesions such as lentigo solaris, speckled lentiginous nevus (nevus spilus), ephelides (freckles), and café-au-lait patches, and benign nevus cell tumors such as junctional nevi.

Epidermal-dermal lesions include compound nevi (nevus cell tumors), Becker's nevus, disorders such as melasma, and infraorbital skin discoloration. *Dermal lesions* include nevus of Ota, blue nevus, nevus of Ito, and intradermal nevi. The pigment in most tattoos (professional, amateur, or traumatic) is also intradermal. Postinflammatory pigmentation is mostly dermal melanin and hemosiderin.

Treatments to date have been varied and the formulary applied differs depending principally on the level of the pigment. Chemical depigmenting agents such as topical hydroquinone or tretinoin[6] may be used. Epidermal lesions, in particular, may be approached with a destructive modality used to remove the epidermis containing the lesion—cryotherapy, cauterization, dermabrasion, or chemical peel.[4, 5] Recently, the carbon dioxide (CO_2) (continuous-wave, 10,600 nm)[2] and neodymium:yttrium-aluminum-garnet (Nd:YAG) (continuous-wave, 1064 nm)[3] lasers have been used with good results for individual lentigos or freckles. All these methods are essentially nonspecific in their destruction of the epidermis. As a consequence, they cause side effects such as permanent hypopigmentation, atrophy, scarring, and skin surface textural changes.

More targeted treatment modalities attempt to remove only the offending pigment within the lesion. As with less specific treatments, however, permanent hypopigmentation that is often difficult to limit to the lesion being treated is a common side effect. Another laser used is the continuous-wave (CW) argon laser (514 nm ± 488 nm), melanin being an important target in this case.[8–10]

Many of these lasers are also used to treat lesions with both dermal and epidermal pigment components, again with some satisfactory results and occasional cosmetically unacceptable side effects.[4, 5] Any attempt to remove a purely dermal lesion with nonspecific forms of treatment is risky: cryosurgery and dermabrasion yield variable results, and microsurgical techniques require absolute precision.[7] Nonetheless, treatment of dermal lesions with cryosurgery, dermabrasion, and microsurgery has been reported.[11–13]

For all lesions, the clinical objective is selective destruction of the offending pigment without cosmetically unacceptable side effects; that is, while preserving otherwise normal skin. The targeting of a subcellular chromophore and inducing specific thermal injury to it resulting in its ultimate removal without damaging surrounding structures, is known as *selective photothermolysis.* This principle was first described by Anderson and Parish[14] in 1983, and is discussed more fully in Chapter 1. Melanin, present in many of the pigmented lesions mentioned above, is an ideal target chromophore for this process. Its absorption spectrum is well-understood.[15] Melanin is packed within melanosomes, which in turn are found within melanocytes and pigmented basal keratinocytes.[4, 16] Selective injury to these subcellular organelles has been observed with pulsed laser irradiation at wavelengths from 351 (excimer laser) to 1064 nm (Nd:YAG).[17–21]

At wavelengths up to approximately 600 nm, radiation is significantly absorbed by both hemoglobin and melanin, seen clinically as increased incidence of purpura. Also, such wavelengths penetrate only a short distance into the skin, reaching the superficial dermis at commonly used fluences and spot sizes.[17, 22–24] At wavelengths of 600 to 1200 nm melanin absorption remains significant, whereas that of hemoglobin is much reduced. Above these wavelengths absorption by both chromophores is reduced and injury becomes increasingly nonspecific.[15, 17, 20] Lasers operating at 600 to 1200 nm can specifically target melanosomes, and their longer wavelength allows penetration to a significant depth into the dermis at appropriate fluences.[17, 20, 22]

Neighboring tissue remains unchanged because the chosen pulse width is less than or equal to the target's thermal relaxation time. This interval is the time taken for induced heat to be dissipated by 50% of its initial value.[14, 20, 25] Melanosomes are known to have short relaxation times on the order of hundred(s) of nanoseconds (the exact value is not known).[24–26]

The Q-switched ruby laser (QSRL) produces very narrow pulse widths (20 to 50 nsecs) and operates at a wavelength of 694.3 nm. Theoretically, this is an obvious choice for selective destruction of either epidermal or dermal pigment. In practice, the laser has been shown to be melanin specific and melanin dependent. In guinea pig skin it causes specific melanosome damage at fluences as low as 0.3 J/cm^2 with minimal absorption by oxyhemoglobin.[27]

Q-Switched Ruby Laser

The laser used to treat patients in our practice is the Spectrum Medical RD-1200 QSRL. Its active medium, a single synthetic ruby crystal (aluminum trioxide doped with chromium), is optically pumped with high-intensity flashlamps. The laser beam produced is red light of wavelength 694.3 nm. Q-switching with an electro-optical switch (called a *Pockles cell*) results in a pulsed emission of coherent light. The pulse widths achievable with this arrangement are 20 to 50 nsec. The laser used in this study produced an output with 28-nsec pulses and high-energy fluences from 3 to 10 J/cm^2. The pulse repetition rate used was 0.5 to 1 Hz (user controlled). The light energy was transmitted to the target area through an articulated arm delivery system to an optical lens capable of focusing the beam to a spot size of 5 to 6.5 mm at the surface of the skin.

During a 36-month period 140 patients were selected for treatment. These patients had 307 lesions of four common types. Patients with purely epidermal lesions—lentigo solaris (51 patients, 216 lesions) and café-au-lait macules (20 patients, 21 lesions)—formed the largest group. Sixteen patients with 16 melasma lesions (epidermal-dermal pigment) were also treated. Patients with nevi of Ota (18 patients, 19 lesions; one had bilateral involvement) and with postinflammatory hypopigmented (PIHP) lesions (35 patients) were also treated. In a separate 8-month study,[36] 17 patients with infraorbital hyperpigmentation were treated.

All patients were treated as outpatients, and none had had any previous treatment of their respective complaints. Patients were photographed before the initial treatment and at each subsequent visit. At re-treatment sessions outcome was assessed and the subjects were questioned about and examined for adverse sequelae. This was undertaken by an independent observer not involved in treatment and unaware of the stage of treatment or fluences used.

The sensation of treatment with the QSRL has been likened to being gently flicked with a rubber band. Thus, most adults do not need anesthesia. For some facial lesions, however (e.g., nevus of Ota, melasma, infraorbital lesions), particularly when higher fluences were to be used, anesthesia was given, either as topical cream (eutectic mixture of local anesthetic [EMLA]), by local infiltration with 1% lignocaine plus epinephrine, or by direct infiltration with 1% lidocaine without epinephrine. All patients received test irradiations with fluences of 7.5 J/cm^2 for infraorbital pigmented lesions, 5 to 7.5 J/cm^2 for lentigo, and 6 to 10 J/cm^2 for café-au-lait lesions, melasma, and nevi of Ota. For smaller lesions a single pulse often covered the entire treatment area; however, for larger lesions several pulses were required and irradiated sites were overlapped by 10% to 20%.

At fluences above the "threshold response" an ash-white discoloration of the irradiated area was observed. Below this, no such reaction was seen. The discoloration resolved within a few hours, occasionally leaving some erythema and edema, which gradually subsided over 24 hours. Postprocedural pain was limited to a transient burning sensation lasting 60 to 80 minutes. At higher fluences scaling and some minor bleeding occurred, often followed by crusting that resolved over 3 to 6 days.

Postprocedural treatments included routine use of topical polymyxin-bacitracin ointment, and a broad-spectrum sunscreen. All patients were advised to continue antibiotic treatment so long as any scaling or crusting persisted, and at minimum 5 days, and to use the sunscreen for at least 1 month. After treatment, treated areas were covered with nonadherent dressings.

Treatments for most lesions were repeated at a minimum of 6 weeks (range 6 to 26), 4 weeks for infraorbital pigmented lesions.[36] Responses, regardless of the lesion, were graded on a scale of I to IV: grade IV, greater than 75% improvement; grade III, 50% to 75% improvement; grade II, 25% to 49% improvement; grade I, less than 25% improvement by comparison with the original photograph.

The largest single group of patients were those with lentigo—51 patients with a total of 216 lesions (range 1 to 8) treated (Table 8–1). The mean age of patients was 43 years (range 25 to 75); 49 were female and 2 male. The ethnic background comprised 40 Caucasians, 7 Hispanics, and 4 Asians.

By the end of the study every lesion showed at least grade III response, and the majority showed better than 75% clearance, grade IV response (69%, or 150 lesions). In a significant proportion of cases, lesions cleared to grade IV after 1 treatment (44%, or 96 lesions). The average number of treatments was 1.5 (range 1 to 3), and the mean treatment interval was 11.5 weeks (range 6 to 26).

No permanent adverse sequelae were detected at the end of the study, although 14 patients had transient hyperpigmentation. This cleared in seven cases without further treatment (grade IV results) and with one more treatment in the remaining seven cases (again grade IV results). Six cases of transient hypopigmentation all cleared to grade IV

Table 8–1. Treatment of Lentigo Solaris

SITE	RESPONSE GRADE	NUMBER OF TREATMENTS (RANGE)	MEAN FLUENCE* (J/CM²)	MEAN TREATMENT INTERVAL† (WK)	NUMBER OF LESIONS
Head, neck	IV	1.5 (1–3)	6.8	8	75
	III	1.8 (1-3)	6.7	7	40
Trunk	IV	1.3 (1–2)	6.9	9	23
	III	2.0 (2)	6.5	10	5
Upper limbs	IV	1.2 (1–2)	6.5	18	43
	III	2.0 (1–3)	6.3	16	14
Lower limbs	IV	1.6 (1–2)	6.9	15	9
	III	2.0 (2)	6.6	18	7
All sites combined	IV	1.44 (1–3)	6.8	11	150
	III	1.88 (1–3)	6.7	12	66
	I & II				
Overall		1.5 (1–3)	6.8	11.5	216

Response scores: I, 0–25% improvement; II, 26–50% improvement; III, 51–75% improvement; IV, 76–100% improvement.
*Range 5–7.5.
†Range 6–26.

over a period of weeks to months. No hypertrophic scars were seen.

In our study, no patients with café-au-lait patches had an associated condition such as neurofibromatosis or Albright's syndrome. Café-au-lait patches were treated in 20 patients, only one of whom had more than one lesion treated (21 lesions). Patients were younger on average than those with other lesions (mean 22 years; range 4 to 45), but as usual there were more females than males—14 and 6, respectively. The ethnic mix was ten Caucasians, three Hispanics, one black, and six Asians.

The results of treatment are shown in Table 8–2. Lesions were treated at various anatomic sites: eight head and neck, four trunk, one upper limb, and eight lower limb. Patients required an average of 2.2 treatments (range 1 to 4). After the first treatment, 9% (two lesions) showed grade IV response and 24% (five lesions), grade I response. With one more treatment, however, 19% (four lesions) were grade IV and 43% (nine lesions) were grade III. Thus, the majority showed better than 50% improvement (19%, or four lesions, were grade I). Unfortunately, not all patients with grade III responses (three lesions) returned for further treatments, as they considered their responses satisfactory (they were close to 75% clear). However, after one or two more treatments of the remaining patients the results were as shown (all patients included) in Table 8–2. Three patients had hypopigmentation at initial follow-up (one Caucasian, one black, one Asian); however, within 4 months this had resolved to a grade IV response in all but one case (the black patient). Even in this case, the hypopigmentation had improved considerably and will probably continue to do so. One case of transient hyperpigmentation was noted to resolve in 3 months. No scarring, skin texture changes, or other side effects occurred.

Patients with melasma compose the smallest group, 16 in all and all female. Each had only a single facial lesion (11 centrofacial, 4 malar, and 1 mandibular). The average age was 34 years (range 27 to 46) and the ethnic mix seven Caucasians, seven Hispanics, and two Asians. Classification by skin type according to Fitzpatrick[28] showed five patients had type II; seven, type III; three, type IV; and one, type V. Not all patients in the study had completed their course of treatment at the time of publication (six ongoing). The overall results of all treatments to date are shown in Table 8–3.

Of the six patients with grade III response, five achieved this in one or two treatments. Also worth noting is that of the eight patients with grade I response, four had had three or more treatments (and three were ongoing cases treated only once to date).

Table 8–2. Treatment of Café-au-Lait Patches by the End of the Study

RESPONSE GRADE	NUMBER OF TREATMENTS (RANGE)	MEAN FLUENCE* (J/CM²)	MEAN TREATMENT INTERVAL† (WK)	NUMBER OF LESIONS (%)
IV	2.2 (1–4)	7.0	12	5 (24)
III	2.3 (1–4)	7.3	10	9 (43)
II	2.0 (1–3)	7.1	11	4 (19)
I	2.3 (1–3)	7.2	13	3 (14)
Overall	2.2 (1–4)	7.1	11	21 (100)

Response scores: I, 0–25% improvement; II, 26–50% improvement; III, 51–75% improvement; IV, 76–100% improvement.
*Range 6–10.
†Range 6–26.

Table 8-3. Treatment of Melasma by the End of the Study

RESPONSE GRADE	NUMBER OF TREATMENTS (RANGE)	MEAN FLUENCE* (J/CM²)	MEAN TREATMENT INTERVAL† (WK)	NUMBER OF LESIONS %
IV	—	—	—	0 (0)
III	2.5 (1–6)	6.9	13	6 (38)
II	1.5 (1–2)	6.3	20	2 (12)
I	2.3 (1–5)	6.6	9	8 (50)
Overall	2.3 (1–6)	6.7	12	16 (100)

Response scores: I, 0–25% improvement; II, 26–50% improvement; III, 51–75% improvement; IV, 76–100% improvement.
*Range 6–10.
†Range 6–26.

Six cases of hyperpigmentation were detected, and no other adverse sequelae were seen. Of these, five were cases with grade I response and one had grade III response. The latter was transient: it resolved after one more treatment. Of the five cases, only one remained at the most recent follow-up (12 weeks). Of interest, three of the five cases of hyperpigmentation occurred in patients who had had three treatments or more.

The final condition considered in this study was nevus of Ota (19 lesions on 18 patients). This group comprised 14 females and 4 males of mean age of 34 years (range 17 to 75). Twelve had lesions from birth or at an early age, and six reported onset during adolescence or early adult life. The ethnic mix was two Caucasians, two Hispanics, three blacks, and eleven Asians. Classification according to Fitzpatrick's sun-reactive skin types[28] showed that the group comprised two with skin type II; three with type III; twelve with type IV; and one with type V. Again, not all patients had completed their course of treatment at publication. Table 8–4 shows the results to date.

Nevus of Ota is typically slow to respond, usually requiring several treatments to achieve satisfactory results. Some patients continued to improve for as long as a year after their final treatment. All 10 patients treated four times or more showed a grade III (two patients) or grade IV (eight patients) response. Of the 13 patients treated three times or more, all but one had a grade III (four patients) or grade IV (eight patients) response. All patients with grades I, II, and III are continuing with their treatment sessions.

No patients experienced permanent adverse pigment changes or other side effects such as scarring. One case of hyperpigmentation and one case of hypopigmentation were seen; both were transient and resolved within 2 months.

The infraorbital pigmented lesions[36] were considered in a separate study. The maximum improvement in most patients occurred 3 to 4 months after the laser treatment; less often, maximum improvement was noted 6 months after the treatment. The group consisted of 15 females and 2 males. Their ages ranged from 32 to 75 years (average 44.4). Three women were taking oral contraceptives, and four were taking progesterone plus estrogen for hormone replacement. Fitzpatrick skin types were II (eight patients), III (six), IV (one), and V (two) (mean, 2.5).

After one treatment, 6 of 17 patients (35%) had a grade I response; seven (41%), a grade II response; and four (24%), a grade III response. Eight patients had at least two treatment sessions. One (11%) achieved a grade II response; six (67%), grade III; and two (22%), grade IV response. Of those treated twice, 88% achieved a grade III or IV response (Table 8–5). Subsequently, we have treated a total of 25 more patients with this problem. The results seem long lasting.

Side effects included transient hyperpigmentation in 29.4%, which resolved in 4 to 8 weeks when treated with 4% hydroquinone solution. Transient hypopigmentation was seen in 5.9%. No permanent textural changes or scarring was noted.

Table 8-4. Treatment of Nevus of Ota

RESPONSE GRADE	NUMBER OF TREATMENTS (RANGE)	MEAN FLUENCE* (J/CM²)	MEAN TREATMENT INTERVAL† (WK)	NUMBER OF LESIONS %
IV	5.3 (3–9)	9.3	10	9 (47)
III	2.9 (1–5)	9.0	12	7 (37)
II	2.5 (2–3)	10.0	8	2 (11)
I	1.0 (1)	10.0	—	1 (5)
Overall	3.9 (1–9)	9.3	10	19 (100)

Response scores: I, 0–25% improvement; II, 26–50% improvement; III, 51–75% improvement; IV, 76–100% improvement.
*Range 6–10.
†Range 6–24.

Table 8–5. Melanocyte-Type Infraorbital Pigmentation

PATIENT	AGE (YR)	SKIN TYPE	TREATMENTS (NO.)	RESPONSE SCORE AFTER LAST TREATMENT
1	49	V	1	III
2	75	II	1	I
3	32	II	3	IV
4	48	II	2	II
5	55	II	2	III
6	66	II	2	IV
7	36	III	1	I
8	39	III	2	III
9	39	IV	2	III
10	37	V	2	IV
11	36	II	1	II
12	42	III	1	I
13	37	III	2	III
14	34	III	2	III
15	48	II	1	II
16	41	II	1	III
17	41	III	1	I

Response scores: I, 0–25% improvement; II, 26–50% improvement; III, 51–75% improvement; IV, 76–100% improvement.
From Lowe NJ, Wieder JM, Shorr N, et al.: Infraorbital pigmented skin. Dermatol Surg 1995;21:767–770.

Discussion

Lentigo is clearly amenable to treatment with QSRL. We observed excellent results with one or two treatments. No permanent adverse effects were seen, and we were able to treat multiple lesions at a single visit. Analysis of the data by site, fluence, and treatment interval did not reveal any convincing differences in outcomes. Caucasians and Asians showed roughly the same proportions of grade III and IV responses (Figs. 8–1 and 8–2). For Hispanic patients it proved harder to achieve the ideal grade IV response: significant reversals in numbers were observed in both grades. The QSRL should be used with caution in these patients, but it should not disqualify them from treatment; since for all groups, the QSRL was more successful than any nonpulsed laser modality and had significantly fewer side effects.[2–10]

Compared with other pulsed laser systems such as the 510-nm pigmented lesion dye laser, the QSRL produced comparable results in treating lentigo.[23, 24, 29]

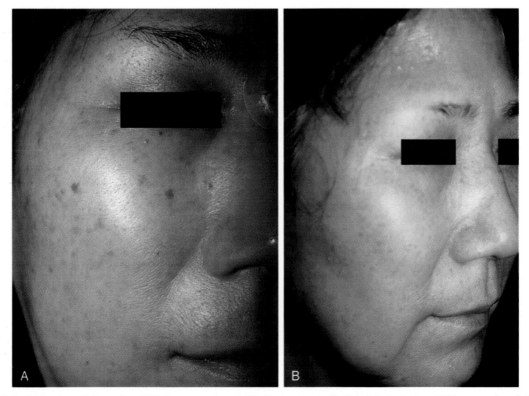

Figure 8–1. Solar lentigo in an Asian patient *(A)* before treatment and *(B)* after treatment with Q-switched ruby laser (694-nm wavelength, 28-nsec pulse, 6 J/cm², 5-mm spot size).

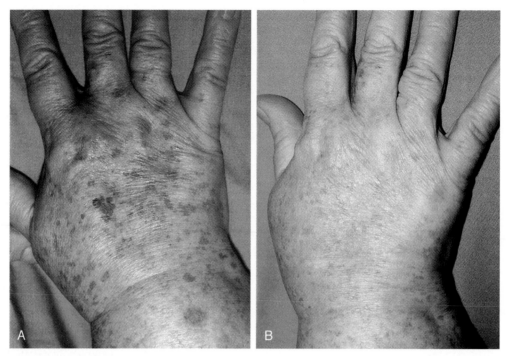

Figure 8–2. Extensive solar lentigo lesions of the dorsal hand *(A)* before treatment and *(B)* after two treatments with Q-switched ruby laser (694-nm wavelength, 28-nsec pulse, 5 and 6 J/cm², 6.5-mm spot size).

Café-au-lait patches are notoriously difficult to treat. The QSRL produced good results at fluences of 6 to 10 J/cm²: approximately 66% of patients had better than 50% improvement and 25% better than 75% improvement. These results are not as impressive as those for lentigos, but they do represent an improvement over nonpulsed laser therapies, particularly when the low incidence of side effects is considered. The lower efficacy of the QSRL for treating café-au-lait patches as compared with lentigos may be due to the presence of active melanocytes in the café-au-lait lesions.[16] The laser acts by selectively disrupting melanosomes rather than directly damaging the melanocytes, and activated melanocytes may be more resistant to subsequent destruction.[20, 27, 30]

For café-au-lait lesions, our results with the pulsed-dye laser (PDL) are not as consistent in terms of improvement as those reported by others.[23, 24, 29] Lesions that do not respond to QSRL may respond to the PDL, and it has been suggested the effects may be additive.[30] Analysis of data by site, ethnic group, and fluence did not predict which patients are likely to respond and which are not.

The mechanism behind the ultimate lightening of lesions is qualitatively the same, regardless of wavelength of irradiation. The process depends either on extreme temperature gradients created across melanosomes or shockwave or cavitation damage resulting from rapid thermal expansion.[27] Melanosomes are disrupted, and selective pigment cell destruction follows. Differences in laser wavelength affect depth of penetration, as, to some extent, do fluence and spot size.[15] The "shorter-wavelength" lasers such as the 510-nm PDL penetrates some 0.25 to 0.5 mm into the skin at commonly used fluences[24] and thus reaches only to the upper dermis in most areas. The "longer-wavelength" of the QSRL at 694.3 nm allows greater depth of penetration—to over 1 mm at typical fluences.[15, 31] This difference in penetration depth—or more importantly the volume profile of energy deposition within the irradiated area—may contribute to the difference in efficacy of the two lasers in the treatment of café-au-lait lesions. It may also help to explain the differences in efficacy of treatment of lentigo and café-au-lait with the QSRL mentioned earlier. Most certainly it explains why treatment of epidermal-dermal and purely dermal lesions is more efficacious with the QSRL.

Melasma, an epidermal-dermal pigmentary process, gave variable results with the QSRL, a problem noted by other authors.[30] Analysis of the outcome by skin type and ethnic group (along with the other possible variables) in our experience did not reveal any difference in outcomes. This does not confirm the observation that response may be better in fair-complexioned patients than in those with olive skin, although our study group is small. Subjectively, there appeared to be three groups of patients identifiable by response to treatment. Approximately 40% achieved early grade III response after only one or two treatments and had fewer side effects. About 50% failed to improve beyond grade I response, despite three treatments or more. Some 10% of responses were neither of these types. Although it is not yet possible to identify which patients will respond well before treatment is begun, these data imply that it may be possible to do so after only a short cautious trial of treatment. Alternative methods may then be applied to nonresponders. Larger study groups are needed for future investigations. We agree that in this photosensitive, hormonally dependent condition the activated melanocytes appear

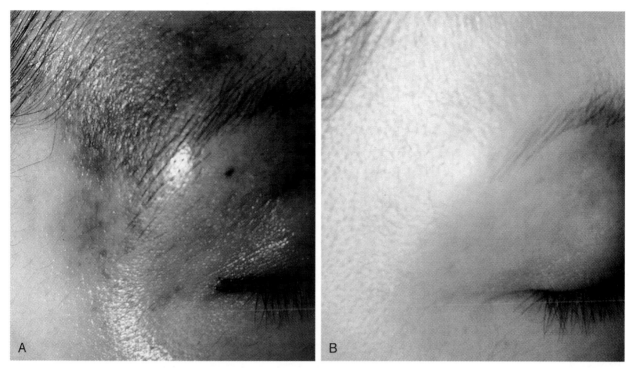

Figure 8–3. Nevus of Ota *(A)* before treatment. *(B)* Results are excellent after five treatments with Q-switched ruby laser (694-nm wavelength, 28-nsec pulse, 10 J/cm², 5-mm spot size). (From Lowe NJ, Wieder JM, Sawcer DE, et al: Nevus of Ota: Treatment with high energy fluences of the Q-switched ruby laser. J Am Acad Dermatol 1993;29:997–1001.)

only to be slowed after treatment.[30] The condition recurs after a time, and use of broad-spectrum sunscreen, and possibly pharmacologic skin-lightening agents, is mandatory after treatment.

Successful treatment of nevus of Ota with the QSRL has been reported by several authors.[30–35] These results are con-

firmed by our experience. The use of narrow pulse widths (28 nsec rather than the 40 nsec of previous trials) allows for use of even higher-energy fluences (up to 10 J/cm² as compared with the previous upper limit of 9 J/cm²), without an increase in adverse sequelae and with a reduction in the number of treatment sessions required (Figs. 8–3 and 8–4).

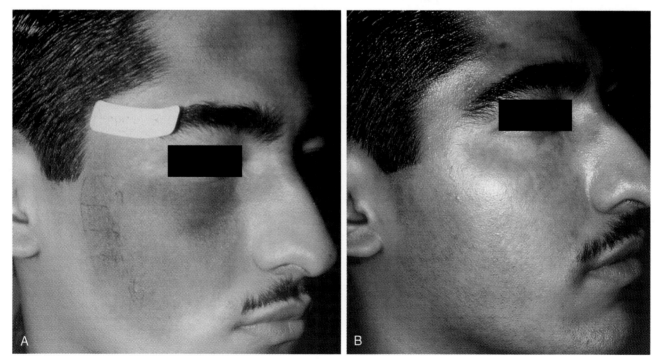

Figure 8–4. Nevus of Ota *(A)* before treatment and *(B)* after four treatments with Q-switched ruby laser (694-nm wavelength, 28-nsec pulse, 10 J/cm², 5-mm spot size).

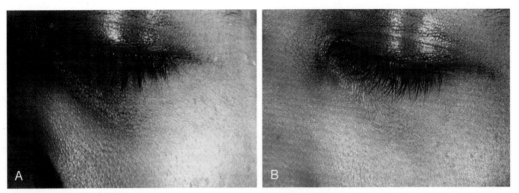

Figure 8–5. Infraorbital dark circle *(A)* before treatment. *(B)* After two treatments with Q-switched ruby laser (7.5 J/cm^2) grade II improvement was realized. (From Lowe NJ, Wieder JM, Shorr N, et al: Infraorbital pigmented skin. Preliminary observations of laser therapy. Dermatol Surg 1995;21:767–770.)

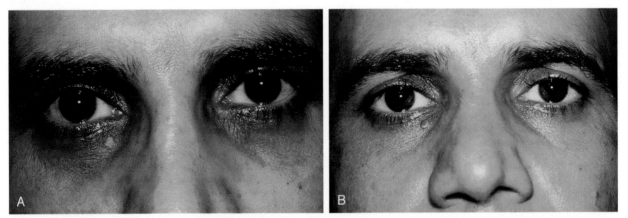

Figure 8–6. Infraorbital dark circle. *(A)* Before treatment. *(B)* After two treatments with Q-switched ruby laser (7.5 J/cm^2). Grade III improvement. (From Lowe NJ, Wieder JM, Shorr N, et al: Infraorbital pigmented skin. Preliminary observations of laser therapy. Dermatol Surg 1995;21:767–770.)

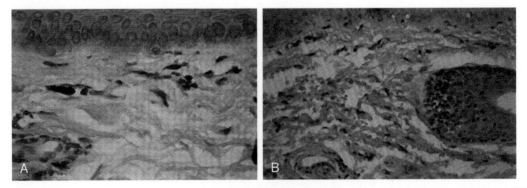

Figure 8–7. *(A)* Skin biopsy taken prior to treatment showing melanin pigment granules within mid and upper dermal macrophages (×200). *(B)* Twelve weeks post-laser treatment. There has been a marked reduction of dermal pigment. Occasional vacuolated basal epidermal cells are observed (×200). (From Lowe NJ, Wieder JM, Sawcer DE, et al: Nevus of Ota: Treatment with high energy fluences of the Q-switched ruby laser. J Am Acad Dermatol 1993;29:997–1001.)

Although multiple treatments are needed, the results are invariably excellent.

Recently, the QSRL has been shown to be effective in the treatment of infraorbital skin darkening (Figs. 8–5 and 8–6).[36] Patients in whom the darkening is assessed clinically to be due to melanin are suitable candidates for treatment with this laser. Other lasers that might be effective for this category of lesions include the Q-switched frequency-doubled Nd:YAG and the Q-switched alexandrite laser. One advantage of the QSRL is the lack of permanent textural changes or scarring and the absence of postlaser scarring.

The QSRL is a highly effective tool for the treatment of a whole gamut of benign pigmented lesions. Although other available pulsed lasers may produce comparable or slightly better results for some epidermal lesions, the increased flexibility of this laser, which can also treat epidermal-dermal and purely dermal lesions, is noteworthy (Fig. 8–7).

Nd:YAG Laser

The QS-Nd:YAG laser has been very effective in the treatment of pigmented lesions and tattoos. Its high-power pulses and short exposure time (pulse width 10 nsec) allow for precise treatment of target tissue with minimal thermal damage and involvement to adjacent tissues.

Because of the absorption characteristics of melanin and the superficial location of the pigmentation of both lentigines and ephelides, the QS-Nd:YAG laser at a wavelength of 532 nm is an ideal treatment modality. Energy densities should range from 2.5 to 3.5 J/cm^2 for a 2-mm spot size.[37] The immediate tissue response at this wavelength is whitening, but purpura (due to absorption in hemoglobin) can also develop and usually lasts 5 to 7 days.

With both of these lesions only one treatment usually is required.[37] The patient should be advised to avoid repeated reexposure to the sun, because these lesions, especially ephelides, can recur.

Successful treatment of café-au-lait macules has been reported after three or fewer treatments with QS-Nd:YAG and QSRL. The pigment in café-au-lait is also superficial; thus, QS-Nd:YAG (wavelength 532 nm) with energy levels ranging between 2.5 and 4 J/cm^2 using a 2-mm spot size is suitable.[37] Unlike lentigines and ephelides, however, these benign pigmented lesions respond variably to laser therapy: they may darken, lighten, or clear. Several treatments might be required for maximum lightening or clearing. Café-au-lait spots can become hyperpigmented if the fluences are too low or scar if they are too high. In addition, the patient should be prepared for the possibility that a lesion might darken after a promising initial result.[37]

Becker's nevus, which is usually located on the shoulder or chest of a man, is a pigmented patch with areas of increased hair growth. The pigment in this lesion is located primarily along the basal cell layer of the epidermis. These lesions usually respond well to a few treatments with QS-Nd:YAG laser at energies ranging from 2.5 to 3.5 J/cm^2 using a 2-mm spot size.[37]

Responses of postinflammatory hyperpigmentation to treatment with QS-Nd:YAG laser are variable and inconsistent. Moreover, quite frequently hyperpigmentation can be observed after treatments. Energy densities used for these lesions should range between 2.5 and 4.0 J/cm^2 at 532 nm and a 2-mm spot size.[37] Such treatment is not advised routinely.

The epidermal type of melasma responds to the 532-nm wavelength at 2.5 to 3.5 J/cm^2 and 2-mm spot size.[37] The risk of recurrence is unpredictable. The dermal type of melasma, on the other hand, does not tend to respond to the QS-Nd:YAG laser at 532 or 1064 nm.

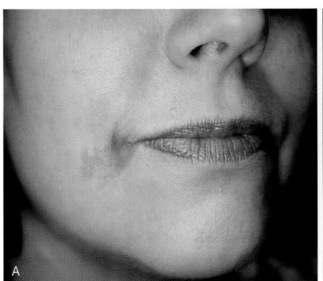 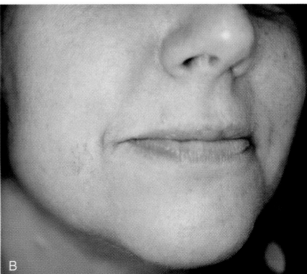

Figure 8–8. *(A)* Café-au-lait macule of right cheek. *(B)* After four treatments with 510-nm pulsed dye laser.

The 510-nm Pulsed Dye Laser

The PDL at 510 nm, with a duration of 300 nsec and 3-mm spot size, was developed specifically for removal of pigmented lesions confined to the epidermis. This laser has been recommended for treatment of café-au-lait spots (Fig. 8–8), lentigines, Becker's nevus, nevus of Ota, nevus of Ito, melasma, and postinflammatory hyperpigmentation.

Alexandrite Laser

The alexandrite laser (760 nm), designed to penetrate into the dermis, became a natural candidate for the treatment of dermal pigmented lesions. Despite the fact that the wavelength of this laser is fairly different from that of the PDL (510 nm) and could appear to match less selective melanin absorption, it has sometimes proven effective in removing dermal pigmentation such as that of postinflammatory hyperpigmentation.

REFERENCES

1. De-Coste S, Stern R: Diagnosis and treatment of nevomelanocytic lesions of the skin: A community based study. Arch Dermatol 1993; 129:57–62.
2. Dover JS, Smoller BR, Stern RS, et al.: Low-fluence carbon dioxide laser irradiation of lentigines. Arch Dermatol 1988;124:1219–1224.
3. Goldman L, Nath G, Schindler G, et al.: High-power neodymium-YAG laser surgery. Acta Derm Venerol (Stockh) 1987;53:45–49.
4. Habif T: Clinical Dermatology: A Color Guide to Diagnosis and Therapy. St. Louis: Mosby–Year Book, 1990.
5. Hunter JA, Savis JA, Dhal MV: Clinical Dermatology. Oxford: Blackwell Scientific, 1989.
6. Rafal ES, Griffiths CE, Ditre CM, et al.: Topical tretinoin (retinoic acid) treatment for liver spots associated with photo damage. N Engl J Med 1992;326:368–374.
7. Gage AA, Meennaghan MA, Nateilla JR: Sensitivity of pigmented mucosa and skin to freezing injury. Cryobiology 1979;16:384.
8. Apfelberg DB, Maser MR, Lash H, et al.: The argon laser for cutaneous lesions. JAMA 1981;245:2073–2075.
9. Trelles MA, Verkuysse W, Pickering JW, et al.: Mono-line argon laser (514 nm) treatment of benign pigmented lesions with long pulse widths. J Photochem Photobiol 1992;16:357–365.
10. Ohishiro T, Maruyana Y: The ruby and argon lasers in the treatment of neavi. Ann Acad Med Singapore 1983;12:385–395.
11. Jay B: Malignant melanoma of the orbit in a case of oculodermal melanosis (neavus of Ota). Br J Ophthalmol 1965;49:359–363.
12. Fujimori Y: Treatment of Neavus of Ota and Neavus Spilus in Skin Surface Surgery. Tokyo: Kokuseido, 1990:181–188.
13. Kobayashi T: Microsurgical treatment of neavus of Ota. J Dermatol Surg Oncol 1991;17:936–941.
14. Anderson RR, Parish JA: Selective photothermolysis: Precise microsurgery by selective absorption of pulsed radiation. Science 1983;220: 524–527.
15. Anderson RR, Parish JA: The optics of human skin. J Invest Dermatol 1981;77:13–19.
16. Lever WF, Schaumburg-Lever G: Histopathology of the Skin, 7th ed. Philadelphia: JB Lippincott, 1990.
17. Sherwood K, Murray S, Kurban K, et al.: Effects of wavelength on cutaneous pigment using pulsed irradiation. J Invest Dermatol 1989; 92:717–720.
18. Anderson RR, Margolis RJ, Watanabe S, et al.: Selective photothermolysis of cutaneous pigment by Q-switched Nd:YAG laser pulsed at 1064, 532, and 355 nm. J Invest Dermatol 1989;93:28–32.
19. Ara G, Anderson RR, Mandel KG, et al.: Irradiation of pigmented melanoma cells with high intensity pulsed irradiation generates acoustic waves and kills cells. Lasers Surg Med 1990;10:52–59.
20. Murphy GF, Shepard RS, Paul BS, et al.: Organelle specific injury to melanin containing cell in human skin by pulsed irradiation. Lab Invest 1983;49:680–685.
21. Margolis RJ, Dover JS, Polla LL, et al.: Visible action spectrum for melanin specific selective photothermolysis. Lasers Surg Med 1989; 9:389–397.
22. Nelson JS, Applebaum J: Treatment of superficial cutaneous pigmented lesions by melanin specific selective photothermolysis using the Q-switched ruby laser. Ann Plast Surg 1992;29:231–237.
23. Fitzpatrick RE, Goldman MP, Ruiz-Esparza J: Laser treatment of benign pigmented epidermal lesions using a 300 ns pulse and 510 nm wavelength. J Dermatol Surg Oncol 1993;18:341–347.
24. Grekin RC, Shelton RM, Geisse JK, et al.: 510 nm Pigmented lesion dye laser. J Dermatol Surg Oncol 1993;19:380–387.
25. Kurbao AK, Morrison P, Trainor S, et al.: Pulse duration effects on cutaneous pigment. Lasers Surg Med 1992;12:282–287.
26. Watanabe S, Anderson RR, Bruson S, et al.: Comparative studies of femtosecond to microsecond laser pulses on selective pigmented cell injury in skin. J Photochem Photobiol 1991;9:389–397.
27. Polla LL, Margolis RJ, Dover JS: Melanosomes are a primary target of Q-switched ruby laser irradiation in guinea pig skin. J Invest Dermatol 1987;89:281–286.
28. Fitzpatrick TB: The validity and practicality of sun-reactive skin types I through VI. Arch Dermatol 1988;127:869–871.
29. Tan OT, Morelli JG, Kurban AK: Pulsed dye laser treatment of benign cutaneous pigmented lesions. Lasers Surg Med 1992;12:538–542.
30. Stafford TJ, Tan OT: 510 nm Pulsed dye laser and alexandrite crystal laser for the treatment of pigmented lesions and tattoos. Clin Dermatol 1995;13:69–71.
31. Levins PC, Anderson RR: Q-switched ruby laser for the treatment of pigmented lesions and tattoos. Clin Dermatol 1995;13:75–79.
32. Goldberg DJ: Benign pigmented lesions of the skin: Treatment with the Q-switched ruby laser. J Dermatol Surg Oncol 1998;19:376–379.
33. Taylor CR, Anderson RR: Treatment of benign pigmented epidermal lesions by Q-switched ruby laser. Int J Dermatol 1993;32:908–912.
34. Lowe NJ, Wieder JM, Sawcer DE, et al.: Nevus of Ota: Treatment with high energy fluences of the Q-switched ruby laser. J Am Acad Dermatol 1993;29:997–1001.
35. Goldberg DJ, Nychay SG: Q-switched ruby laser treatment of nevus of Ota. J Dermatol Surg Oncol 1992;18:817–821.
36. Lowe NJ, Wieder JM, Shorr N, et al.: Infraorbital pigmented skin. Dermatol Surg 1995;21:767–770.
37. Lask GP, Glassberg E: Neodymium:yttrium-aluminum-garnet laser for the treatment of cutaneous lesions. Clin Dermatol 1995;13:81–86.
38. Grossman MC, Anderson RR, Farinelli W, et al.: Treatment of café-au-lait macules with lasers: Clinicopathologic correlation. Arch Dermatol 1995;131:1416.

9

BLEPHAROPLASTY

Sterling Baker

Patel[1] developed the carbon dioxide (CO_2) laser in 1964. Emitting in the fundamental mode at 10,600 nm, the CO_2 laser incorporates a coaxial helium-neon (He-Ne) laser for visualization. The concept of selective photothermolysis[2] promotes an understanding of the clinical application of this laser. The target component in tissue (or chromophore) for the energy emitted by the CO_2 laser is water. The effect on tissue of radiation from far infrared lasers is explained by combining this concept of a target chromophore with the concept of extinction length, which is that depth of water that effectively absorbs the incident radiation. Since the extinction length for the CO_2 laser is about 0.03 mm in water and since periorbital soft tissues are 80% to 90% water, the water component of both intracellular and extracellular tissue rapidly absorbs the energy of the applied laser beam. This energy heats the water to vapor, which creates a wound in an explosive fashion. The thermal effects of this vaporization are conducted to adjacent tissue, cauterizing small blood vessels, nerves, and lymphatics. Thermal damage is controlled to produce clinically acceptable results with the appropriate choice of output power, mode of application, focus of the incident beam, and duration of application.

Clinical investigations using the CO_2 laser and the applications that followed were extensively developed in the 1970s, predominantly by gynecologists, otolaryngologists, and dermatologists.[3–6] Early ophthalmic investigations addressed safety standards and the effect of the laser on ocular structures.[7–19] Baker and colleagues[20] reported the first series of CO_2 laser blepharoplasties at the American Academy of Ophthalmology in 1983. Subsequently, David and colleagues and others published their series, beginning in 1987.[21–23] These early reports were greeted with little enthusiasm.[17, 24–26] By the 1990s, though, worldwide interest in periorbital CO_2 laser incisional applications had significantly expanded.[27–34] The 1994 publication of Goldman and Fitzpatrick's landmark text, *Cutaneous Laser Surgery,*[35] gave the voice of the international community of laser surgeons a clear expression and an established presence.

Blepharoplasty techniques have been developed that use existing CO_2 laser equipment. The basic application for upper lids has changed little since it was described in 1984.[20] In contrast, lower lid laser blepharoplasty has evolved from the initial transcutaneous application[20] to a laser adaptation of the transconjunctival approach.[22, 36, 37]

Carbon Dioxide Laser Blepharoplasty: Upper Lid Technique

Preoperative sedation is helpful before establishing anesthesia. Under direct observation to avoid small vessels, 2 to 3 ml of 2% lidocaine with 1 : 100,000 epinephrine mixed with 0.75% bupivacaine is infiltrated subcutaneously. The anesthetic is injected as a bolus laterally in the area of the planned excision and then massaged across the lid with either digital pressure or a cotton-tipped applicator. This maneuver minimizes ecchymosis during the injection. Hyaluronidase may be added to the anesthetic solution to facilitate its distribution.

The lower margin of the incision is marked in the lid crease with attention to the aesthetic considerations affecting the distance from the lid margin. The general guidelines for placing incisions are followed: 6 mm ± 2 mm for Asians; 8 mm ± 2 mm for males; 10 mm ± 2 mm for females (Fig. 9–1). The amount of skin and orbicularis to be resected is determined by a pinch or overlap method. Care is taken to respect the transition zone between thin palpebral skin and thick orbital skin superiorly (Fig. 9–2), thus minimizing the potential for postoperative lagophthalmos secondary to the lid being tethered to the brow. Medially, the incision stops at an imaginary vertical line connecting the puncta, to avoid a "bowstring"-type contracture scar. If removal of excess skin or orbicularis medial to this imaginary line is desired, a small triangle is based on the upper limb of the incision in the superonasal area (Fig. 9–3). Care must be taken during this step because overly aggressive resection can produce iatrogenic medial brow ptosis. The inferior margin of the incision should be kept at least 4 mm above the lid margin medially and laterally (Fig. 9–4), to minimize the risk of transecting the marginal palpebral artery. The lateral incision is extended as far as necessary to produce the desired resection without causing brow ptosis. The incision can be hidden laterally in a laugh line. The medial

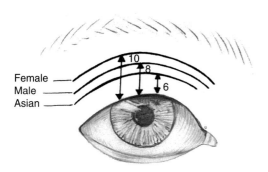

Figure 9–1. Incision guidelines.

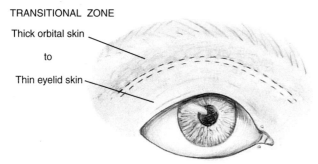

Figure 9–2. Transitional zone between thin palpebral skin and thick orbital skin.

and lateral margins of the incision are not joined at one point but rather overlap by 1 to 2 mm, to minimize the creation of a "dog ear" (Fig. 9–5).

The entire face is prepared in the usual fashion with a nonflammable solution. Nonflammable materials such as wet towels are used as drapes, to minimize the fire hazard. Supplemental oxygen is avoided for the same reason. The globe is protected with either an oversized, laser-safe, metallic shield that covers the entire globe or a David-Baker lid clamp (Fig. 9–6).[38] Adequate smoke evacuation is used to remove the potentially toxic laser plume.[39]

The margins of the skin and orbicularis flap may be incised with the laser in either a focused, continuous-wave (CW) or a pulsed mode. The laser setting most often recommended for CW incisional applications for the eyelids is 6 W with a 0.2-mm focused delivery system. In the pulsed mode a low-power rapid-delivery application is most often suggested (e.g., 5 to 8 mJ at 8 W for the Coherent Ultrapulse). The pulsed delivery systems reduce conduction of thermal energy to adjacent tissue, producing less tissue devitalization at the wound margin than CW lasering. In theory, a smaller zone of devitalized tissue should produce a smaller scar. Investigations of wound healing, however, have shown the process to be a complicated one that depends only in part on the amount of devitalized tissue.[40] Furthermore, clinical comparisons of scar tissue have consistently failed to demonstrate a cosmetically significant difference between wounds produced by a scalpel and ones produced by a CO_2 laser in a CW application.[21, 23]

The skin and orbicularis flap is removed by grasping

the lateral margin with stout forceps (e.g., Brown-Addison) (Fig. 9–7) and elevating it with force while applying the laser beam parallel to the plane of the lid in a side-to-side fashion. Skin only is removed outside the orbit, to preserve the lateral palpebral artery. Within the orbit, the dissection is conducted in the preseptal plane. The medial end of the incision is protected with a laser-safe Jaeger plate or wet gauze. Defocused laser application usually provides additional hemostasis as needed. Bipolar cautery may be used for the unusual brisk or persistent bleeder that fails to respond to the laser.

The septum is divided over the area of maximum prolapse of the preaponeurotic fat pad when the globe is gently tamponaded by direct digital pressure on the lid clamp (Fig. 9–8). Only the yellow preaponeurotic fat that with gentle

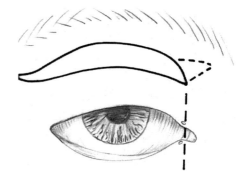

Figure 9–3. Excisional triangle placed in superonasal orbit.

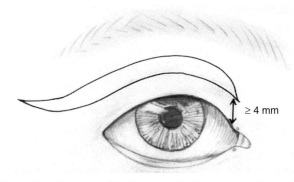

Figure 9–4. Placement of incision at medial lid margin avoids palpebral artery.

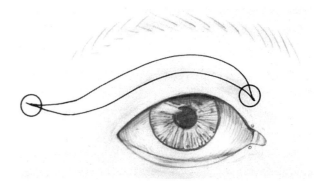

Figure 9–5. Design of incision avoids "dog ears" by overlapping superior and inferior limbs of the incisions, both medially and laterally.

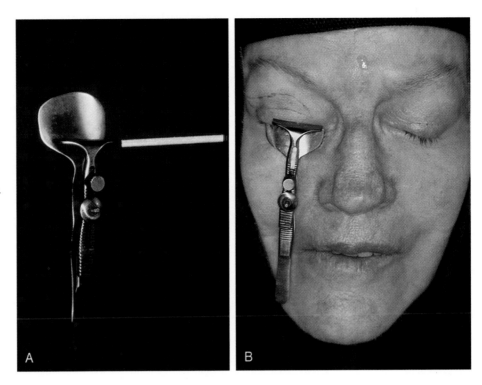

Figure 9–6. *(A)* David-Baker lid clamp. *(B)* Clamp in place prior to surgery.

pressure can be prolapsed anterior to the orbital rim is resected. Clamping the fat is not necessary. This conservative approach helps to avoid an iatrogenic ptosis caused by disruption of Whitnall's suspensory ligaments and superior sulcus deformity caused by overly aggressive resection of fat. The nasal fat compartment is entered via the superonasal orbit, to avoid the infratrochlear artery. The fascial investments covering the white orbital fat are cut, and the fat that prolapses on gentle pressure is removed, with special attention being given to maintaining hemostasis. Resection of fat

is accomplished by cutting against a soaking-wet cotton tip or another laser-safe instrument.

The lids are closed with interrupted or running sutures. Central sutures may be placed deep to the tarsus or aponeurosis to emphasize a lid crease. Sutures may be absorbable or permanent and may be reinforced with glue. Gross vision in each eye separately is checked and recorded at the end of the procedure. During the early postoperative period (24 to 48 hours) ice packs are applied as much as possible. The head is elevated at bedtime if possible, and vision is

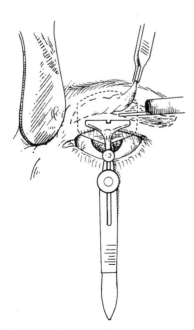

Figure 9–7. Diagram of skin muscle flap being removed from central lid with sharp upper traction of forceps.

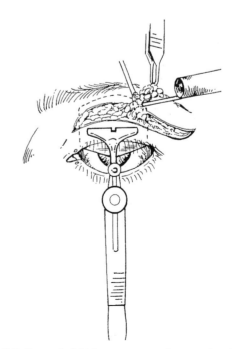

Figure 9–8. Removal of fat from preaponeurotic compartment.

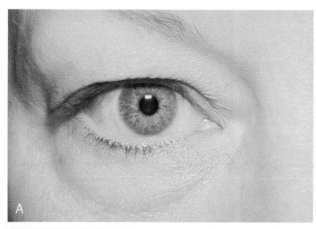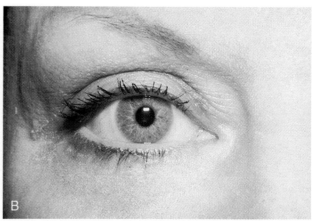

Figure 9–9. A 35-year-old patient preoperatively *(A)* and 3 months after *(B)* upper lid blepharoplasty, transconjunctival lower lid blepharoplasty, and resurfacing.

checked frequently. The patient avoids strenuous activity for about 7 days. Sutures are removed in 5 to 7 days, if applicable (Fig. 9–9).

Carbon Dioxide Laser Blepharoplasty: Transconjunctival Lower Lid Technique

Preoperative intravenous sedation is helpful before inducing anesthesia. Several drops of topical anesthetic are instilled in the inferior cul-de-sac. The anesthetic is 2% lidocaine with 1:100,000 epinephrine mixed with 0.75% bupivacaine. Hyaluronidase is optional. The lower lid is everted and the upper lid retracted. With gentle pressure on the globe, the orbital fat prolapses against the exposed conjunctival surface (Fig. 9–10). The bulge is greatest 7 to 8 mm below the lid margin centrally, which is 2 to 4 mm below the inferior margin of the tarsus and at least 2 to 3 mm above the transverse plexus of subconjunctival vessels visible in the depth of the inferior fornix. The injection is made transconjunctivally in the center of the lid at the point of maximum bulge. The surgeon sits at the patient's head, aims

at the orbital rim, and injects 1 to 2 ml of anesthetic as a bolus. The anesthetic is then massaged into the retroseptal tissues.

The incision is planned over the point of maximum bulge of the prolapsed orbital fat and extends from the caruncle medially to the lateral canthus laterally. The globe is protected by a laser-safe Jaeger plate. The lashes of the upper lid are everted during placement of the plate, to avoid a corneal abrasion. Topical anesthetic drops or an ocular ointment may be used to lubricate the plate. Adequate smoke evacuation is necessary to remove the potentially toxic laser plume. The CO_2 laser is set at 6 W in the continuous mode with a 0.2-mm focused delivery.

The conjunctiva and lower lid retractors are cut in one or two passes. Gentle pressure on the Jaeger plate enhances prolapse of orbital fat from the nasal, middle, and lateral fat pads. That fat that extends anterior to the orbital rim is removed in a sculpting fashion by cutting against a Desmarres lid retractor or another laser-safe instrument such as a soaking-wet cotton tip. Cutting is done in a slightly defocused fashion to maximize hemostasis. Large vessels are visualized and thus directly avoided. Clamping

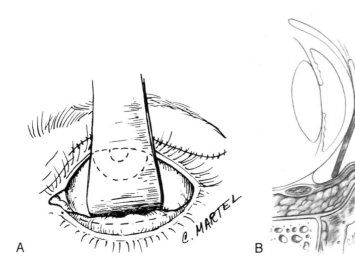

Figure 9–10. *(A,B)* Position for transconjunctival resection of prolapsed orbital fat.

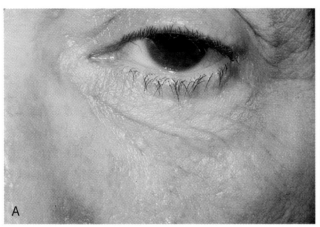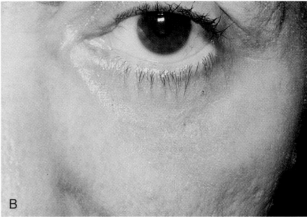

Figure 9–11. A 58-year-old woman *(A)* preoperatively and *(B)* 2 months after upper lid blepharoplasty, transconjunctival lower lid blepharoplasty resurfacing.

the fat before cutting is not necessary. Meticulous attention is given to hemostasis by defocused laser applications, or electrocautery if needed. The wound is not sutured. The lower lid is redraped or repositioned by removing instruments and digitally manipulating the lid superiorly. This maneuver helps to reveal any remaining orbital fat and restores normal anatomic relationships, thus avoiding possible postoperative cicatricial ectropion. Gross vision is checked in each eye separately and recorded.

As with the upper lids, during the first 24 to 48 hours after the procedure, ice packs are used continuously. The head is elevated during sleep if possible. Periodically, vision is checked in each eye separately. Strenuous activity is avoided for about 7 days. Topical antibiotics are used for 5 to 7 days while the transconjunctival wound closes (Fig. 9–11).

REFERENCES

1. Patel CKN: Continuous-wave laser action on vibrational-rotational transitions of carbon dioxide. Phys Rev 1964;136:A1187–A1193.
2. Anderson RR, Parrish JA: Selective photothermolysis: Precise microsurgery by selective absorption of pulsed radiation. Science 1983; 220:524.
3. Cochrane JPS, Beacon JP, Creasy GH, Russell RCG: Wound healing after laser surgery: An experimental study. Br J Surg 1980;67: 740–743.
4. Ben-Bassat MI, Ben-Bassat MO, Kaplan I: A study of the ultrastructural features of the cut margin of skin and mucous membrane specimens excised by carbon dioxide laser incision. Res Exp Med (Berl) 1979;176:69–79.
5. Shepanek NA, Kaplan BJ, Townsend D: In vitro cell changes in laser-exposed tissue. Acta Cytol 1980;24:244–246.
6. Kaplan I, Raif J: The Sharplan carbon dioxide laser in clinical surgery: Seven years' experience. In Goldman L (ed): The Biomedical Laser. New York: Springer-Verlag, 1981.
7. Fine BS, Fine S, Peacock GR, et al.: Preliminary observations on ocular effects of high-power, continuous CO_2 laser irradiation. Am J Ophthalmol 1967;64:209–222.
8. Geeraets WJ, Fine BS, Fine S: Ocular injury from CO_2 laser irradiation. Acta Ophthalmol 1969;47:80–91.
9. Beckman H, Rota A, Barraco R, et al.: Limbectomies, keratectomies and keratostomies performed with a rapid-pulsed carbon dioxide laser. Am J Ophthalmol 1971;71:1277–1283.
10. Karlin DB, Patel CKN, Wood OR, Llovera I: Carbon dioxide laser in vitreoretinal surgery. I. Quantitative investigation of the effects of carbon dioxide laser radiation on ocular tissue. Ophthalmology 1979; 86:290–298.
11. Mainster MA: Ophthalmic applications of infrared lasers—thermal considerations. Invest Ophthalmol Vis Sci 1979;18:414–420.
12. Peyman GA, Larson B, Raichand M, Andrews AH: Modification of rabbit corneal curvature with use of carbon dioxide laser burns. Ophthalmic Surg 1980;11:325–329.
13. Miller JB, Smith MR, Pincus F, Stockert M: Intraocular carbon dioxide laser photocautery. I. Animal experimentation. Arch Ophthalmol 1979; 97:2157–2162.
14. Miller JB, Smith MR, Boyer DS: Intraocular carbon dioxide laser photocautery. II. Preliminary report of clinical trials. Arch Ophthalmol 1979;97:2123–2127.
15. Beckman H, Fuller TA: Carbon dioxide laser scleral dissection and filtering procedure for glaucoma. Am J Ophthalmol 1979;88:73–77.
16. Beckman H, Fuller TA, Boyman R, et al.: Carbon dioxide laser surgery of the eye and adnexa. Ophthalmology 1980;87:990–1000.
17. Wesley RE, Bond JB: Carbon dioxide laser in ophthalmic plastic and orbital surgery. Ophthalmic Surg 1985;16:631–633.
18. Chopdar A: Carbon dioxide laser treatment of eye lid lesions. Trans Ophthalmol Soc UK 1985;104:176–180.
19. Hornblass A, Herschorn BJ: Carbon dioxide laser surgery in hemophilia. Am J Ophthalmol 1983;96:689–690.
20. Baker SS, Muenzler WS, Small RG, Leonard JE: Carbon dioxide laser blepharoplasty. Ophthalmology 1984;91:238–243.
21. David LM, Sanders G: CO_2 laser blepharoplasty: A comparison to cold-steel and electrocautery. J Dermatol Surg Oncol 1987;13: 110–114.
22. David LM: The laser approach to blepharoplasty. J Dermatol Surg Oncol 1988;14:741–746.
23. Morrow DM, Morrow LB: CO_2 laser blepharoplasty: A comparison with cold-steel surgery. J Dermatol Surg Oncol 1992;18:307–313.
24. Gregory RO: Letter to the editor. Ophthalmology 1985;92:52A.
25. Mittleman H, Apfelberg DB: Carbon dioxide laser blepharoplasty: Advantages and disadvantages. Ann Plastic Surg 1990;24:1–6.
26. Flaharty PM, Anderson RL: Lasers in oculoplastic surgery. In Benson WE, Marshall J, Spaeth GL (eds): Annual of Ophthalmic Laser Surgery. Philadelphia: Current Medicine, 1992.
27. David LM, Abergel RP: CO_2 laser blepharoplasty. In Coleman WP, Hanke CW, Alt TH, Asken S (eds): Cosmetic Surgery of the Skin: Principles, and Techniques. Philadelphia: BC Decker, 1991.
28. Baker SS: Carbon dioxide laser upper lid blepharoplasty. Am J Cosmetic Surg 1992;9(2):141–145.
29. Trelles MA, Sanchez J, Sala P, Elspas S: Surgical removal of lower eyelid fat using the carbon dioxide laser. Am J Cosmetic Surg 1992; 9(2):149–152.
30. Baker SS, Gregory RO: Laser blepharoplasty. Aesth Surg Q 1995; Summer:12–15.
31. Baker SS: Carbon dioxide laser ptosis surgery combined with blepharoplasty. Dermatol Surg 1995;21:1065–1070.

32. Baker SS, Pham RTH: Lateral canthal suspension using the carbon dioxide laser. Dermatol Surg 1995;21:1071–1073.

33. Glassberg E, Babapour R, Lask G: Current trends in blepharoplasty. Dermatol Surg 1995;21:1060–1063.

34. Baker SS, Glaser DA: Periorbital and Facial Laser Applications. St. Louis: Medical Video Productions, 1996.

35. Goldman MP, Fitzpatrick RE: Cutaneous Laser Surgery. St. Louis: Mosby–Year Book, 1994.

36. Bourguet: Les hernies graisseuses de l'orbite: Notre trâitement chirurgical. Bull Acad Med (Paris) 1924;92:1270.

37. Baylis HI, Sutcliffe RT: Conjunctival approach in lower eyelid blepharoplasty. Adv Ophthalmol Plastic Reconstr Surg 1983; 2:43–54.

38. David LM, Baker SS: David-Baker eyelid retractor. Am J Cosmetic Surg 1992;9(2):142–148.

39. Garden JM, O'Banion MK, Schelnitz LS, et al.: Papillomavirus in the vapor of carbon dioxide laser treated verrucae. JAMA 1988;259:1199–1202.

40. Monafo WW: Initial management of burns. N Engl J Med 1996; 335:1581–1586.

10

SKIN RESURFACING

Nicholas J. Lowe
C. Anne Maxwell
Philippa Lowe

Quan Nguyen
Christopher Ho
Gary P. Lask

Looking young and beautiful forever has been the dream of millions of people throughout the ages. From the time of Cleopatra, privileged women and men alike have tried various natural extracts to beautify their skin against the natural elements of time and aging. Within the past two decades, there have been many scientific discoveries regarding the mechanism of the skin aging process. Coupled with this new information has been an explosion of cosmetic products and procedures offered to repair the damages of age. Billions of dollars are spent annually by the public on various sunscreens, retinoids, alpha-hydroxy acids and antioxidants. Their therapeutic effects require time, and these products have their limitations; therefore, many people opt to seek more rapid surgical methods of facial rejuvenation. Chemical exfoliation and dermabrasion have been the cosmetic surgeon's mainstays of treatment for photodamaged skin. Because of the lack of control of the depth of tissue removal, these procedures have variable results and can cause complications such as scarring and depigmentation.

Indications

Laser skin resurfacing has been suggested as a promising new treatment for solar elastosis. Carbon dioxide (CO_2) laser skin resurfacing for treatment for aging facial skin was first introduced in the late 1980s with impressive results.[1,2] The continuous-wave CO_2 laser, however, is associated with a risk of unwanted thermal injury to the surrounding dermis and adnexal structures. Recent advances in rapidly pulsed lasers and flashscan techniques allow more precise control of tissue ablation, reducing the risk of scarring.[1-7] The ultrapulsed carbon dioxide ($UPCO_2$) laser has been shown to be effective treatment for aging facial skin.

Laser skin resurfacing can remove thin layers of old, damaged skin and replace them with newly formed, healthy skin. It also offers a clinical advantage in the treatment of superficial skin lesions for which surgery may leave scars. Table 10–1 lists some of the lesions or diseases for which CO_2 lasers have been reported to be successful. Pulsed CO_2 lasers have been claimed to offer advantages over cold-steel surgery for incisional procedures such as rhytidectomy and blepharoplasty[8]; these techniques are discussed in Chapters 13 and 9, respectively.

Types of CO_2 Lasers

Because of the popular demand for laser resurfacing, many CO_2 lasers are available. These can be divided into two groups: pulsed laser systems and continuous-wave systems. Table 10–2 summarizes the features of the laser systems currently available.

The first pulsed laser system, introduced by Coherent Medical, Inc., Palo Alto, CA, was the Ultrapulse laser. This laser produces high-energy pulses of very short duration, which allows controlled, char-free tissue ablation with a thermal injury depth of 70 μm. It has a pulse width of less than 1 msec and a pulse energy of up to 500 mJ. The energy is delivered through an articulated handle connected to a 3-mm collimated handpiece. This handpiece allows the user to precisely deliver consistent energy at any distance from the skin. This laser was developed to be operated with a computer controlled scanner called a computer pattern generator.

The Sharplan Surgilase 150 XJ is another first-generation pulsed laser. It produces a double pulse in 1.8 msec, but each pulse is within the limit of the thermal relaxation time. The first pulse partially ablates the tissue, and, during the resting period that follows, steam, debris, and thermal buildup from the first pulse is dispersed. Subsequently, the second pulse fires, which completely vaporizes the tissue. The pulse energy is calculated to be 400 mJ, with each pulse producing 200 mJ, and the depth of thermal injury is 150 μm.

Luxar Corporation introduced the Novapulse laser, which allows the delivery of laser through a lightweight flexible, hollow fiber arm. This is advantageous over the articulated arm, which is frequently bulky and difficult to maneuver. The Novapulse superpulsed laser delivers laser energy to tissue in high-amplitude, short-duration pulses of 800 μsec. Each pulse is followed by a laser period of off-time, when the tissue is allowed to cool down. This minimizes unwanted charring and thermal necrosis. In

Table 10–1. Some Other Clinical Applications for Carbon Dioxide Laser Resurfacing

CATEGORY	APPLICATIONS
Epidermal lesions	Actinic keratosis, seborrheic keratosis, verrucae, epidermal nevi
Skin tumors	Superficial basal cell carcinoma, Bowen's disease, benign pigmented nevi
Dermal lesions	Syringomata,[23] sebaceous hyperplasia, xanthelasma, neurofibroma,[24] adenoma sebaceum,[25] trichoepithelioma
Inflammatory dermatoses	Rhynophyma, psoriasis,*[26] Hailey-Hailey disease[27]

*Not considered clinically practical.

addition, the Novapulse features the "top hat" beam geometry, providing even distribution of laser energy up to 500 mJ, unlike the gaussian beam of other pulsed laser systems.

The Clearpulse laser produced by LaserSonics delivers single pulses of 500 mJ. Unlike other pulsed laser systems, the Clearpulse has a pulse duration of 6 msec, which is six times that of thermal relaxation time. However, the manufacturer states that the "histological testing has shown that the Clearpulse laser effectively ablates the epidermis to a level of 100 μm, with collateral damage limited to only 25 μm."

One addition to the pulsed laser system is the Tru-Pulse by Tissue Technologies and Palomar Medical Technologies. The Tru-Pulse was specifically designed to reduce postoperative erythema and expedite healing time after laser resurfacing. Erythema due to thermal damage is minimized through use of a pulse width of only 65 μsec. The ability to deliver high energy of up to 500 mJ rapidly may account for the shorter healing time and less erythema. The amount of tissue removed per pass may also be less, however, so it requires more passes for areas of deep rhytides.

The Sharplan SilkTouch laser, unlike the pulsed laser system, is an optomechanical device, is microprocessor controlled, and consists of rotating mirrors at a rapid speed, resulting in a spiral scan beam. The resulting dwell time of the laser beam at any particular point is less than the thermal relaxation time. The time for one cycle of beam rotation ranges from 0.2 to 0.45 second, and the spot sizes vary from 2 to 16 mm. The SilkTouch device can be adapted to a

Table 10–2. Some Carbon Dioxide Laser Systems Used for Skin Resurfacing

LASER	PULSE WIDTH	PULSE ENERGY (mJ)	COLLIMATION
SilkTouch	600 μsec	>500	No
FeatherTouch	300 μsec	>500	No
Surgilase	1.8 msec	400	Yes
Ultrapulse	<1 msec	500	Yes
Novapulse	800 μsec	500	No
Clearpulse	6 msec	500	Yes
Tru-Pulse	65 μsec	500	No

conventional continuous-wave CO_2 laser. More recently, Sharplan added the FeatherTouch to its family of flashscanner devices. The FeatherTouch laser has a shorter dwell time than the SilkTouch, which allows more superficial ablation of the epidermis and reduces postoperative erythema. By switching between the SilkTouch and FeatherTouch modes, the user can select the depth of skin resurfacing in accordance with the rhytid or scar.

Computer Pattern Generators

The technique of CO_2 laser surgery has been modified with the development of scanning systems such as the computer pattern generator (CPG). This device, which is available for a number of laser systems, allows areas of skin of any size and pattern to be treated rapidly and with precision (Fig. 10–1). The time for a full-face resurfacing procedure is reduced with the use of a CPG, and the result is more uniform (Fig. 10–2).

Laser–Skin Interaction

The CO_2 laser emits a beam of infrared light with a wavelength of 10,600 nm. This light is absorbed by all biologic tissue containing water, its target chromophore. Approximately 90% of the laser energy is absorbed by 30 μm of tissue, resulting in intracellular boiling to 100°C and vaporization. In earlier use of the CO_2 laser in the continuous mode, the tissue became progressively desiccated and heat accumulated to a temperature of 600°C. This heat would then conduct away from the treating site, leading to a surrounding zone of thermal necrosis 200 μm to 1 mm thick. The nonselective thermal damage can leave scars and discoloration.

Newer laser systems can reduce the collateral thermal injury by shortening the duration the laser beam spends on the target site. According to Beer's law, laser energy heats a critical volume of tissue until the temperature exceeds the vaporization threshold. This threshold for human skin—the *thermal relaxation time,* defined as the time required for the heated tissue to lose 50% of its heat through surrounding diffusion—is approximately 695 to 950 μsec. Thus, if the laser energy is delivered in less than the thermal relaxation time, heat dissipates rather than accumulates around the treatment area. A variety of CO_2 lasers can now be pulsed or scanned across the tissue, allowing the tissue dwell time or exposure time to be less than the thermal relaxation time.[9–13]

General Considerations

The energy density, or *fluence,* needed to ablate tissue has been estimated to be 4.5 to 5.0 J/cm². By using a laser system with a fluence above 5 J/cm² and a pulse duration

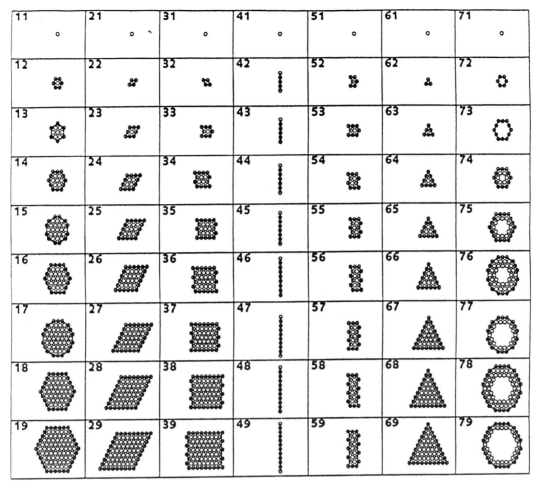

Figure 10–1. Representative scan patterns for the Coherent ultrapulse CO_2 delivery system.

less than 1 msec, an effective depth of 30 μm of tissue can be vaporized, leaving a shallow residual zone of thermal damage of 40 to 100 μm. This zone of necrosis is responsible for the sealing of small blood vessels, resulting in hemostasis. It has been hypothesized that collagen shrinkage also takes place below this zone, which accounts for the skin tightening effect seen during laser surgery.[4–7]

Recent clinical and histologic comparisons among

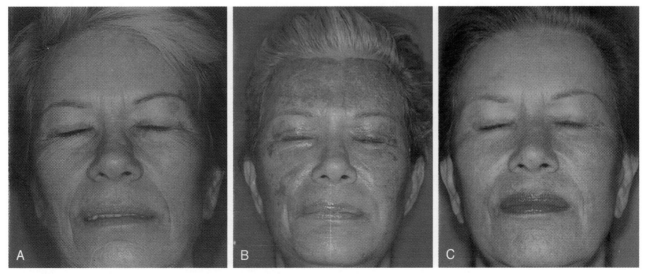

Figure 10–2. Photoaged facial skin. *A,* Before treatment. *B,* Three days after treatment with the UPCO₂ laser (300 mJ, 60 W, CPG 6, three passes). *C,* Twelve months after treatment.

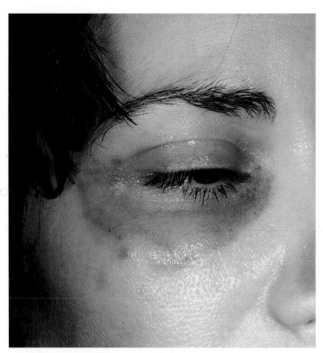

Figure 10–3. Immediately after UPCO$_2$ laser treatment (single pass, 250 mJ, 60 W, CPG 5). The lesion is protected with petroleum ointment.

pulsed CO$_2$ laser, medium-strength trichloroacetic acid peel, and dermabrasion have shown comparable results, with the exception of Baker's phenol peel, which may give deeper dermal injury.[14] Healing from medium-strength trichloro-acetic acid peel and dermabrasion was similar to that after one to three passes of pulsed laser treatment. The phenol-treatment caused a deeper wound and required a longer recovery time.

In the past, most studies had been performed on facial skin caucasian phototypes I and II. There have been few reports on the use of these lasers for the rejuvenation of photoaged neck skin. The neck is often considered to be an area of potential complication with treatments such as dermabrasion and chemical peels. In a recent study, 200 patients with facial photoaging and 40 patients with neck skin photoaging, skin types I, II, III, and IV, were treated. All patients were treated with Ultrapulse CO$_2$ laser with CPG handpiece. An energy setting of 250 W/cm^2 was used with a low density CPG setting of 3, using a single pass, no wiping technique.

Facial photoaging was improved between 50% and 75% with a single treatment and occasionally a second treatment. The result after a single treatment continues to improve for 6 months to 2 years.

Successful rejuvenation of the neck skin is very dependent on appropriate low density settings and the skill and caution of the laser surgeon.

Preoperative Preparation

For optimal results with laser skin resurfacing, carefully selected skin care regimens are needed both before and after

treatment.[16, 17] This is especially important in the treatment of patients with darker complexions.[16, 17] The pretreatment regimen consists of use of daily broad-spectrum sunscreens, application of bleaching agents such as hydroquinone or azelaic acid, and nightly application of tretinoin cream or glycolic acid cream. This regimen is usually started after the initial consultation, about 2 to 4 weeks before the procedure.

The day before laser surgery, the patient is started on therapy with oral antibiotics and antiherpes medications. Use of these drugs is continued for 5 to 7 days postoperatively. Wound care consists of petroleum ointment (petroleum jelly, solid vegetable shortening) applied for 2 weeks; hydrogel surgical dressings (Vigilon, Silon) applied for 3 days; diluted acetic acid soaks from days 4 to 7, and soap-free wash (Aquanil, Cetaphol) thereafter (Fig. 10–3). The sunscreen, bleaching, and tretinoin cream regimen is started again 2 to 4 weeks after treatment.

Complications of CO$_2$ Laser Resurfacing

Complications of laser surgery include infection, contact dermatitis, swelling, prolonged erythema, depigmentation, and scarring. Recurrence of herpes infection can be prevented with prophylactic medication. Topical antibiotic use is no longer recommended because of the common occurrence of contact dermatitis. Postoperative swelling, especially around periorificial areas, is managed with ice compresses or a short course of systemic corticosteroid. Prolonged erythema can last from several weeks to several months (Fig. 10–4). Postinflammatory hyperpigmentation sometimes follows the erythema, so all patients with prolonged erythema are treated with bleaching agent. Hyperpigmentation is most common in the infraorbital areas, where direct sunlight exposure can play a role. Hypopigmentation can also occur and tends to be delayed, occurring 6 months to 1 year after the procedure. Although laser skin resurfacing is precise, thermal damage accumulates with multiple passes of the laser, and hypertrophic scars have been reported. Scarring is related to the depth of resurfacing as well as the location of treatment. The perioral areas usually require more passes, and a few incidences of scarring have been reported.[17]

Laser Techniques

Anesthesia Anesthesia for a cosmetic unit (perioral, malar areas) can be achieved with topical EMLA cream applied at least 1 hour before nerve blocks (infraorbital or mental), using lidocaine 1% with 1:100,000 epinephrine. Additional ring blocks are usually necessary for the periorbital and lateral face areas, since these are innervated by more than one nerve branch. Topical anesthesia can work for up to two laser passes for a full-face procedure.[18] Sedation with 5 mg of diazepam (Valium) or intramuscular injection with 50 mg meperidine (Demerol)

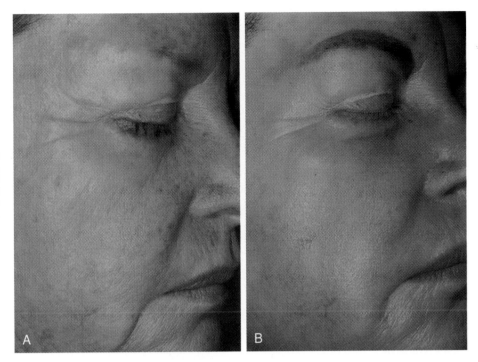

Figure 10–4. Photoaged skin. *A*, Before treatment. *B*, Three months after $UPCO_2$ laser resurfacing (two passes on each cheek; three passes periorally). There is some persistent erythema. See Figure 10–5 for further views of this patient.

is necessary in some patients. For patients with a low pain threshold, sedational anesthesia is required with appropriate monitoring by an anesthesiologist. Many laser surgeons prefer sedational over topical anesthesia because of the pain patients experience during large area laser resurfacing.

The technique for treating rhytides consists of laser ablation of a particular cosmetic unit. A series of multiple side-by-side laser impacts with minimal overlap is laid down. The areas are subsequently wiped off with saline-soaked gauzes. Repeated passes are made, emphasizing the shoulders of the deep rhytides. In general, it takes three or four passes to get significant improvement of the perioral rhytides. The periorbital areas, in contrast, require fewer laser passes because the dermis is thinner. Treatment of icepick scars sometimes necessitates punch excisions of these scars 1 month before laser resurfacing. Feathering of the margins of the treated areas can be performed by decreasing the power or decreasing the density of the scanner pattern to reduce the obvious change of skin texture and color during the healing phase.

It can be helpful to use the visual signs of laser depth penetration to decrease the chance of scarring. If used inappropriately, even char-free ablation lasers can cause

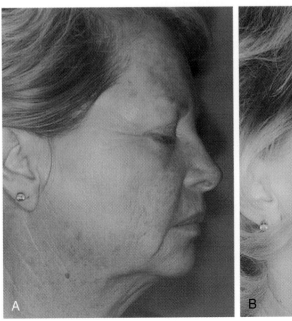
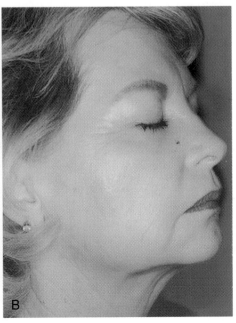

Figure 10–5. Same patient as shown in Figure 10–4. *A*, Before treatment. *B*, After treatment. Ultrapulse CO_2 laser settings used were as follows: for the face—first pass, 300 mJ, 60 W, CPG 3.9.6; second pass, 250 mJ, 60 W, CPG 3.9.5; for the neck—single pass, 250 mJ, 60 W, CPG 3.9.3.

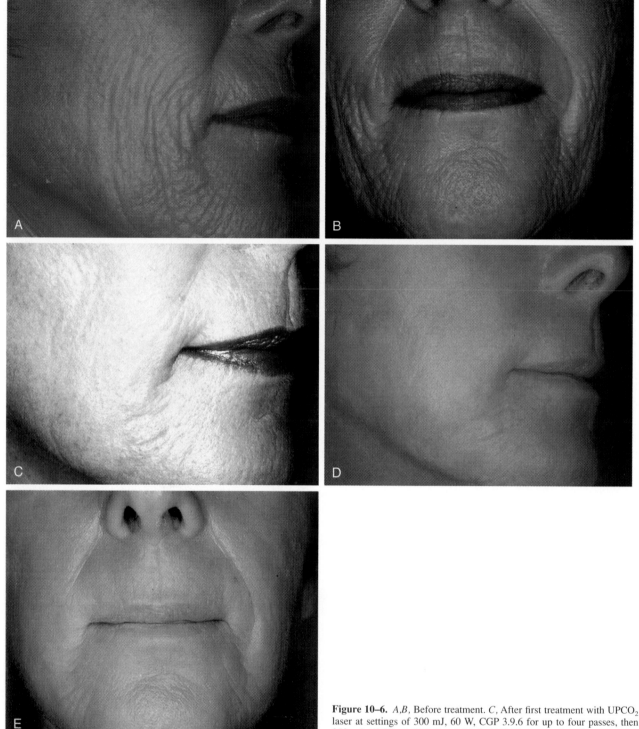

Figure 10–6. *A,B,* Before treatment. *C,* After first treatment with UPCO$_2$ laser at settings of 300 mJ, 60 W, CGP 3.9.6 for up to four passes, then 250 mJ, 60 W, at CPG 3 and 5.9.5. *D,E,* Three months after treatment.

scars despite their minimal thermal injury. The signs of depth penetration of the skin are as follows:

1. Pink, erythematous appearance—ablating of the epidermis with effacing of the papillary dermis
2. Yellow chamois cloth appearance—deep papillary dermis

The authors do not wipe the final laser pass as we have found removal led to more prolonged erythema. These are helpful guides but are not always consistent and should not be used as the sole end point determination.

Results

Skin resurfacing with CO$_2$ lasers is an effective form of skin rejuvenation (Figs. 10–5 to 10–10). In our recent study, we used an Ultrapulse 5000C CO$_2$ laser with a CPG of

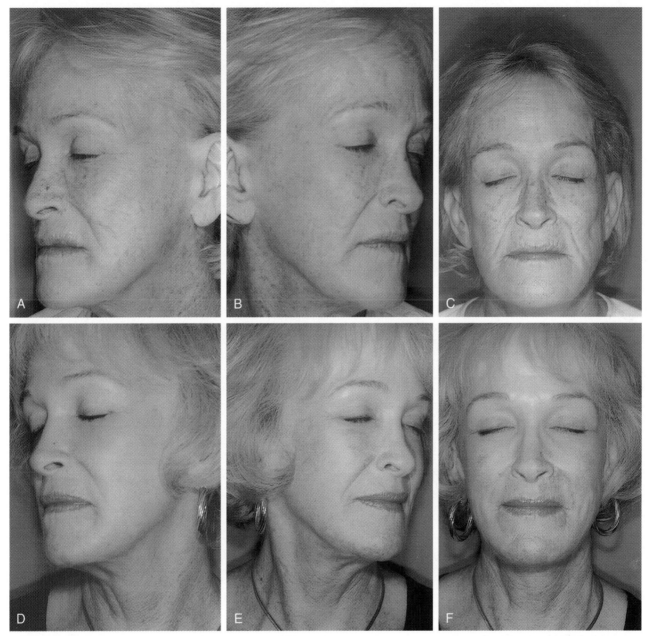

Figure 10–7. Pretreatment *(A,B)* side views and *(C)* frontal view. Three months after UPCO$_2$ laser treatment *(D,E)* side views and *(F)* frontal view. For the face: first pass, 300 mJ, 60 W, CPG setting of 3.9.6; second pass: 250 mJ, 60 W, CPG 3.9.5. For the neck: Single pass, 250 mJ, 60 W, CPG 3.9.3.

either pattern 3, for most areas of the face, or pattern 5, for the periorbital and perioral skin. For the central and main areas of the face, the maximum size setting was 9, with the density setting of either 5 or 6, depending on the degree of photodamage. For the subsequent laser pulses on the face, the settings were 250 mJ and 60 W, with pattern 3 or 5 determined as above; densities of 4 or 5 were used. Laser settings for neck rejuvenation were as follows: a single pass with the laser was used for treatment of the neck area; laser energy settings of 225 mJ, 100 W were used, with density settings of 3 (Table 10–3). For the face, the vaporized skin was wiped after each pass except for the final pass, which was left unwiped. For the neck treatment, no wiping of the vaporized skin was performed after the single low-density CPG laser ablation.

Results of the treatment of facial photoaging are shown in Figure 10–11. Between 50% and 75% improvement was eventually achieved 12 to 24 months after a single laser treatment. A small number of patients were successfully treated either completely or partially after a second laser treatment. In these patients (see Table 10–3), the final improvement was 25% to 50% improved over the first treatment. In general, the patients received fewer passes during their second treatment than during their first.

The global responses after a single neck rejuvenation treatment varied between 40% and 75% improvement (Fig. 10–12). The neck is at much greater risk for scarring than the face. The risk increases the more interior one goes, in part because of the decreasing amount of adnexal structures (see Figs. 10–5 and 10–8). The temporary side effects were

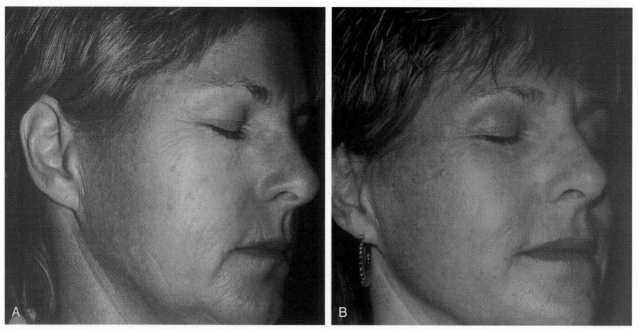

Figure 10–8. *A,* Before treatment. *B,* Twelve months after treatment with $UPCO_2$ laser at settings of 300 mJ, 60 W, CPG 3.9.6 for the first pass and 250 mJ, 60 W, CPG 3.9.5 for the second pass.

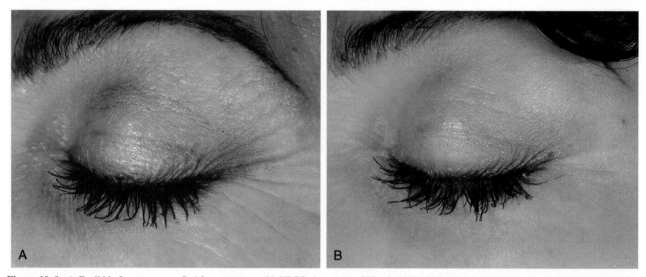

Figure 10–9. *A,* Eyelid before treatment. *B,* After treatment with $UPCO_2$ laser set at 300 mJ, 60 W, CPG 5.9.5 for the first pass, and 250 mJ, 60 W, CPG 5.6.4 for the second pass.

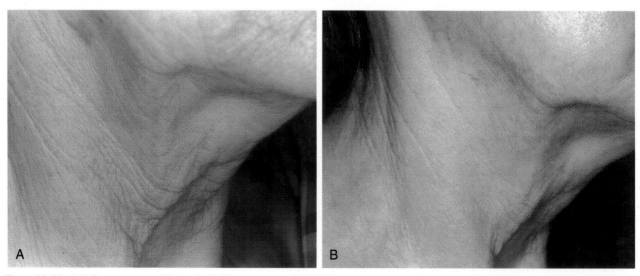

Figure 10–10. *A,* Before treatment of the neck. *B,* After treatment with $UPCO_2$ laser at settings of 250 mJ, 60 W, CPG 3.9.3, single pass, no wipe.

Table 10–3. Laser Settings for Use at Different Skin Sites (Coherent Ultrapulse 5000 CO$_2$ Laser)

	FIRST PASS		REPEAT PASSES		NUMBER OF PASSES
	Laser Energy Settings	CPG Density	Laser Energy Settings	CPG Density	
Cheeks	300 mJ 60 W	4–6	250 mJ 60 W	4–6	1–3
Perioral	300 mJ 60 W	5–6	250 mJ 60 W	5–6	2–5
Acne scars (cheeks, forehead)	300 mJ 60 W	6–7	250 mJ 60 W	6–7	2–5
Eyelids	250 mJ 60 W	4–5	250 mJ 60 W	4	1–3
Neck	250 mJ 60 W	2–3	0	0	1 (no wiping)

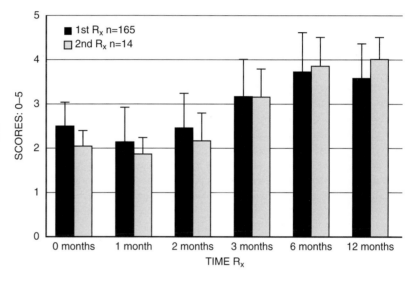

Figure 10–11. Histogram showing improvement scores in 165 patients with photodamaged facial skin treated with UPCO$_2$ laser resurfacing.

exudation, scaling, erythema, and discomfort. After the 7th to 10th day, complete reepithelization was seen. A smaller percentage of patients had postoperative erythema that lasted up to 6 months. After the second month, however, this was generally of a relatively mild degree and was frequently more pronounced after exercise or exposure to hot weather.

In skin types II and IV, transient hyperpigmentation lasted up to 7 to 9 months in some patients. It is important

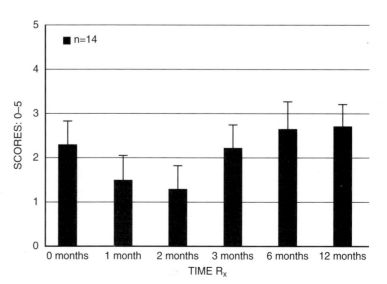

Figure 10–12. Histogram showing improvement scores in 14 patients with photodamaged neck skin treated with UPCO$_2$ laser resurfacing.

to use extreme caution in treatment of the neck with the use of a low density with a single pass and no wiping. Great care must be taken in the performance of laser rejuvenation on the neck, and it is advisable that the laser be tested in a small area before general treatment is undertaken.

Improvement from laser skin rejuvenation was observed to last during the entire study period for these patients. For patients who have severe photodamage (e.g., perioral rhytides), it is perhaps best to treat a second time to avoid an overaggressive single treatment. The patients treated for a second time show a significant improvement. Potential mechanisms of action include in vivo dermal collagen shrinkage and remodeling, as noted by Ross and colleagues.[19] In addition, it is likely that the epidermal proliferative regrowth seen after laser skin rejuvenation also releases a variety of growth factors that aid in formation of new dermal connective tissue.

The new observations on the successful treatment of photodamaged neck skin are encouraging, but the advice given here about superficial use and low-density laser settings should be heeded. Further patient studies are needed before laser neck rejuvenation can be considered safe and effective.

Er:YAG Laser

Another laser system being evaluated for skin resurfacing is the erbium:yttrium-aluminum-garnet (Er:YAG) laser. It may be of value for more superficial skin resurfacing such as neck and eyelid skin. The last few years have seen an increased use for skin resurfacing.

The Er:YAG laser has a high affinity for water absorption. The wavelength of 2940 nm is at the peak of water absorption (ten times greater than the CO_2 laser).[20] The available Er:YAG lasers have a pulse duration of 250 to 350 μsec. This, along with its high affinity for water absorption, allows for ablation with much less residual thermal damage than with CO_2 laser systems. Initial studies show that a single pass with some Er:YAG lasers ablates 20 to 25 μm of epidermis. The minimal thermal damage of Er:YAG lasers has been claimed to allow quicker healing and less erythema than CO_2 lasers. This is entirely dependent on the aggressiveness of the laser resurfacing. With the small amount of coagulation, however, bleeding can be a problem, and more passes are required to attain adequate depth for clinical improvement. The question of equivalent results with equal depth but less thermal effect with the Er:YAG laser versus the CO_2 laser system, as well as long-term equivalency, remains to be seen.

Recently Er:YAG lasers have been developed to reduce bleeding either by using longer pulse duration or by combining with CO_2 systems.

The Er:YAG laser is potentially of benefit in areas at high risk for scarring, such as the neck and dorsum of the hands. In dealing with deep rhytides and extensively sun-damaged skin, investigators are evaluating variations in parameters,

Table 10–4. Typical Laser Settings and Passes for Er:YAG Lasers at Different Skin Sites

	EACH PASS LASER SETTINGS	NUMBER OF PASSES
Cheeks	700 to 900 mJ	5 to 10
Perioral	700 to 900 mJ	5 to 10
Acne scars (cheeks, forehead)	700 to 900 mJ	5 to 10
Eyelids	500 mJ	Usually 3
Neck	500 mJ	Usually 3

scanning patterns, and repetition rates that will allow them to increase penetration and thermal damage when necessary.[21]

One study comparing the Er:YAG laser with the UPCO$_2$ laser found seven passes with the former and three passes with the latter produced tissue vaporization of 50 to 80 μm. Residual thermal damage was none to 20 μm with the Er:YAG laser and 80 to 150 μm with the CO_2 laser. Regardless of the number of passes, the Er:YAG laser had more rapid reepithelization and decreased erythema than the CO_2 laser. However, with an equal number of passes, the CO_2 laser resulted in greater wrinkle improvement.[22]

In addition to the lasers used, the outcome of laser skin rejuvenation depends on many factors, including the laser settings and pre- and post-treatment skin care provided (Table 10–4).

The rapidly advancing technological development in the area of laser resurfacing, with the need for long-term follow-up, makes this a constantly evolving area, so physicians require frequent updates to perform the most efficacious and safest procedures possible.

REFERENCES

1. David LM, Lask GP, Glassberg E, et al.: CO_2 laser ablation for cosmetic and therapeutic treatment of facial actinic damage. Cutis 1989;43:583–587.
2. Fitzpatrick RE, Ruiz-Exparaza J, Goldman MP: The depth of thermal necrosis using the CO_2 laser: A comparison of the superpulsed mode and the conventional mode. J Dermatol Surg Oncol 1991;17:340–344.
3. Fitzpatrick RE, Goldman MP: Advances in carbon dioxide laser surgery. Clin Dermatol 1995;13:35–47.
4. Lowe NJ, Lask G, Griffin ME, et al.: Skin resurfacing with the ultrapulsed carbon dioxide laser: Observation on 100 patients. Dermatol Surg 1995;21:1025–1029.
5. Hruza GJ: Skin resurfacing with lasers. J Clin Dermatol 1995;3:38–41.
6. Waldorf HA, Kauvar A, Geronemus RG: Skin resurfacing of fine to deep rhytides using a char-free carbon dioxide laser in 47 patients. Dermatol Surg 1995;21:940–946.
7. Lask G, Keller G, Lowe N, et al.: Laser skin resurfacing with the SilkTouch flashscanner for facial rhytides. Dermatol Surg 1995;21:1021–1024.
8. Serkel BR: Anesthetic Laser Surgery. Boston: Little, Brown and Co, 1996.
9. Trost D, Zacheri A, Smith M: Surgical laser properties and their tissue interaction. Chicago: Mosby–Year Book 1992;131–162.
10. McKenzie AL: How far does thermal damage extend beneath the surface of CO_2 laser incisions? Phys Med Biol 1983;28:905–912.
11. Hobbs E, Bailin P, Wheeland R, Ratz J: Superpulsed lasers: Minimizing thermal damage with short duration high irradiance pulses. J Dermatol Surg Oncol 1987;13:9.

12. Verschueren RCJ, Koudstaal J, Oldhoff J: CO_2 laser surgery. In Hillencamp F, Pratesi R, Sacni CA (eds): Lasers in Biology and Medicine. New York: Plenum, 1980.

13. Von Gernert MJC, Welch AJ: Time constants in thermal medicine. Lasers Surg Med 1989;9:405.

14. Fitzpatrick RE, Tope WD, Goldman MP, et al.: Pulsed carbon dioxide laser, trichloroacetic acid, Baker-Gordon phenol, and dermabrasion: A comparative clinical and histological study in a porcine model. Arch Dermatol 1996;132:469–471.

15. Lowe NJ, et al.: Scientific exhibit, American Academy of Dermatology 1996 annual meeting.

16. Cotton J, Hood AF, Gonin R, et al.: Histologic evaluation of preauricular and postauricular human skin after high-energy short-pulsed carbon dioxide laser. Arch Dermatol 1996;132:425–428.

17. Lowe NJ, Lask G, Griffin ME: Laser skin resurfacing: Pre and posttreatment guidelines. Dermatol Surg 1995;21:1017–1019.

18. Ho C, Nguyen Q, Lowe NJ, et al.: Laser resurfacing in pigmented skin. Dermatol Surg 1995;21:1035–1037.

19. Ross EV: Symposium on laser resurfacing. Presentation at the American Academy of Dermatology Meeting, Orlando, July 16, 1996.

20. Kaufman R, Hirbot R: Pulsed erbium:YAG laser ablation in cutaneous surgery. Laser Surg Med 1996;19:324.

21. Hirst R, Stock K, Kaufman R: Ablation and controlled heating of skin with the Er:YAG laser. Laser Surg Med 1997(Suppl);9:40.

22. Khatri K, Ross V, Grevelink J, et al.: Comparison of erbium:YAG and CO_2 lasers in wrinkle removal. Laser Surg Med 1997(Suppl); 9:37.

23. Apfelberg DB, Maser MR, Lash H, et al.: Superpulsed CO_2 laser treatment of facial syringomata. Laser Surg Med 1987;7:533.

24. Roenigk RK, Ratz JL: CO_2 laser treatment of cutaneous neurofibromas. J Dermatol Surg Oncol 1987;13:187.

25. Wheeland RG, Bailin PL, Kantor GR, et al.: Treatment of adenoma sebaceum with carbon dioxide laser vaporization. J Dermatol Surg Oncol 1985;13:149.

26. Morelli M, Anselmi C, Farinelli F, et al.: CO_2 laser peeling for psoriasis. Laser Surg Med 1987;7:97.

27. Don PC, Carney PS, Lynch WS, et al.: Carbon dioxide laser abrasion: A new approach to management of familial benign pemphigus. J Dermatol Surg Oncol 1987;13:1187.

11

HAIR TRANSPLANTATION: AN OVERVIEW

Walter P. Unger

The original technique of hair transplantation involved hair-bearing grafts approximately 4 mm in diameter that were placed into recipient site holes made with punches approximately 3.5 mm in diameter. It has been gradually but steadily replaced by "minigrafting" in which grafts containing only one to six hairs are used.[1] These smaller grafts are placed into holes made with (1) an ordinary 16- to 18-gauge hypodermic needle or Nokor needle (one- to two-hair *micrografts*) and (2) 1- to 2-mm-diameter punches *(round minigrafts),* or into slits made with a scalpel blade *(slit grafts).* Micrografts and slit grafts do not remove any existing original hair, since the recipient sites are made *between* the existing hairs. In addition, although round minigrafts are far less "pluggy" looking than, for example, 4-mm round grafts, because of the cosmetic advantage of a linear shape over a round shape, many hair transplant surgeons prefer slit grafts over round minigrafts. Slit grafting has a number of potential drawbacks of its own, however:

1. The darker, coarser, or more dense the hair, the more potential there is to produce dense, dark lines of hair that are at least as unsightly as round grafting. This effect is referred to as *compression.*
2. With round grafts of whatever size, alopecic or potentially alopecic skin is being removed at the same time as hair is being added. With scalpel slit grafting, no alopecic or potentially alopecic skin is being eliminated and skin surface is actually being increased. Thus, if one is moving the same amount of donor tissue, slit grafting does not produce the same hair density as does round grafting.
3. Because a 0.5- to 1-mm-wide graft is being squeezed into a narrow slit, there is an increased opportunity for graft elevation or depression.

All of these three potential drawbacks of slit grafting—compression, decreased density, and graft elevation or depression—are avoided if the linear recipient site can itself be made 0.5 to 1 mm wide, such as by using a laser to ablate tissue in a line. Unfortunately, until recently, carbon dioxide (CO_2) lasers were associated with unacceptably wide zones

of thermal damage adjacent to the lines of incision or ablation.

In the autumn of 1993, Dr. Larry David and I began a series of studies using the new Ultrapulse laser developed by Coherent Medical, Inc, of Santa Monica, CA. This laser produces high-energy pulses that are delivered in ultrabrief bursts shorter than 695 msec (the thermal relaxation time of skin). Photomicrographs of incisions made to the depth of superficial subcutaneous tissue showed zones of thermal damage less than 70 μm wide at the level of the hair matrix. Adjacent hair follicles, whether original or previously transplanted, could be expected to be spared injury with such narrow zones of thermal damage. The studies involved the use of different handpieces, laser energy, power, and time settings, and hair counts in grafts transplanted into laser- and scalpel-prepared sites in similar but contralateral locations in the subject's recipient area. Results seen in the first ten patients were reported in 1994 and revealed better hair survival in laser-prepared slit sites in four of ten patients, equal survival in five patients, and less hair yield in one patient.[2] In addition, hair growth occurred earlier (7.5 to 9.0 weeks) in the laser grafts in five patients. Each time a specific number of grafts showed good hair growth, I increased that number in the next study patients. Contrary to the initial study, with larger numbers of grafts, a delay in hair regrowth rather than accelerated hair regrowth was noted at the laser sites.

The most important finding in these later studies was a more "even" distribution of hair in laser-prepared areas and therefore a more natural-appearing distribution of hair when compared with the conventionally treated control side.[3, 4] In addition, there was total absence of compression. Added advantages of using the laser included complete control of bleeding in the recipient area and control of the depth of ablation. However, although one can eliminate all bleeding by decreasing the energy density (millijoules [mJ]) of the laser, the goal should not be the absence of all blood. A small amount of bleeding increases the likelihood that the grafts are getting adequate and rapid revascularization. Blood also acts as a "biologic glue." One or two grafts fell out several days after surgery in two of the early study patients because there wasn't enough bleeding to "glue" them in place.[3] About a year and a half after our studies began with the Ultrapulse laser, other investigators began using a Sharplan CO_2 laser to produce round holes for minigrafts.[5, 6] I began my own studies with this laser in late 1995. Histologic findings with it have been previously published.[4]

Technique

Planning

The same principles that guide planning in conventional hair transplantation are used for laser transplantation and have been described in great detail elsewhere.[7] In particular, one assesses the long-range donor and recipient area ratio when deciding how much of the bald or potentially bald area one can reasonably hope to treat. A hairline is chosen by beginning and ending the line where one expects the *ultimate* anterior-most, superior-most points of the temporal hair will be, and by joining them to a midline point that is chosen so that the hairline runs more or less parallel to the ground when viewed laterally. I believe in the wisdom of placing transplants not only in alopecic areas but also through hair-bearing areas that can reasonably be expected to eventually become bald. This minimizes the likelihood of having to chase an enlarging bald area (Fig. 11–1).

Notwithstanding the foregoing, I reserve laser transplantation for individuals whose recipient areas are alopecic or nearly alopecic. Existing hair is ablated as the laser lines are being produced, and thus treating hair-bearing areas with the laser results in less hair for the first 3 months. This must be contrasted with the likelihood of minimal immediate postoperative change in hair density if scalpel slits or needle holes are made between existing hairs. However, patients initially treated with conventional micrografting and slit grafting because of existing hair in the recipient area can be treated with laser transplantation between the previously transplanted grafts when more of the existing hair has been lost with the progression of male pattern baldness. Thus, such individuals will ultimately be treated with a mixture of conventional and laser transplantation. I often choose (with the patient's concurrence) to treat only a portion of the recipient area with the laser and the bulk of the site conventionally. Waiting 5 or 6 months allows both the doctor and the patient to assess the difference in postoperative course and results in conventionally transplanted and laser-treated sites. Subsequent treatment can be decided upon on the basis of what is seen. If cosmetic results are superior at the laser sites, the laser is used for the entire second session. If they are the same or inferior, the laser may not be used at all during second and subsequent sessions.

Anesthesia

Tumescent anesthesia is used in the donor area by employing an anesthetic solution that consists of 5.0 mL of 2% lidocaine without epinephrine and 0.4 mL of fresh epinephrine 1:1000 added to 100 ml of normal saline. Usually between 70 and 100 mL of this mixture is infiltrated slowly into the donor area using a single injection site and an 18×3.5–inch spinal needle.[8] A recipient area field block is produced with 1.0% lidocaine with 1:100,000 epinephrine and 50 mEq/L of sodium bicarbonate. The sodium bicarbonate is added to minimize the pain of infiltration. Unbuffered 2% lidocaine with 1:50,000 epinephrine is used to produce a field block superior to the first one, and a 1:50,000 solution of epinephrine is used in the rest of the recipient area. I do not use tumescent anesthesia in the recipient area because of the difficulty of accurately estimating graft spacing once the distention caused by the tumescent anesthesia has disappeared, and the increased likelihood of "losing" a graft beneath the surface of the

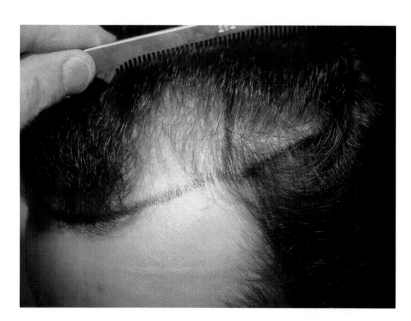

Figure 11–1. In many patients with less than complete alopecia, a triangle-shaped corner area is present, with some hair persisting within it that is eventually lost. This area is marked in the photograph and should be transplanted at the same time as the obviously bald areas more anteriorly so as to avoid constantly "chasing" an enlarging area of alopecia.

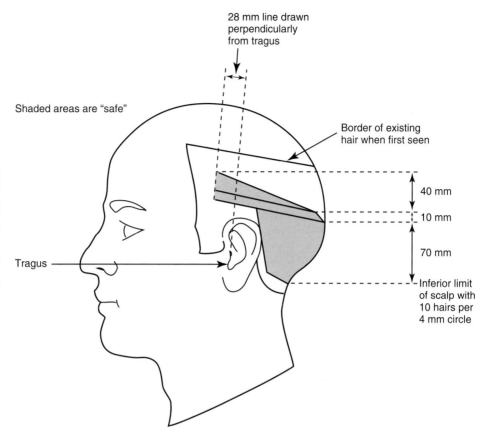

28 mm line drawn
perpendicularly
from tragus

Shaded areas are "safe"

Border of existing
hair when first seen

40 mm

10 mm

70 mm

Tragus

Inferior limit
of scalp with
10 hairs per
4 mm circle

Figure 11–2. A study in which 328 men aged 65 years and older were included revealed good hair density in over 80% of those less than 80 years of age when transplants were within the parameters shown in this schematic drawing. (Reprinted with permission from Unger W: The donor site. In Hair Transplantation, 3rd ed. New York: Marcel Dekker, 1995;184.)

skin. Tumescent anesthesia in the recipient area can also cause more postoperative edema.

The Donor Area

A "safe" donor area for 80% of patients under the age of 80 years was established by a study in which persisting rim hair was recorded in 328 men who were 65 to 79 years of age[9] (Fig. 11–2). A quadruple- or quintuple-bladed knife is used to excise strips of skin, each of which is 2.0 to 2.5 mm wide, from the donor area.[10] The strips are later carefully sectioned into grafts containing one to six hairs each. A donor area running from ear to ear that is only 44 mm high is sufficient in most patients to produce six sessions consisting of 350 to 400 slit grafts and 250 micrografts per session (Fig. 11–3). Larger bleeding vessels are cauterized before the wound is closed in a single layer using a simple running suture and 2-0 Supramid on a CL20 needle.

Different sites in the donor area produce grafts with different hair densities, textures, and often color. I therefore usually prefer to use two donor zones for each session (Fig. 11–3) to get grafts with a variety of hair characteristics that are advantageous for specific areas in the recipient site. Fine hair in the inferior occipital area and temporal hair, for example, work well for producing soft, natural-looking hairlines. Coarse or denser hair from more superior occipital and parietal areas is more suitable for creating greater

density in the remainder of the recipient area. In subsequent sessions, new donor areas are harvested immediately superior or inferior to the scars from previous donor areas. These old scars are excised as part of the new "donor strip" so that no matter how many procedures are carried out, only two narrow donor site scars are produced. As mentioned earlier, it is rare to be unable to obtain enough donor material from the parietal occipital areas for six *or more* sessions.

The Recipient Area

Natural-looking results in the recipient area depend on hair being as evenly distributed as possible while having an irregular or random pattern. To this end, I have always advocated an "organized disorganized" pattern for each session of transplanting.[11] For laser transplantation, I recommend the following four parameters:

1. Grafts in session 1 should be 3 mm apart.
2. They should be 1 mm anterior or posterior to their neighboring graft.
3. The angle of incision should be approximately 45 degrees.
4. The direction of the incision should follow the direction of the original hair in that area.[12, 13]

The "art" of hair transplantation to a large extent depends on learning how to consistently accomplish these four goals.

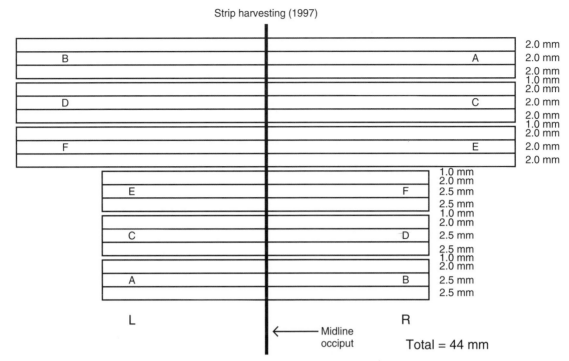

Strip harvesting (1997)

Figure 11–3. Schematic drawing showing organization of the donor area for strip harvesting sessions of micrografts and minigrafts. A, B, C, D, E, and F represent donor strips excised in sessions 1, 2, 3, 4, 5, and 6, respectively. The 1-mm gap between each of the session areas represents a typical 1-mm-wide band of scar from the previous sessions that is excised as part of subsequent ones. This donor area is well within the parameters of the "safe donor area" shown in Figure 11–2. (Reprinted with permission from Unger W [ed]: Hair Transplantation, 3rd ed. New York: Marcel Dekker, 1995.)

One of the advantages of using a laser is that a computer-driven "scanner" that moves the laser beam in an accurate and consistent fashion can be added to it. The Ultrapulse laser comes with a scanner that can produce the pattern described here, among others (Fig. 11–4). Thus, relative novices can accomplish spacing and positioning like an expert.

During session 2, the slits should be made midway between those of the first session. In session 3, conventional slit grafting is recommended to fill the spaces between previously transplanted grafts (Fig. 11–5). Although three sessions usually produce excellent cosmetic results, if hair characteristics are particularly good (e.g., fine or light colored or dense), even one or two sessions may produce a satisfactory one.

The graph shown in Figure 11–6 is a schematic summary of the findings of more than 500 biopsies of laser slits carried out in four centers. It indicates that optimal settings for adequate depth of incision appear to be 300 to 325 mJ and 40 to 60 W with the Coherent Ultrapulse CO_2 laser with its scanner set at pattern 4, which ablates a line 3 mm long with 22 0.2-mm collimated spots laid down in a *nonsequential* order (Fig. 11–7). The line is produced in less than 0.5 second and is approximately 2 mm deep. Zones of thermal damage are 50 to 70 µm wide at the level of the hair matrices. I have also produced excellent cosmetic results using pattern 1, 300 mJ and 12 to 15 W.

As mentioned earlier, other lasers have been used in hair transplantation. I previously reported on a Sharplan handpiece designed to create lines for slit grafts.[4] Unfortunately, because the beam of light is not collimated, lines of equal depth can be produced only with the handpiece held perpendicular to the skin. Hairs growing in grafts placed into such sites are cosmetically unacceptable because of their too-vertical orientation. For those patients or physicians who prefer round minigrafts to slit grafts, however, the Sharplan CO_2 laser with flashscanner attachment can be used to create a round hole by rapid movement of the spot in a spiral fashion.[4] Histologic assessment in 48 of my patients revealed that the optimal setting varies from 0.1 to 0.15 second and 50 to 80 W when the "minus" size setting is used. With these parameters, a round hole approximately 0.8 mm in diameter is produced to the level of superficial subcutaneous tissue with zones of thermal damage that are approximately 50 µm wide. I prefer to use the Sharplan instead of the Ultrapulse laser for making round holes because the holes produced by the former are of more or less equal depth throughout the entire hole, whereas the Ultrapulse holes are more saucer shaped (Fig. 11–8).

New, more user-friendly or otherwise better lasers will inevitably be developed for laser transplantation. The most promising of these is the iridium:yttrium-aluminum-garnet (Ir:YAG) laser. It is claimed that its energy is absorbed by water 17 times better than that of a CO_2 laser, so theoretically it should produce substantially less thermal damage than either of the two lasers previously discussed. Unfortunately, despite extensive conversations with several manufacturers over the last 2 years, I have yet to receive a suitable unit to test.

Graft Insertion and Bandaging

Grafts are placed into the laser sites with their hair directed and angled in the same direction and angle as the original hair at that site. It is important that care be taken to ensure that no hair is accidentally trapped under a graft and that the grafts sit flush with the surrounding skin. Bacitracin ointment (Baciguent) is applied in both the recipient area and the donor area. The recipient area is then covered with Telfa, and an overnight pressure bandage is applied.[14] The next morning, the patient returns to have his bandage removed. Bleeding is usually minimal when a laser has been used, but any blood that is present can be gently washed away with hydrogen peroxide. The patient's hair is then carefully washed, blown dry, and styled.

Postoperative Course

Patients are advised to apply bacitracin ointment three times daily to both the recipient and donor areas for 1 week. This is important in that a small amount of superficial de-epithelialization occurs around each laser site, making the area more prone to secondary infection, which could affect hair yield. It is also helpful in decreasing the amount of postoperative crusting over the grafts, which can last up

Representative Example of Pattern Adjustments

Mode	Slit						Mode	Hole			
	16 spots/mm			22 spots/mm							
Pattern Number	1	2	3	4	5	6	Pattern Number	1	2	3	4
Graphic Representation							Graphic Representation				

The pattern push buttons control the shape of the incisions.

Representative Example of Size Adjustments

Mode	Slit			Mode	Hole		
Size Number	1	5	9	Size Number	1	5	9
Graphic Representation				Graphic Representation			
Approximate Slit Spacing (millimeters)	2.0	3.0	4.0	Approximate Hole Diameter (millimeters)	0.4	1.2	2.0

The size push buttons control the slit length or hole diameter.

Figure 11–4. Schematic depiction of the various patterns produced by the scanner attachment for the Ultrapulse laser. (Courtesy of Coherent Laser, Inc.)

Representative Example of Density Adjustments

Mode	Slit			Mode	Hole		
Density Number	1	5	9	Density Number	1	5	9
Graphic Representation				Graphic Representation			
Approximate Slit Spacing (millimeters)	3.0	2.5	2.2	Approximate Hole Diameter (millimeters)	4.0	3.0	2.0

In slit mode, the density push buttons are used to select horizontal spacing between slits.
In hole mode, the density push buttons are used to select horizontal and vertical spacing between spots. The density push buttons have no effect on single slit or single hole patterns (i.e., pattern family 1).

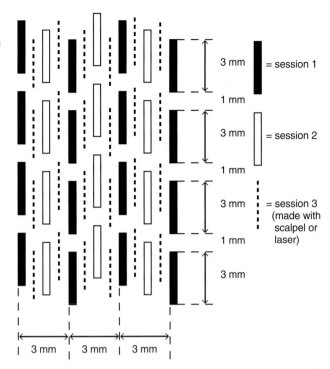

Figure 11–5. Schematic depiction of the pattern of slits recommended for laser transplantation of hair. The laser slits are produced with a 0.2-mm spot in focus and result in a wound that is about 0.5 mm wide. The distance between adjacent slits made in the same session is 3 mm, and slits are 1 mm anterior or posterior to their nearest neighbors. Angle and direction should mimic that of the original hair in the area. (Reprinted with permission from Unger W [ed]: Hair Transplantation, 3rd ed. New York: Marcel Dekker, 1995.)

to 14 days. Sutures are removed from donor sites in 7 to 10 days. When 75 or more grafts have been transplanted, hair regrowth usually occurs 2 to 6 weeks later at laser-prepared areas than is normally seen with conventional slit grafting. Use of a 3% minoxidil solution twice daily for the first 5 postoperative weeks is recommended to counterbalance the effect of sealing of blood vessels by the laser. Minoxidil can help to shorten the dormant period.

Patients are given acetaminophen with 16 mg codeine (Tylenol #3), oxycodone 2.5 mg with acetaminophen 325 mg (Percocet), and 50 mg meperidine hydrochloride (Demerol) to take as required for postoperative pain. Few patients use anything more than Tylenol #3 and usually only for the first 24 to 48 hours. Aside from a slightly increased tendency for development of postoperative infection as a result of laser-induced adjacent de-epithelialization, all complications that can occur with conventional transplantation can also occur with laser transplantation but are equally infrequent.[15]

Clinical Results

In the studies done to date, cosmetic results were superior on the laser-treated side in 285 of 357 patients in whom Ultrapulse laser slit grafts were used on one side of the recipient area and conventionally prepared slit grafts containing five or six hairs on the contralateral side. As in the earliest studies, the transplanted hair appeared as dense but was more evenly distributed and looked far more natural on the laser treated side (Figs. 11–9 and 11–10). Unfortunately, however, the cosmetic results have not been consistent. I continue to view laser transplantation as an incompletely developed technique. Sixty-nine of the study patients appeared no better on the laser side than on the conventionally prepared side, and three patients looked worse. Those three individuals were treated in the earliest studies when we were still experimenting with different laser energy, power, and time settings.

Other authors have reported that one- to three-hair grafts placed into round recipient sites created with CO_2 lasers have shown good hair survival.[5, 6] The advantages of using a laser for round holes include less bleeding, increased speed of preparation, less danger of epidermal cysts from tissue accidentally left in recipient sites, and potentially less postoperative pain and edema. However, superior *cosmetic*

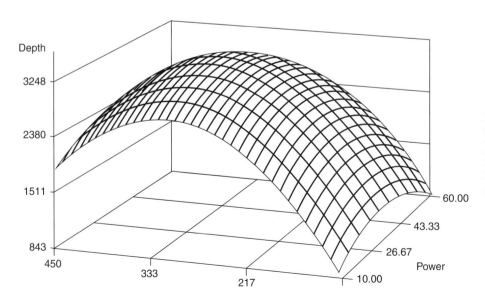

Figure 11–6. Schematic depiction of the findings from 500 patient biopsies using the Ultrapulse laser with scanner set at pattern 4 and various millijoule and watt parameters. The optimal settings appear to be 300 mJ and 40 to 60 W. (Courtesy of Coherent Laser, Inc.)

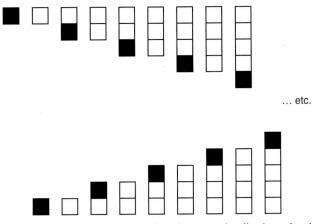

... etc.

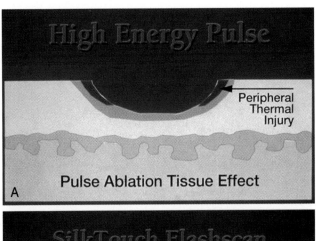

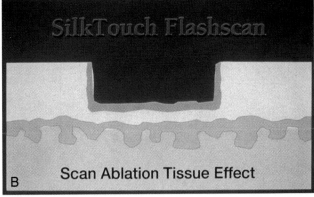

Figure 11–7. Using the Ultrapulse laser in pattern 4, a line is produced with the spot skipping from one end of the preselected line length to the other end, then back to just inside the first spot before returning to just inside the spot on the other end of the line, and so on, until the last pulse occurs at the midpoint of the line. The "random" ablation pattern results in longer intervals between adjacent spots than would a sequential pattern and therefore produces less thermal damage. (Reprinted with permission from Unger W [ed]: Hair Transplantation, 3rd ed. New York: Marcel Dekker, 1995.)

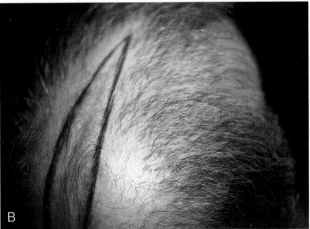

Figure 11–8. *A,* The Ultrapulse laser produces a saucer-shaped round defect. *B,* The Sharplan laser produces a round defect of equal depth throughout the entire hole. (Courtesy of Sharplan Laser, Inc.)

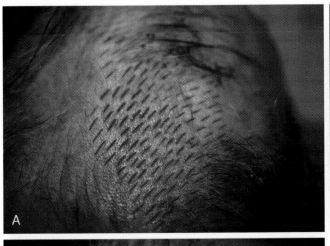

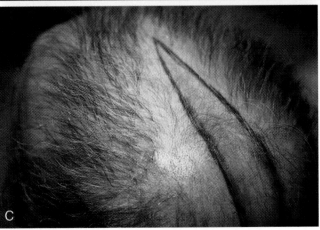

Figure 11–9. *A,* Intraoperative photograph showing 77 laser-produced sites on the right side and control scalpel slits on the left. *B,* Photograph taken 7.5 months after *A* reveals relatively dense, even, natural-looking hair growth on the laser-treated side. *C,* Photograph of the control scalpel-slit side, taken at the same time as *B,* shows a more stringy distribution of hair.

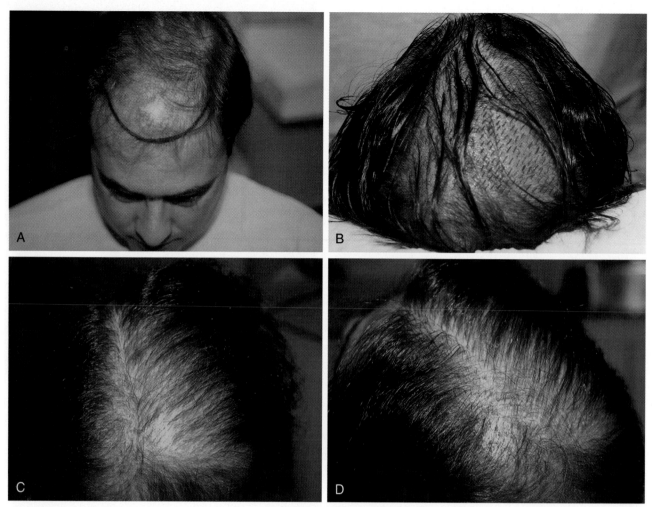

Figure 11–10. *A,* Before treatment. *B,* Intraoperative photo shows 110 laser-slit sites on the right side of the midline frontal area, and a similar number of scalpel-slit sites on the left side. Hair growth from two earlier conventional transplants can be seen more anteriorly. *C,* The same area as in *B* 9 months later. Hair distribution is denser and more even on the laser-treated side. The results in the zone treated with only a single session of hair transplanting looked so natural that the patient and his wife thought that it had never been treated until they were shown the "before" photographs. *D,* Another view from the left side of the study area shows greater hair density in the laser side as well as some mild "compression" on the scalpel-prepared side, which probably would not be noticeable without the laser-treated side being available for comparison.

results cannot be expected if the laser is used to make round holes, whereas this does occur in most of those treated with laser slits.

A New Photographic Computer-Assisted Study

A recent study used a specially designed photographic apparatus consisting of a Nikon N6006 camera with a Nikkor 60-mm micro lens held on a metal arm that swings in various positions but is always equidistant from the subject. With this unit, a constant light source is used, and the patient's chin is placed in a "cradle" while the forehead lies against a curved "arm." This apparatus produces high-quality photos of the head in four easily and accurately reproducible specific positions and views, all with a constant distance and light intensity. The results were analyzed by Canfield Scientific, Inc., using computers to count the numbers of hairs in grafts on laser-treated and conventionally treated contralateral sites. (A similar photographic

apparatus is being used in our continuing studies on finasteride for Merck Canada, Inc.) The study was carried out in four centers (California, New Jersey, Georgia, and Norway), and 45 patients who were initially bald or nearly bald were included in this protocol. Hair yield was no more than 2% less at laser sites and frequently was equal to the conventionally prepared control sites. However, laser sites seemed to heal faster and consistently produced hair with a more natural texture and distribution. Patients who were treated with the laser in one session and conventionally in the next also consistently preferred the results from the laser procedure because of greater postoperative comfort, absence of any complications, and appearance. Dr. Barry DiBernardo is at present writing a report for publication.[16]

Summary

It is easy to believe that laser transplantation is more a marketing tool than a true advance—certainly it is being used widely for this purpose. To view it simply as a marketing tool, however, ignores the advantages of nearly bloodless ablation of tissue and superior cosmetic results in most patients undergoing laser slit grafting. There is no doubt in my mind that laser hair transplantation will play an important role in the future of hair transplanting, but it is also *not yet* state of the art.

REFERENCES

1. Unger W: Surgical approach to hair loss. In Olsen E (ed): Diagnosis of Hair Growth, Diagnosis and Treatment. New York: McGraw-Hill, 1994;353–374.

2. Unger W, David L: Laser hair transplantation. J Dermatol Surg Oncol 1994;20:515–521.

3. Unger W: Laser hair transplantation II. Dermatol Surg 1995;21:759–765.

4. Unger W: Laser hair transplantation III. Computer-assisted laser transplanting. Dermatol Surg, 1995;21:1047–1055.

5. Villnow M, Slatkine M, Strobele B, et al.: Laser assisted hair transplanting. In Stough D, Haber R (eds): Hair Replacement, Surgical and Medical. St Louis: CV Mosby, 1995;365–370.

6. Avrom M: The Role of the Laser in Hair Transplantation. Presented at the Annual Meeting of the International Society of Hair Restoration Surgery, Nashville, September 21, 1996.

7. Unger WP, Knudsen R: General principles of recipient site organization and planning. In Unger W (ed): Hair Transplantation, 3rd ed. New York: Marcel Dekker, 1995;105–158.

8. Unger W: Anesthesia. In Unger W (ed): Hair Transplantation, 3rd ed. New York: Marcel Dekker, 1995;165–181.

9. Unger W: Delineating the "safe" donor area for hair transplanting. Am J Cosm Surg 1994;11:239–243.

10. Unger W: The donor site. In Unger W (ed): Hair Transplantation, 3rd ed. New York: Marcel Dekker, 1995;183–214.

11. Unger W: The recipient area. In Unger W (ed): Hair Transplantation, 3rd ed. New York: Marcel Dekker, 1995;215–322.

12. Unger W: Laser hair transplantation. In Alster TS, Apfelberg D (eds): Cosmetic Laser Surgery. New York: Wiley–Liss, 1996;55–66.

13. Unger W: Laser hair transplanting. J Am Acad Cosm Surg 1997; 14:143–148.

14. McKeown M: Preparation and insertion of grafts. In Unger W (ed): Hair Transplantation, 3rd ed. New York: Marcel Dekker, 1995;331–348.

15. Unger W: Complications of hair transplantation. In Unger W (ed): Hair Transplantation, 3rd ed. New York: Marcel Dekker, 1995;363–374.

16. DiBernardo B: Laser Assisted Hair Transplantation. Didactic Workshop, 6th Annual Meeting of The International Society of Hair Restoration Surgery, Washington D.C., September 18, 1998.

12

HAIR TRANSPLANTATION WITH CARBON DIOXIDE AND Er:YAG LASER DONOR INCISIONS

Nicholas J. Lowe
Gary P. Lask
Christopher Ho

The increasing popularity of hair transplantation has led many cosmetic surgeons to search for more innovative techniques to enhance their results. Advances in surgical hair replacement include approaches to minigrafting, micrografting, and slit grafting to improve aesthetic results (Figs. 12–1, 12–2). In 1992, Unger and colleagues first demonstrated the use of Ultrapulse carbon dioxide (CO_2) laser in hair transplantation. The Ultrapulse produces ultrashort, high-energy pulses that result in far less thermal damage to adjacent tissues than earlier types of CO_2 lasers. Laser was used to create recipient site slits, with preliminary results showing less bleeding, pain, and postoperative edema than with conventional hair transplantation. The ablation of tissue along the slit line results in a trough that eliminates the two major potential drawbacks of conventional slit grafting—compression and less hair density with comparable amounts of donor material. Laser-assisted slit grafting produced results that, in the opinion of Unger and associates, were cosmetically superior to those seen with conventional slit grafting.

The major potential drawback of laser-assisted hair transplant lies in the possible adjacent thermal damage. If the zone of damage is too wide, there may be impairment of the revascularization of the grafts with subsequent poor "take" of the grafts. In addition, thermal damage can destroy existing hair adjacent to the grafted areas, resulting in less hair density. The conventional continuous CO_2 laser produced too much thermal damage, which made it impractical for delicate procedures such as hair transplantation. With the advent of pulsed laser systems, thermal damage could be minimized with optimal laser setting. Multicenter experiences and histologic studies of the laser-assisted slit sites show adjacent thermal damage ranging from 80 to 150 μm. Within this range, there is minimal damage to the adjacent hair follicles, allowing laser hair transplantation to be safe and effective.

Earlier studies by Ho and associates included the use of slit handpiece using the Ultrapulsed CO_2 laser. Figure 12–3 shows this laser, and the slit handpiece is shown in Figure 12–4). Before this handpiece was developed, slits were created freehand, which required experience and finesse. In addition, slits created freehand were often inconsistent and difficult to reproduce. The slit handpiece consistently created 2×0.2-mm slits to allow easy placement of hair minigrafts. The operative time with two surgeons was about 2.5 to 3 hours for 200- to 400-minigraft procedures. Intraoperatively, there was minimal bleeding and charring. The grafts fit into the laser-created slits with minimal compression. Postoperatively, in a small series of patients, there was less pain and swelling than with conventional hair transplants. Short-term follow-up visits showed that over 98% of grafts took and revealed crusting, which lasted up to 2 weeks. Long-term follow-up of 4 to 6 months demonstrated good regrowth of hair at the laser sites.

To further reduce possible thermal damage and consistently create slit recipient sites with ease and speed, developers of the Ultrapulse laser created a scanning device similar to the computer pattern generator used for skin resurfacing. The scanner further decreased thermal damage by controlling the duration of each pulse at the site of recipient slits. It can also be programmed so that multiple slits are created with each pass, resulting in decreased operative time. This is truly an added benefit.

Sharplan has also introduced laser hair transplantation using the SilkTouch flashscanner. Unlike the pulsed CO_2 laser, the SilkTouch uses an optomechanical scanner that allows the laser beam to dwell at a particular point less than the thermal relaxation time of the skin with high peak powers. Because the SilkTouch uses software technology, it allows the surgeon to select either a slit or a hole for the recipient sites in addition to offering a variation of recipient sizes. Studies we have done using the SilkTouch laser with the slit recipient mode showed thermal damage to be limited to 80 μm at the base of the recipient sites when the parameter was set at 80 W and 0.1-second

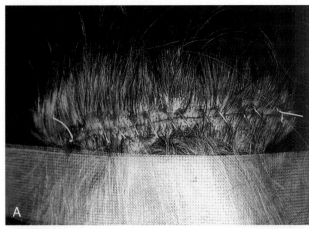

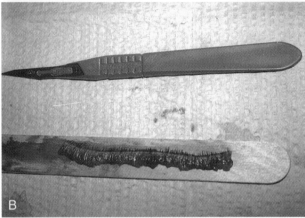

Figure 12–1. *A,* Donor site scar after excision of strip using parallel scalpel blades. *B,* A 3-mm wide strip of donor tissue from the above patient, harvested from the posterior scalp.

dwelling time. The pulsed CO_2 laser and the flashscanner appear to produce a similar amount of thermal damage, and both are suitable for laser hair transplantation.

CO_2 laser hair transplantation offers some advantages over the conventional slit grafting with the scalpel. First, there is minimal bleeding so the hair transplant surgeon is permitted a near-bloodless surgical field. Cutaneous vessels on the scalp are partially sealed as incisions are made with the laser. Thus, the surgeon can easily visualize the recipient sites and spend less time handling the hair grafts. The overall operative time is reduced by at least one third as compared with the conventional scalpel technique. The scanner device further decreases the operative time, especially in long sessions in which more than 1000 slit grafts are placed. This benefits both the surgeon and the patient since it reduces the risks for contamination and infection and reduces patient discomfort. Patients who had previous scalpel hair transplantation prefer the laser procedure because of less postoperative pain and swelling.

Second, laser hair transplantation using the slit handpiece or the scanner device enables the surgeon to produce uniform slits consistently for slit grafts. Previously, laser hair transplantations were done freehand, a procedure that requires greater skill and a great deal of experience by the surgeon. Unlike conventional scalpel slit grafting, in which the scalp is stabbed to create slits, the laser vaporizes and removes excess tissue to create slit spaces. Grafts planted into the laser-treated slits are inserted more easily, and there is virtually no graft compression. In addition, graft handling is minimized, and there is no need for dilators. Theoreti-

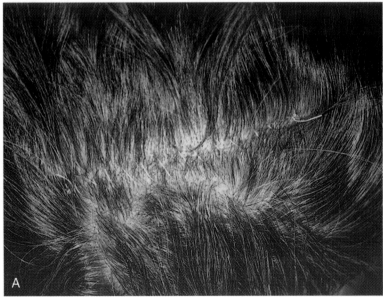

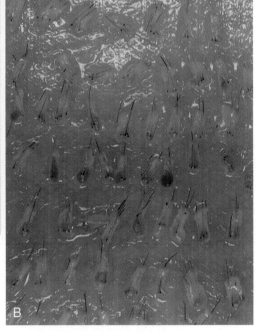

Figure 12–2. *A,* A posterior scalp donor site from the patient in Figure 12–1, healed 1 week before suture removal. *B,* Two- and three-hair minigrafts.

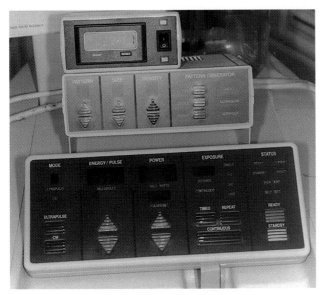

Figure 12–3. Coherent Ultrapulse CO_2 laser with additional control unit for hair transplant system on top.

cally, grafts should survive better with less compression, and the aesthetic result should be more acceptable. There is less cobblestoning or punctate scarring due to graft compression, and since some alopecic skin is removed, hair density is increased.

Finally, because the pulsed laser system delivers high-intensity energy in ultrashort pulses and the flashscanner produces a high peak power with a short dwell time, there is minimal adjacent tissue damage. An optimal laser setting allows superior hair transplantation. Any setting too low produces more bleeding and more superficial slits; any setting too high produces excessive charring and scarring.

Computer-Controlled Incision for Ultrapulsed Laser Hair Transplantation

Because of the initial success with the slit handpiece using the Ultrapulse laser, Coherent Medical developed a computer-controlled handpiece that modifies the Ultrapulse CO_2 laser to make circular or slit scalp incisions to receive hair micrografts. The advantages of computer-controlled delivery with the Ultrapulsed CO_2 laser include the following:

1. Consistent depth of slits or holes.
2. Consistent width of slits or holes.
3. Minimized bleeding.
4. Consistently minimal lateral thermal damage.
5. With bald or relatively bald scalps, multiple laser

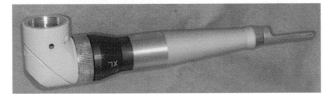

Figure 12–4. Ultrapulse CO_2 laser slit handpiece.

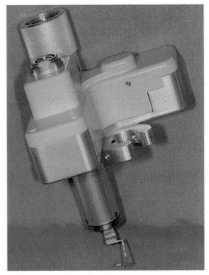

Figure 12–5. Computer pattern generator (CPG) handpiece.

incisions can be made rapidly and at predetermined patterns.

Laser settings with this device usually are energy 250 mJ, power 40 to 60 W, and pattern 4. This device is shown in Figure 12–5. The laser incision is shown in Figure 12–6. Minimal lateral thermal injury is seen in Figure 12–7. Examples of patients before and after Ultrapulsed CO_2 laser–assisted hair transplantation are shown in Figures 12–8 to 12–10.

CO_2 laser hair transplantation is not without disadvantages. Beside the high cost of the laser, there are safety and fire hazard requirements. In addition, there is prolonged crusting in the grafts probably because of some deepithelization at the slit edges. There was some delay in hair growth, but long-term follow-up showed good hair regrowth. Laser hair transplantation has many potential and promising results. Further studies and experiences will provide additional data in the use of laser for hair transplantation.

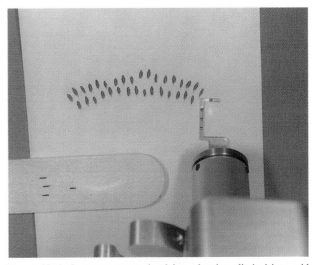

Figure 12–6. Computer pattern handpiece showing slit incisions with ultrapulsed CO_2 laser.

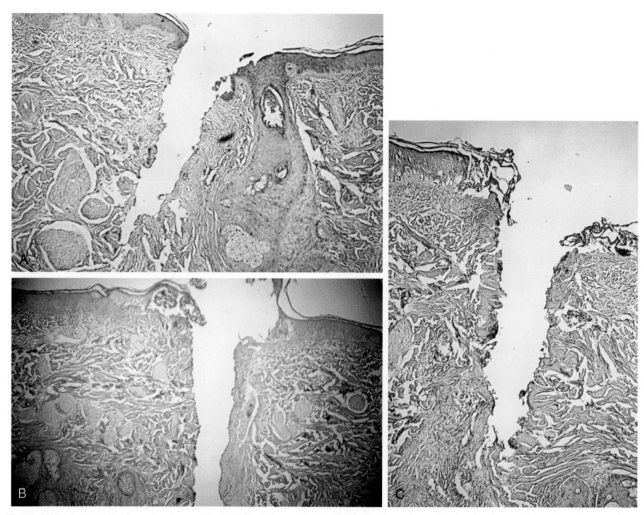

Figure 12–7. *A,* Blade incision using Swann-Mortin SP91 blade set at 5-mm depth. *B,* Photomicrograph showing laser incision with minimal adjacent tissue thermal injury (hematoxylin & eosin, ×16). Slit handpiece. Laser energy 350 mJ, 12 W, 0.8-second duration. *C,* Computer pattern generator Ultrapulse CO_2 Coherent laser; setting 4, size 4. Laser energy 300 mJ, 60 W. The site shows minimal lateral thermal injury, including epidermal (mini) resurfacing adjacent to the laser incision.

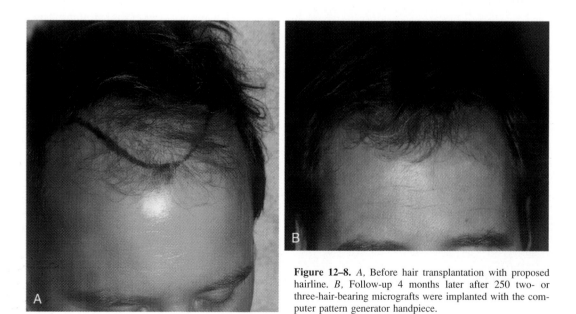

Figure 12–8. *A,* Before hair transplantation with proposed hairline. *B,* Follow-up 4 months later after 250 two- or three-hair-bearing micrografts were implanted with the computer pattern generator handpiece.

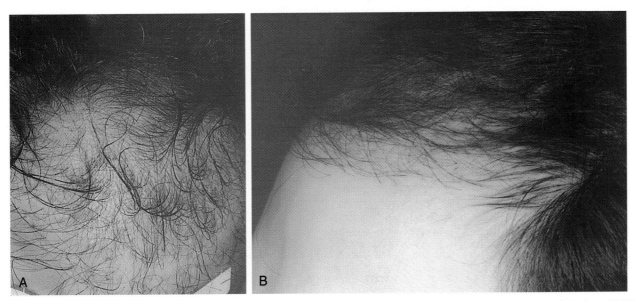

Figure 12–9. *A,* Patient before hair transplantation. *B,* After two sessions (first session 300 micrographs, second session 200 micrographs) using a UPCO$_2$ laser with slit handpiece set at 350 mJ, 13 W, 0.9-second duration.

Observations of Scalp Reduction Using Ultrapulse Carbon Dioxide Laser Incision

During the course of a bilateral comparison study of laser-incised versus Swann-Mortin SP91 blade cold steel incisions, one of us (NJL) observed that the laser-incised scalp areas were significantly reduced compared with the blade incised scalp. These results are shown in Figures 12–11 and 12–12. These observations are being explored and may be another reason to consider laser-assisted hair transplantation.

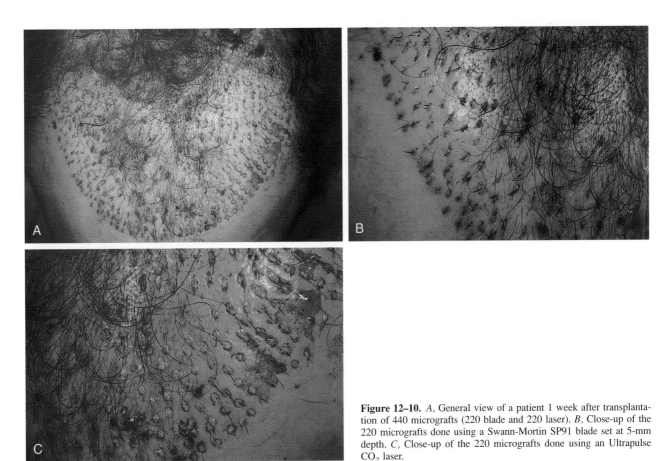

Figure 12–10. *A,* General view of a patient 1 week after transplantation of 440 micrografts (220 blade and 220 laser). *B,* Close-up of the 220 micrografts done using a Swann-Mortin SP91 blade set at 5-mm depth. *C,* Close-up of the 220 micrografts done using an Ultrapulse CO$_2$ laser.

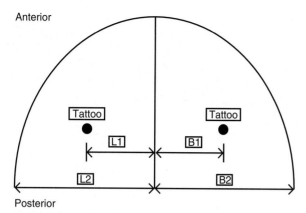

Figure 12–11. Diagram of study examining influence of laser incision on scalp dimensions. L1 and L2 refer to distances measured before and after laser donor hair transplant incisions. B1 and B2 refer to distances measured before and after blade donor hair transplant incisions. L1 and B1: from midscalp to tattoo; L2 and B2: from midscalp to lateral side of transplanted area.

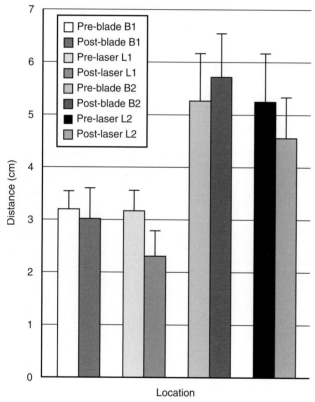

Figure 12–12. Histogram demonstrating reduction of scalp after laser micrograph incisions.

Er:YAG Laser Assisted Hair Transplantation

Recent observations suggest that Er:YAG lasers may be used to make donor scalp incisions for hair transplantation. There is less lateral thermal injury seen with Er:YAG incisions; however, because there is less coagulation, bleeding remains a problem. Methods to reduce bleeding with the Er:YAG laser include using a combined Er:YAG plus CO_2 laser (Derma-K™, Sharplan-ESC systems). These and other laser systems may have a role for hair transplantation.

BIBLIOGRAPHY

Bisaccia E, Scarborough D: Hair transplant by incisional strip harvesting. J Dermatol Surg Oncol 1994;20:443–448.

Fitzpatrick RE: Laser hair transplantation. Tissue effects of laser parameters. J Dermatol Surg Oncol 1995;21:1042–1046.

Ho C, Nguyen Q, Lask G, Lowe NJ: Mini-slit graft hair transplantation using the Ultrapulse carbon dioxide laser handpiece. J Dermatol Surg Oncol 1995;21:1056–1059.

Hugeneck J, Kokott R, Wagner KH, et al.: Nontufted incisional slit grafting. J Dermatol Surg Oncol 1994;20:718–723.

Rassman WR, Carson S: Micrografting in extensive quantities: The ideal hair restoration procedure. J Dermatol Surg Oncol 1995;21:306–311.

Unger WP: Laser hair transplantation III. J Dermatol Surg Oncol 1995;21:1047–1055.

Unger WP, David LM: Laser hair transplantation. J Dermatol Surg Oncol 1994;20:515–521.

13

ENDOSCOPIC LASER SURGERY OF THE AGING FACE

Robert W. Hutcherson
Gregory S. Keller
Julene E. Cray

Advances in carbon dioxide (CO_2) laser technology have resulted in the production of a high-energy laser beam that cuts with negligible char and excellent coagulation. These lasers produce invisible light of 10,600 nm (far infrared) and are strongly absorbed by water in all tissues. Because of this property, they have shallow penetration through tissue when compared with other laser systems and allow surgical precision. The additional development of a fiber delivery system has facilitated the applicability of the CO_2 laser to endoscopic procedures.

The high-output pulsed fiber CO_2 laser produces high-energy pulse pairs of up to 400 mJ. No component of the pulse pair is delivered for longer than 600 msec, which is approximately the thermal relaxation time of skin. The resultant effects on tissue of this high-energy pulse are char-free cutting and vaporization using spot sizes of less than 1 mm and tissue dehydration with spot sizes above 2 mm. The significant degree of localized energy produces coagulation of most blood vessels encountered in this type of surgery, allowing undermining of flaps and bloodless incision of muscles.

The endoscopic procedures discussed in this chapter require a laser, special instrumentation, an endoscope, a television monitor, and a video camera. Several satisfactory systems of this type are available, but we prefer endoscopic equipment manufactured by Karl Storz because of the quality of their optics.

Endolaser Procedures

Endoscopic procedures are designed to use smaller incisions and less dissection than conventional procedures to modify anatomic areas of concern. We have used the endoscopic approach for virtually all areas of facial rejuvenation surgery but have found that the most consistently useful endolaser techniques are oriented toward the forehead, midface, and anterior neck.

Forehead

Endoscopic forehead-lift techniques are the most popular of endoscopic facial plastic surgery procedures. The accessible dissection planes and brow musculature are ideally suited for endoscopic modification. Although a myriad of techniques have been developed to endoscopically alter the forehead, they have in common the intent to elevate the brow, reduce horizontal forehead rhytides and vertical glabellar lines, elevate lateral canthal hooding, and improve infrabrow overhand produced by sagging of the forehead tissues (Fig. 13–1). In most forehead procedures, myotomy of the brow depressor muscles with subsequent backward elevation of the forehead and brow accomplishes surgical goals. By sufficiently weakening the depressor musculature, the elevator muscles of the forehead work with less opposition and elevate the brow without posterior fixation of the scalp.

The use of a series of small incisions allows access to the forehead and brow for the endoscope and laser. The small incisions minimize soft tissue trauma and result in significantly less damage to sensory nerves while diminishing hair loss associated with large incisions that resect hair-bearing scalp. Although there are many variations in the placement of these small incisions, we prefer four vertical incisions (two central and two lateral frontal) in the frontal area and a diagonally placed incision in each temporal area (Fig. 13–2).

The two central incisions are vertically placed behind the frontal hairline in the plane of the medial brow. They are approximately 1 cm in length. The lateral frontal fixation incisions are similarly placed behind the hairline and are oriented in line with the lateral canthus or the lateral limbus. The former orientation allows maximal upward pull on the tail of the brow. The lateral limbus incision exerts a more powerful pull on the medial brow and is useful in ameliorating the "fallen in" look of the glabellar area.

The temple incisions are approximately 2 cm long and diagonal in orientation. The inferior extent of the incision is

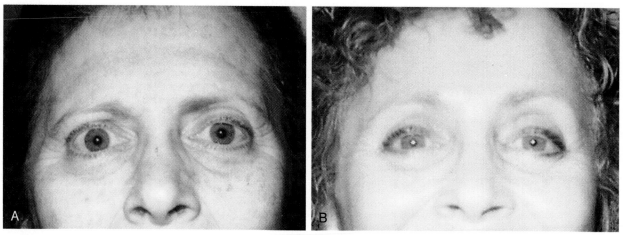

Figure 13–1. *A,* Frontal view of patient before endoscopic forehead lift. *B,* Postoperative view.

at the level of the superior orbital rim, allowing for additional outward and upward movement of the tail of the brow. This is important because the frontal musculature does not suspend the brow tail as effectively.

In male pattern baldness, modification of the incisions is necessary, with 1 cm vertical incisions usually being placed along the fringe. A single 1-cm incision can also be placed in the midline if a frontal tuft is present or is going to be created with hair transplantation. If the frontal tuft is missing, the frontal area can also be approached through a blepharoplasty incision.

Once the incisions are made, an optical cavity must be created over the frontal bone to allow the work on the musculature to be accomplished. This cavity can be formed in a subcutaneous, subgaleal, or subperiosteal plane. Typically, a combination of these planes is used. The subperiosteal plane is easier to dissect, and because of the thickness and resultant stiffness of the overlying tissue, a fairly reliable degree of brow elevation is attainable. One centimeter of brow elevation is often achieved for every 1.2 cm

of backward pull on the subperiosteal flap. The targeted musculature of the forehead lies in the subgaleal plane, however, and a transition to this plane must be made to allow appropriate exposure. This transition is usually created at the level of the brow by means of a horizontal cut through the periosteum in the midline. Subsequent supraperiosteal dissection allows visualization of the procerus, depressor supercilii, corrugator, and orbicularis muscles.

Transition to the supraperiosteal plane is also necessary over the lateral aspect of the orbital rim in the region of the zygomatic process of the frontal bone. Dissection in this plane allows the surgeon to complete exposure over the malar eminence if desired.

In the temporal region, an optical cavity is formed through the diagonally placed 2-cm temporal incisions. Dissection is easily carried out in a plane overlying the superficial layer of deep temporal fascia. This cavity is joined to the resultant cavity from the frontal dissection at the level of the brow through the temporal line.

Once the optical cavity has been created, the release of

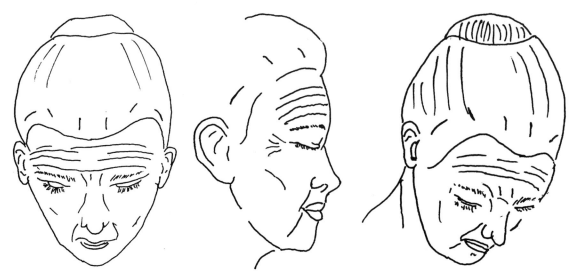

Figure 13–2. Incisions for endoscopic forehead and midface lifting.

the brows' attachments to the orbit can be performed. Some surgeons believe that selective denervation of the depressor musculature is adequate to allow brow elevation. However, our results have been better using myotomies of these muscles near their bony attachments. Depending on the configuration of the brow ptosis, the release can be generalized or selective. Medial to the supraorbital nerve, the brow is held downward by the periosteum and the procerus, depressor supercilii, orbicularis oculi, and corrugator muscles. The collective depressor function of these muscles can be inactivated by the myotomies. In the mid-frontal portion of the brow, between the supraorbital nerve and the lateral orbital rim, the periosteum below the orbital rim and the orbicularis oculi are potentially subject to release. In the lateral temporal region, the conjoint tendon region at the level of the brow can be released, along with the orbital rim periosteum and the soft tissue overlying the malar eminence.

After the described steps have been completed, the unopposed elevator function of the frontal–galeal–occipitalis sling allows the scalp and periosteum to shift posteriorly, resulting in brow elevation. The amount of brow elevation desired is predetermined according to the presurgical brow anatomy. It is usually 0.75 to 1.75 cm. At the anterior aspect of the frontal incisions, a mark is made with the laser before the periosteum is elevated. Subsequent to release of the brow musculature, another marking is made posterior to the first, corresponding to the desired distance of brow elevation, adding 0.2 cm to compensate for subsequent relaxation. A self-tapping screw is then placed at this point, and the posterior portion of the incision is pulled backward until the screw sits at the anterior edge of the incision. A surgical staple is placed immediately behind the screw, fixing the scalp and brow upward. Fixation can also be performed using plates, sutures, and soft tissue rolls. In the temporal area, fixation is accomplished with sutures. The temporoparietal fascia is grasped in the anterior portion of the temporal incision and sutured posteriorly to the deep temporal fascia. This stabilizes the elevation of the brow tail.

TECHNIQUE

After the central and lateral incisions are made, blind dissection using a slightly curved elevator is performed to create the frontal subperiosteal pocket. The elevation is in a counterclockwise direction and is done through each frontal incision. Once a pocket is formed, the endoscope can be placed and the dissection continued with the laser. Usually, the endoscope is placed in the port to the left of the laser for a right-handed surgeon, beginning with the laser in the right lateral incision and the endoscope in the right central incision. The flap is developed bloodlessly using 8 to 15 W of power and 250- to 300-mJ pulses. At this level, spread of energy to the overlying skin is minimized. In areas where increased speed of dissection is desired, the laser is used at 20 W. In areas where the dissection must proceed more

carefully (i.e., close to nerves or with especially thin skin), the laser is turned down to 8 to 10 W. In the glabella, the supraperiosteal plane is entered and developed approximately 2 cm above the brow. This plane can be followed downward over the dorsum of the nose. The supratrochlear and supraorbital nerves and vessels are identified and preserved. Frequently, multiple branches of these nerves emerge from the supraorbital notch or the accessory foramen above the notch. Laterally, the subperiosteal dissection is carried to the level of the brow and extended to the superior aspect of the zygomatic process of the frontal bone. Visualization is achieved by changing the respective ports for the endoscope and laser, and the right and left frontal dissection is completed.

The procerus muscle is a relatively thin, vertically oriented muscle located between the corrugator muscle insertions. The endoscope is placed through the left central incision, and the CO_2 laser is placed in the right central incision. The muscle is incised with 250 mJ of energy at the level of the nasofrontal suture.

The corrugator muscle is easily visualized in the supraperiosteal dissection pocket over the glabella. Its fibers run horizontally, and it occasionally has a bluish hue when severely hypertrophic. Medially, this muscle is vertically incised with the laser between the supraorbital nerve and branches of the supratrochlear nerve. Laterally, this muscle is often tightly adherent to the bony rim. This attachment is mobilized with the laser as close to its insertion as possible.

The depressor supercilii muscle is fan shaped and is located medial to the insertion of the corrugator. The multiple branches of the supratrochlear nerve are usually interspersed within this muscle. The muscle may be thin or hypertrophic, in which case it too can appear bluish. The muscle is incised with the laser with care to avoid damaging the supratrochlear nerve.

Deep to the depressor supercilii and corrugator muscles is the orbicularis muscle, which adheres to the skin. It is vertically incised medial to the supraorbital nerve. Lateral to the nerve and extending as far as the malar eminence, myotomies can also be performed with the laser circumferentially around the orbital rim.

The area of the confluence of the corrugator and procerus muscles with the frontalis may appear full and demarcated. This supraorbital "wad" of muscle can be cross-hatched or vaporized with the laser. This step is particularly important if prominent glabellar creases are present.

For the temple dissection, both the endoscope and laser are placed in the right temporal incision. The loose areolar tissue (innominate fascia) between the temporoparietal fascia and the superficial layer of the deep temporal fascia is easily identified and forms the dissection plane for this part of the procedure. The innominate fascial plane allows the surgeon to stay clear of the frontal zygomatic branch of the facial nerve, which travels in the lower portions of the temporoparietal fascia. The temporoparietal fat pad is seen above the dissection plane and should be swept upward. Superior to the zygomatic arch, the zygomatic fat pad can be visualized. It is perforated by several veins in its superior portion, the most medial of which is often accompanied by a sensory nerve (zygomaticotemporal). This "sentinel" vein is cauterized by the laser. The vein immediately lateral to this is in the vicinity of the facial nerve where it crosses the zygoma, and precision must be used if this vein is cauterized. The dissection does not proceed inferiorly farther than where fascial layers fuse above the zygoma. Here the dissection is brought medially and inferiorly over the malar eminence if desired.

Communication between the temporal and frontal optical cavities is established with the laser by developing the innominate fascial plane superiorly and medially. When the temporal line is encountered, it is incised and the periosteum is elevated over the frontal bone until the connection is completed. The same procedure is then completed in the left temporal optical cavity.

Neck

The endoscopic laser approach to the neck is particularly useful in a younger patient who has neck ptosis and minimal skin laxity or in an older patient with lax skin who desires correction only of the midline wattle (Fig. 13–3). The small incisions with minimal edema and ecchymosis typically allow a relatively quick recovery and little morbidity, with complications being no more severe than those encountered with liposuction.

TECHNIQUE

Three incisions are usually required, including a 1- to 2-cm submental crease incision and two postauricular sulcus incisions of varying length, depending on skin laxity. If the laser is used to make the skin incisions, a 0.1-mm spot handpiece is used, with the laser set to 250 to 300 mJ at 8 to 10 W. Normally, these incisions are bloodless. The submental skin flap is elevated first, with the laser set to 300 mJ at 15 to 20 W. This skin flap is elevated easily and rapidly if the surgeon is in the correct plane. As the surgeon pulls upward on the skin flap, an assistant applies forward traction ahead of the dissection, delineating the proper dissection plane. Some fat is left attached to the skin to prevent subsequent midline puckering. If liposuction is to be performed, the surgeon can do so after tumescent injection of Klein's solution without using the laser for flap elevation.

Flap elevation is performed in the soft tissue plane lateral to the platysma, using all surgical incisions for access. Laser energy is reduced for undermining over the sternocleidomastoid–platysmal junction because of the thinness of skin. The undermining extends across the midline, with its vertical extent determined based on the pathology present.

If platysmal banding is present and an anterior platysmaplasty is necessary, a conservative vertical strip of platysma is excised with the laser to the level of the hyoid. Only a limited amount of subplatysmal fat should be removed with the laser. When platysma bands are severe, limited horizontal incisions or triangular excisions of

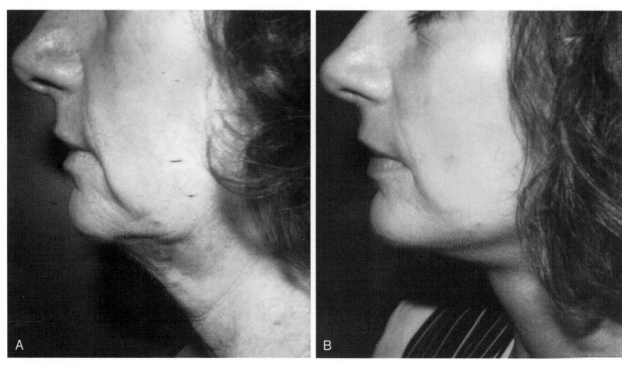

Figure 13–3. *A,* Patient before endoscopic neck lift. *B,* Postoperative view.

muscle are also undertaken. Suturing for the platysmaplasty varies, but we prefer suspension style sutures advocated by Giampapa (Fig. 13–4). These are easily passed under the skin flap and sutured to the mastoid fascia. If the platysmal bands are particularly severe, additional excision or midline suturing can be executed.

The postauricular sulcus incision can be extended if some neck skin is to be resected or if additional exposure is needed for platysma plication. If the laser is used to dissect in the plane of the superficial postauricular fascia, fat should be left on the elevated skin flap, and the fascial covering over the sternocleidomastoid muscle should be preserved. Over the muscle, the laser should be turned down to 8 to 10 W.

Cheek and Midface

The CO_2 laser has been used for some time for dissection in the standard facelift. Advocates of its use indicate that swelling and ecchymosis in the immediate postoperative period are markedly reduced. When the approach to facelift surgery becomes endoscopic, however, the cheek and midface are more of problem than the forehead and neck regions, with a significant limitation on results being related to dealing successfully with excess skin laxity. For this reason, the ideal patient for this procedure is one who is young and who has thick skin, prominent cheekbones, and an early structural laxity of the midface (Fig. 13–5).

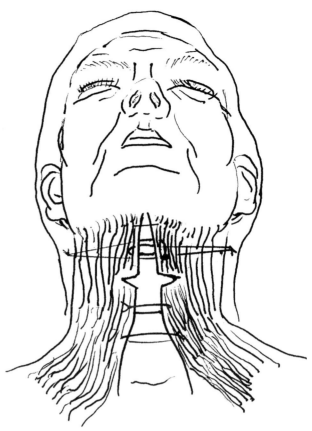

Figure 13–4. Suspension platysmaplasty using interlocking vertical horizontal mattress sutures placed through minimal submental and postauricular sulcus incisions.

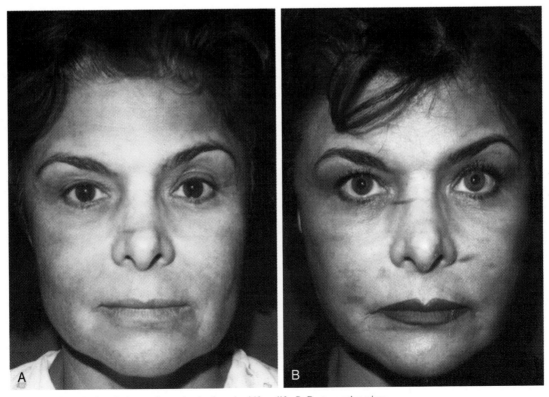

Figure 13–5. *A*, Patient before endoscopic cheek and midface lift. *B*, Postoperative view.

TECHNIQUE

Although there are several procedures described as "endoscopic facelifts" that can be combined with laser techniques, the one we favor is performed by means of a tragal edge incision. The incision can be made with the laser using a 0.1-mm spot size, 250 mJ of energy per laser burst, and a delivery rate of 8 to 10 W. The incision is extended upward anterior to the sideburn or splits the sideburn vertically. A flap is developed in the superficial fascia above the superficial temporal artery, with fat preserved on the flap. Superiorly, the dissection extends over the orbicularis oculi to the lateral margin of the orbit. Inferiorly, the dissection remains in a superficial plane and extends 2.5 to 3 cm preauricularly. The laser is set at 250- to 300-mJ bursts with a delivery rate of 10 to 25 W. Dissection over the malar eminence is continued with a laser delivery rate of 8 to 10 W. Although we used to dissect over the cheek in the sub-SMAS or subplatysmal plane, we have used a suprafibromuscular technique for more than 2 years (Fig. 13–6). This technique allows a more superficial dissection over the soft tissue of the cheek and does not expose the peripheral branches of the facial nerve. The dissection can be extended as far medially as the nasolabial fold and as far inferiorly as the superior margin of the mandible. Because a relatively thin flap is created with medial extension of the dissection, the laser delivery must be kept low. Blunt dissection is used if required. A thin layer of fat is left over the zygomaticus muscles laterally.

Suspension sutures are used as indicated to ameliorate a prominent nasolabial fold, drooping corner of the mouth, or ptotic submalar area. A 3-0 Gore-Tex suspension suture is placed in the overlying fat and fascia of the malar eminence and is then suspended to the suprafibromuscular layer of the cheek (Fig. 13–7). The fascia overlying the buccal fat is then stitched upward to the remaining layer of fat and fascia overlying the malar eminence. These sutures can also be anchored more posteriorly into the deep temporalis fascia just above the ear. If desired, the buccal fat can be dissected

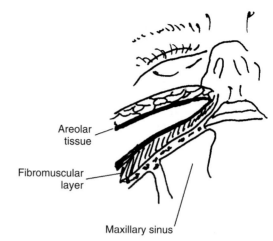

Figure 13–7. The malar fat pad is dissected with overlying skin in the areolar tissue plane overlying the fibromuscular layer. The fibromuscular layer is subsequently sutured upward to the periosteum of the malar bone or is suspended to the superficial layer of the deep temporalis fascia.

free and sutured over the zygoma in the form of a malar implant to augment the zygomatic arch. Additionally, a flap of SMAS and orbicularis muscle can be dissected superiorly and suspended by 3-0 Gore-Tex suture to the fascia at the most anterior point of hair-bearing skin, helping to stabilize the superior portion of the lift.

Summary

Aesthetic surgical procedures are continually being amended and modified in an endeavor to reduce postoperative morbidity and expedite recovery time. The endoscopic approach to facial rejuvenation surgery has been well received because of its contribution toward accomplishing these goals. With particular reference to the forehead, neck, and midface, the endoscope is allowing surgeons to achieve aesthetic results comparable or superior to more conventional procedures. When used in conjunction with the high-output CO_2 laser, we believe that these endoscopic techniques are even more useful in reducing ecchymosis and edema and enhancing the results.

BIBLIOGRAPHY

Ramirez OM: Endoscopic full facelift. Aesthet Plast Surg 1974;18: 363–371.

Hutcherson RW, Keller GS: Endoscopic facial plastic surgery: An overview. Facial Plast Surg Clin North Am 1996;4:247–256.

Giampapa VC: Suture suspension platysmaplasty. Presented at the American Academy of Aesthetic and Restorative Surgery, Philadelphia, May 14, 1993.

Aiache AE: Endoscopic facelift. Aesthet Plast Surg 1994;118:275–278.

Keller GS, Cray J: Laser-assisted surgery of the aging face. Facial Plast Surg Clin North Am 1995;3:319–341.

Keller GS, Cray J: Suprafibromuscular facelift with periosteal suspension of the superficial musculoaponeurotic system and fatpad of Bichat rotation. Arch Otolaryngol Head Neck Surg 1996;122:377–384.

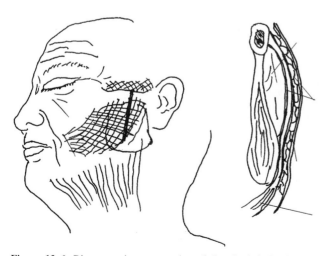

Figure 13–6. Diagrammatic cross section of the cheek indicating the fibromuscular layer used in the suprafibromuscular facelift.

14

FACIAL ACNE SCARS

Nicholas J. Lowe
Gary P. Lask
Philippa Lowe
Vladislav Chizhevsky

Preliminary observations by the authors had suggested that laser resurfacing used together with scar subcision and fat transfer were useful for acne scar improvement.[1-4] It was thought logical to combine these procedures with postacne distensable scars and laser resurfacing to tighten and make the skin surface smoother. Methods of treating acne scarring have included dermabrasion, dermal grafting, dermal grafting plus laser resurfacing, and laser resurfacing alone.

The ultrapulsed carbon dioxide ($UPCO_2$) laser produces high-energy pulses of very short duration, allowing for controlled char-free tissue ablation.[5-8] The use of this machine has been recently modified with the use of a computer pattern generator (CPG).[9-11] This affords significantly more uniform treatment of large areas of skin.

We describe a technique of surgical scar subcision, fat transfer, and laser resurfacing for distensible facial scars.

Methods

Six to twelve weeks before surgery all patients are usually started on tretinoin, 0.05%, hydroquinone, 5%, and desonide, 0.1% cream nightly. They are instructed to apply a broad-spectrum sunscreen each morning. Local anesthesia or conscious sedation anesthesia may be used depending on patient preferences and areas of skin to be treated.

Scar Subcision

The saucer-shaped acne scars and facial lines are defined with gentian violet marking pen (Figs. 14–1, 14–2[9]). The scar subcision is performed with a 16-gauge Nokor needle, which is introduced lateral to the scarred area and passed many times tangentially under the scarred area, cutting fibrous bands, until elevation of the scar is observed. To achieve hemostasis pressure is then applied for 5 to 10 minutes.

Laser Resurfacing

A variety of CO_2 lasers may be used. With the Ultrapulse CO_2 laser, the CPG pattern used for the initial passes around the acne scars can be pattern 7, an annular pattern to outline the acne scars (Fig. 10–3). With smaller scars, pattern 3 size 2 is used to surround the scarred area with the initial passes. Initial power settings are 300 mJ and 60 W (Table 14–1). The skin is then wiped with saline-soaked gauze and subsequent passes are delivered using pattern 3 or 5 with density between 3 and 5 (see Fig. 14–3). The number of subsequent passes is one to three, depending on the depth of the acne scarring.

Results

Thirty-nine patients with post-acne scarring of varying degrees of severity ages 22–45 were treated with the Coherent Ultrapulse 5000C CO_2 laser (Palo Alto, CA) coupled to a CPG handpiece.[12]

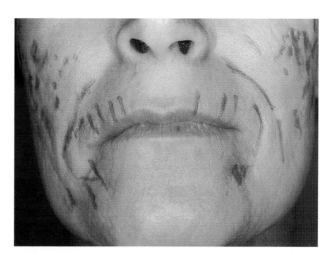

Figure 14–1. Gentian violet marking of scars and lines before scar subcision and laser resurfacing.

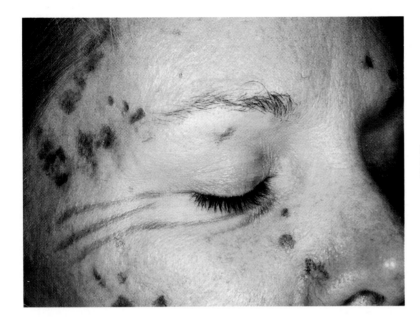

Figure 14–2. Marking of deeper acne scars immediately after scar subcision using 16-gauge Nokor needle followed by Ultrapulse CO_2 laser resurfacing.

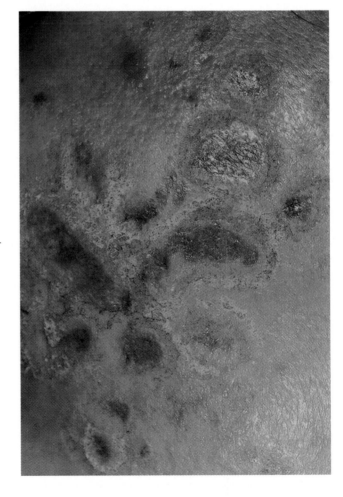

Figure 14–3. The peripheral rim immediately after scar subcision followed by $UPCO_2$ laser with scan pattern of 7.7.

Table 14–1. Laser Settings for Resurfacing

	1ST PASS		REPEAT PASSES		
	Laser Energy Settings	CPG Density	Laser Energy Settings	CPG Density	Number of Passes
Cheeks	300 mJ 60 W	4–6	250 mJ 60 W	4–6	1–3
Perioral	300 mJ 60 W	5–6	250 mJ 60 W	5–6	2–4
Acne scars					
Cheeks Forehead	300 mJ 60 W	6–7	250 mJ 60 W	6–7	2–4
Eyelids	250 mJ 60 W	4–5	250 mJ 60 W	4	1 No wiping
Neck	250 mJ 60 W	2–3	0	0	1 No wiping

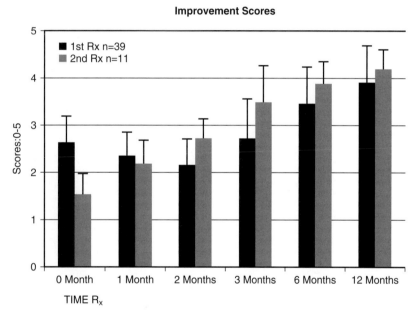

Figure 14–4. Histogram shows improvement scores for 39 patients treated with scar subcision followed by treatment with UPCO$_2$ laser.

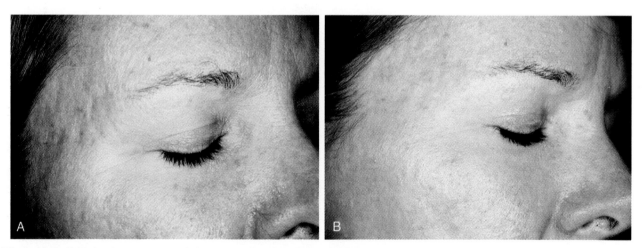

Figure 14–5. *(A)* Before laser treatment. *(B)* Six months after scar subcision using 16-gauge Nokor needle and UPCO$_2$ laser set at periphery of the scar (300 mJ, 60 W, computer pattern generator [CPG] density 7 followed by second and third passes (250 mJ, 60 W, and CPG density 5).

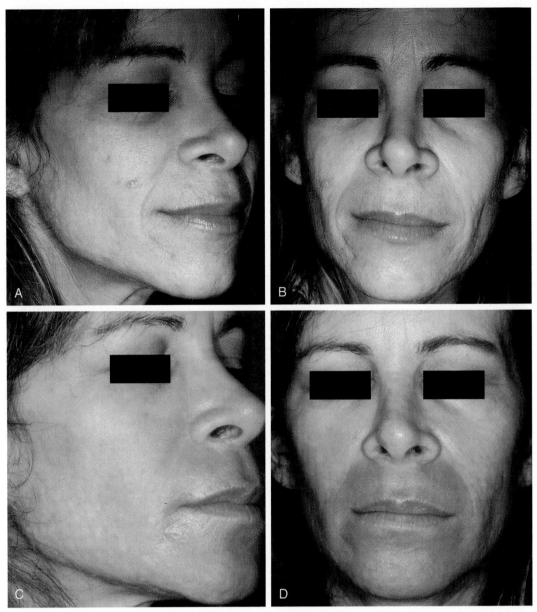

Figure 14–6 . *(A, B)* Before laser treatment. *(C, D)* Six months after treatment with UPCO$_2$ laser set at periphery of the scar (300 mJ, 60 W, CPG density 7).

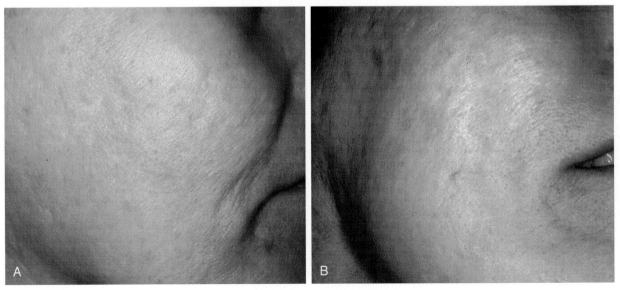

Figure 14–7. *(A)* Before laser treatment. *(B)* Six months after treatment with scar subcision and UPCO$_2$ laser at periphery of the scar (300 mJ, 60 W, CPG density 7), and for second and third passes (250 mJ, 60 W, and CPG density 5).

UPCO$_2$ laser resurfacing alone resulted in significant improvement of acne scarring—approximately 42% over pretreatment severity. Scar subcision resulted in a similar degree of improvement. A combination of scar subcision followed by laser resurfacing resulted in a significantly greater degree of scar elevation. More important perhaps, the resultant skin texture and quality and the scar elevation were preferred by patients utilizing the combination of scar subcision followed by laser resurfacing (Fig. 14–4).

Discussion

The combination of scar subcision and laser skin resurfacing has been shown to be a logical and useful combination for improving certain types of acne scarring (Figs. 14–5 through 14–7). All of the patients treated in our study had saucer-shaped acne scars. Preliminary observations of "ice pick" scars suggest that the combination of punch excision of the scars followed by UPCO$_2$ laser resurfacing might be very beneficial. It appears that the patient's improvement is maintained over at least the period of 12 months.

REFERENCES

1. David LM: Laser vermillion ablation for actinic cheilitis. J Dermatol Surg Oncol 1985; 11:605–608.
2. David LM, Lask GP, Glassberg E, et al.: CO$_2$ laser ablation for cosmetic and therapeutic treatment of facial actinic damage. Cutis 1989; 43:583–587.
3. Ratz J, McGillis S: Treatment of facial acne scarring with the carbon dioxide laser. Am J Cosmetic Surg 1992; 9(2):181–183.
4. Lowe NJ, Lask G, Griffin ME, et al.: Skin resurfacing with the ultrapulsed carbon dioxide laser: Observation on 100 patients. Dermatol Surg 1995; 21:1025–1029.
5. Fitzpatrick RE, Ruiz-Exparaza J, Goldman MP: The depth of thermal necrosis using the CO$_2$ laser, a comparison of the superpulsed mode and the conventional mode. J Dermatol Surg Oncol 1991; 17:340–344.
6. Fitzpatrick RE, Goldman MP: Advances in carbon dioxide laser surgery. Clin Dermatol 1995; 13:35–47.
7. Hruza GJ: Skin resurfacing with lasers. J Clin Dermatol 1995; 3:38–41.
8. Waldorf HA, Kauvar A, Geronemus RG: Skin resurfacing of fine to deep rhytides using a char-free carbon dioxide laser in 47 patients. Dermatol Surg 1995; 21:940–946.
9. Lask G, Keller G, Lowe N, et al.: Laser skin resurfacing with the silktouch flashscanner for facial rhytides. Dermatol Surg 1995; 21: 1021–1024.
10. Hobbs E, Bailin P, Wheeland R, Ratz J: Superpulsed lasers: Minimizing thermal damage with short duration high irradiance pulses. J Dermatol Surg Oncol 1987; 13:9.
11. Verschueren RCJ, Koudstaal J, Oldhoff J: CO$_2$ laser surgery. In Hillencamp F, Pratesi R, Sacni CA (eds): Lasers in Biology and Medicine. New York: Plenum, 1980.
12. Lowe NJ: Unpublished observation.

15

HYPERTROPHIC SCARS AND KELOIDS

Lisa Airan
Gary P. Lask
Nicholas J. Lowe

Physicians have continued to search for a definitive treatment for hypertrophic scars, saucer-shaped scars, and keloids, which are estimated to affect some 4.5% to 16% of the population.[1] Successful revision depends on the dynamics of scar contracture as it affects functional regions, the biology of wound healing, and the aesthetics of the affected region.[2, 3] In the past, cryosurgery,[4–6] intralesional steroids,[7–9] silicone gel sheeting,[10–14] pressure therapy,[15, 16] radiotherapy,[17–24] and surgical excision[25–27] have been used to treat scars. It is important to note that the type of scar is determined by its shape and the degree of elevation. A keloid is a tumor of fibrous tissue that overgrows its incisional scar and invades surrounding normal tissue. A hypertrophic scar represents proliferative scar tissue confined to the site of original trauma.[25] Constant tension on wounds in certain cosmetic units (upper lip, chin) can result in hypertrophic scarring. Also, keloids and hypertrophic scars tend to occur on the anterior chest and in areas of increased mobility or pressure. These scars, which occasionally cause itching or pain, are frequently difficult to treat and sometimes are exacerbated by intervention. The biology of the process is still ill-understood.[25] Fair-skinned persons are less likely to develop keloids and hypertrophic scars; however, their scars tend to have persistent redness. Scar erythema is part of the healing process, secondary to neovascularization, and can be exacerbated by tension.

Initially, lasers, including the argon[28–30] and neodymium:yttrium-aluminum-garnet (Nd:YAG)[31–33] were used to treat scars. The argon laser is a continuous-wave vascular laser that can be used to treat the vascular components of a scar to decrease erythema. Potassium titanyl phosphate (KTP), krypton, copper vapor, and argon dye may also be effective in improving the appearance of scars for this reason.

The 585-nm flashlamp-pumped pulsed-dye laser (450-μm pulse width) has been shown to be effective in treating a variety of benign vascular lesions.[34] Recent studies have indicated that the pulsed-dye laser (PDL) may be effective for treating a variety of scars.[35–38] It has been shown to improve the color, texture, pliability, scar tissue volume, and symptoms (pruritus and dysesthesia) of hypertrophic scars. Most recently, facial acne scars have been treated by the 585-nm PDL (see Chapter 14).[39] It has been theorized that the PDL may alter collagen metabolism by selectively targeting the increased microvascularity of hypertrophic scars.

In a study conducted by the authors with the 585-nm PDL (450-μm pulse width), 17 scars were treated at 5 to 7 J/cm² using a 5-mm spot size. One to four treatments were given at 4-week intervals. Clinical evaluation of the response to PDL was obtained by independent observers and evaluation of pre- and postprocedure photographs. Five scars were evaluated by pre- and posttreatment laser profilometry. A variety of scars were treated, including (1) erythematous and flesh-colored hypertrophic and (2) erythematous and flesh-colored macular ones, and (3) striae. Punch biopsy specimens (3 mm) from pre- and posttreatment scars were evaluated by immunohistochemical staining. Staining was quantified with a computer image analysis system. For evaluation of collagen and elastin fiber morphology, laser scanning confocal microscopy was performed on dual immunofluorescence-labeled sections. The response varied: scars with a significant vascular component had a more dramatic clinical response (Figs. 15–1 to 15–3).

The 585-nm Pulsed-Dye Laser (450-μsec Pulse-Width): Treatment Protocol

The authors' recommended protocol is to treat the entire scar at each session with a 585-nm PDL with a pulse duration of 450 μsec. Single discrete or slightly overlapping laser pulses should be delivered. We recommend a 5-mm spot size with energy fluences ranging between 5.0 and 7.0 J/cm² or a 7-mm spot size and energy fluences of 5.0 to 6.5 J/cm². Usually, no anesthesia is required, although EMLA cream or lidocaine may be applied before treatment. Purpura develops immediately and lasts 7 to 10 days. No specific aftercare is required. If crusting occurs, an antibiotic may be applied twice a day until the area heals. Treatments are performed at intervals of 4 to 6 weeks, to an

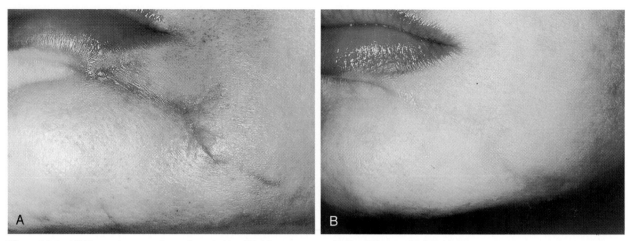

Figure 15–1. *(A)* Traumatic scar to lower lip and chin. *(B)* After treatment with the 585-μm pulsed dye laser.

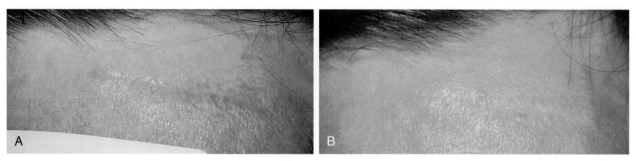

Figure 15–2. *(A)* Hypertrophic scar to the forehead. *(B)* After treatment with the 585-μm pulsed dye laser.

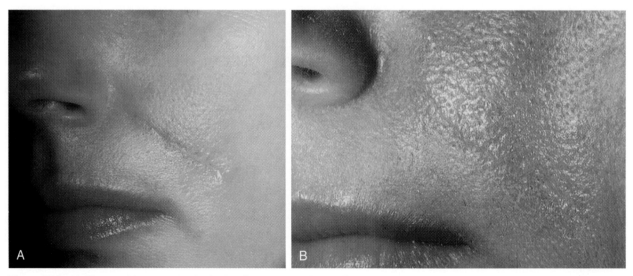

Figure 15–3. *(A)* Hypertrophic scar to the cheek. *(B)* After treatment with the 585-μm pulsed dye laser.

end point of no erythema or hypertrophy. Most scars improve after three treatments, although several more may be required to achieve the desired effect. Also, laser treatment can be alternated with intralesional steroid injections every other month (see Table 15–1).

Discussion

Multiple studies have shown the 585-nm flashlamp-pumped PDL (450-μsec pulse width) is effective in improving the appearance of hypertrophic scars and keloids.[35–39] In the

Table 15–1. **Protocol for 585-nm Pulsed Dye Laser Treatment of Scars**

Anesthesia if required
585-nm Pulsed dye laser (450 μsec pulse width)
Energy density 5.0–7.0 J/cm^2
Spot size 5 or 7 mm with slight or non-overlapping pulses
Treatment interval 4–6 wk

authors' study, improvements in skin surface texture correlate with a decrease in overall volume of the scar as calculated by the computer program used with the optical profilometric method (Table 15–2). This method makes use of an autofocus microscope with a helium-neon laser beam, which generates signals to characterize points at 100-μm intervals on the replica surface in three dimensions. These data are used to calculate the volume of individual surface features using a custom computer program developed by Dr. Gormley (patent #4,569,358). Scar height and pliability are improved. Immunohistochemical staining and confocal laser scanning microscopy for collagen, elastin, fibronectin, hyaluronic acid, and factor VIII were performed on paired tissue samples from treated and untreated skin from the same subjects. Preliminary results with confocal microscopy suggest a decrease in staining for factor VIII–related antigen, which probably represents a decrease in the number of blood vessels (unpublished data L. Airan, G. Lask, E. Bernstein). In addition, there appears to be reorganization of the elastic tissue and perhaps an increase in epidermal and dermal hyaluronic acid staining with a hyaluronic acid probe (Fig. 15–4 A–D).

As expected, macular erythematous scars improve in appearance with PDL treatment because it removes the erythematous component. Hypertrophic erythematous scars improve with PDL treatment by removing erythema and improving texture. Laser profilometry data support the observation of textural improvement (unpublished data L. Airan, G. Lask, N. Lowe). The volume of scars is reduced as measured by profilometry after 585-nm

Table 15–2. Profilometry Results

PATIENT NO.	SCAR SITE	SCAR TYPE	IMPROVEMENT (%)
1	Posterior scalp	Hypertrophic	56.9
2	Right temple	Hypertrophic	47.9
3	Left chest	Hypertrophic	46.5
4	Right chest	Striae	45.1
5	Right temple	Atrophic	(−)54.4

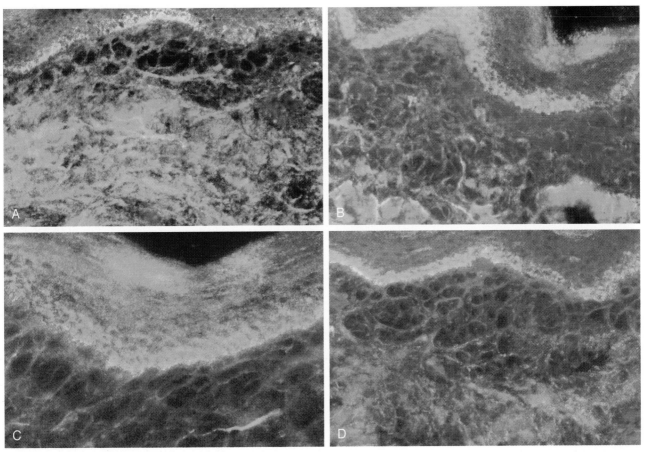

Figure 15–4. Laser scanning confocal microscopy. Laser treated *(A)* and untreated *(B)* samples stained for elastin and factor VIII. Elastin, stained with a monoclonal antibody, stains green; factor VIII, stained with polyclonal antibodies, stains red. *(C)* Laser treated and untreated *(D)* samples stained for fibronectin and hyaluronic acid. Fibronectin, stained with polyclonal antibodies, stains red; hyaluronic acid, stained with a monoclonal antibody, stains green.

PDL (450-μsec pulse width) treatment. The mechanism whereby hypertrophic scars and keloids are improved by a vessel-specific laser system is not understood. Hypertrophic scars with a significant erythematous component have the best response to laser treatment as measured by scar volume using laser profilometry; however, non-erythematous atrophic scars have minimal improvement, if any. Thus, it appears that the specificity of the 585-nm PDL (450-μsec pulse width) for cutaneous microvessels is important in improving the clinical appearance of hypertrophic scars (Table 15–3). Another study reported some return of normal skin markings with atrophic hyperpigmented scars.

The mechanism of action by which the 585-nm PDL alters scar tissue metabolism is thought to be microvascular destruction leading to ischemia and a change in collagen metabolism. Additionally, dermal mast cells are more numerous after laser treatment. The roles of mast cells in normal and in scar tissue metabolism are not understood. Previous studies have demonstrated stimulation of normal and keloid fibroblast growth by histamine.[40]

Future studies include determination of the time to intervene (early or late); frequency of treatments (intervals, energy densities for skin types, site, and scar type); and the role of concomitant treatments (chemical peels, carbon dioxide laser resurfacing, corticosteroid injections, and topical formulations such as silicone gel sheeting and retinoic acid).

There have been reports of striae responding to PDL therapy. The best responses seem to be from large spot sizes and low fluences. The mechanism of action could be similar to that of erythematous hypertrophic scars: targeting the vascular component; however, some reports state that the hypopigmented striae are most responsive rather than the erythematous ones. One study concluded that not all striae respond; that the smaller-diameter striae respond better; and that site, age, and cause of striae had no correlation with responsiveness.[41]

At present, results are inconsistent, and larger long-term studies are needed to evaluate the role of PDL treatment for striae. Transient hyper- and hypopigmentation can result from laser treatment. It remains to be determined how many treatments are needed for improvement and at what intervals.

The role of the longer–pulse duration and longer-wavelength PDLs in treating scars and striae is currently being evaluated. The question remains whether they will offer any significant improvement over the 585-nm 450-μsec pulse width laser, and what the rate of side effects will be.

Table 15–3. Areas of Improvement with Laser Treatment of Hypertropic Scars

Decreased erythema
Improved texture
Increased pliability
Reduced volume
Probable decrease in amount of blood vessels
Reorganization of elastic tissue
Increase in epidermal/dermal hyaluronic acid

REFERENCES

1. Cosman B, Crikelair GF, Ju DM, et al.: The surgical treatment of keloids. Plast Reconstr Surg 1961;27:335–341.
2. Edlich RF, et al.: Biology of sound repair: Its influence on surgical decision. Facial Plast Surg 1984;1:169–180.
3. Reed BR, Clark RAF: Cutaneous tissue repair: Practical implications of current knowledge. J Am Acad Dermatol 1985;13:919.
4. Layton AM, Yip J, Cunliffe WJ: A comparison of intralesional triamcinolone and cryosurgery in the treatment of acne keloids. Br J Dermatol 1994;130:498–501.
5. Zouboulis CC, Blume U, Buttner P, Orfanos CE: Outcomes of cryosurgery in keloids and hypertrophic scars. A prospective consecutive trial of case series. Arch Dermatol 1993;129:1146–1151.
6. Shepherd JP, Dewber RP: The response of keloid scars to cryosurgery. Plast Reconstr Surg 1982;70:677–682.
7. Ketchum LD, Smith J, Robinson DW, Masters FW: Treatment of hypertrophic scars, keloids, and scar contracture by triamcinolone acetonide. Plast Reconstr Surg 1966;38:209–215.
8. Maguire HC Jr: Treatment of keloids with triamcinolone acetonide injected intralesionally. JAMA 1965;192:325–330.
9. Golladay ES: Treatment of keloids by single intraoperative perilesional injection of repository steroid. South Med J 1988;81:736–738.
10. Gold MH: Topical silicone gel sheeting in the treatment of hypertrophic scars and keloids. A dermatologic experience. J Dermatol Surg Oncol 1993;19:912–916.
11. Sproat JE, Dalcin A, Weitauer N, Roberts RS: Hypertrophic sternal scars: Silicone gel sheet versus Kenalog injection treatment. Plast Reconstr Surg 1992;90:988–992.
12. Ahn ST, Monafo WW, Mustoe TA: Topical silicone gel for the prevention and treatment of hypertrophic scar. Arch Surg 1991;126:599–604.
13. Sawada Y, Sone K: Treatment of scars and keloids with a cream containing silicone oil. Br J Plast Surg 1990;43:683–688.
14. Mercer NS: Silicone gel in the treatment of keloid scars. Br J Plast Surg 1989;42:83–87.
15. Carr-Collins JA: Pressure techniques for the prevention of hypertrophic scar. Clin Plast Surg 1992;19:733–743.
16. Ward RS: Pressure technique for the control of hypertrophic scar formation after burn injury. A history and review. J Burn Care Rehab 1991;12:257–262.
17. Klumpar DI, Murray JC, Anscher M: Keloids treated with excision followed by radiation therapy. J Am Acad Dermatol 1994;31:25–31.
18. Ship AG, Weiss PR, Mincer FR, Wolkstein W: Sternal keloids: Successful treatment employing surgery and adjunctive radiation. Ann Plast Surg 1993;31:481–487.
19. Lo TC, Seckel BR, Salzman FA, Wright KA: Single-dose electron beam irradiation in the treatment and prevention of keloids and hypertrophic scars. Radiother Oncol 1990;19:267–272.
20. Sallstrom KO, Larson O, Heden P, et al.: Treatment of keloids with surgical excision and postoperative x-ray radiation. Scand J Plast Surg Hand Surg 1989;23:211–215.
21. Bokor TL, Bray M, Sinclair I, et al.: Role of ionizing irradiation for 393 keloids. J Radiat Oncol Biol Phys 1988;15:865–870.
22. Ollstein RN, Siegel HW, Gillooley JF, Barsa JM: Treatment of keloids by combined surgical excision and immediate postoperative x-ray therapy. Ann Plast Surg 1981;7:281–285.
23. Lukacs S, Braun-Falco O, Goldschmidt H: Radiotherapy of benign dermatoses: Indication, practice, and results. J Dermatol Surg Oncol 1978;4:620–625.
24. Craig RD, Pearson D: Early postoperative irradiation in the treatment of keloid scars. Br J Plast Surg 1965;18:369–376.
25. Brown LA, Pierce HE: Keloids: Scar revision. J Dermatol Surg Oncol 1986;12:51–56.
26. Pollack SV, Goslen JB: The surgical treatment of keloids. J Dermatol Surg Oncol 1982;8:1045–1049.
27. Apfelberg DB, Maser MR, Lash H: The use of epidermis over keloid as an autograft after resection of the keloid. J Dermatol Surg Oncol 1976;2:409–415.

28. Hulsbergen-Henning JP, Roskam Y, van Gemert MJ: Treatment of keloids and hypertrophic scars with an argon laser. Lasers Surg Med 1986;6:72–75.
29. Apfelberg DB, Maser MR, Lash H, et al.: Preliminary results of argon and carbon dioxide laser treatment of keloid scars. Laser Surg Med 1984;4:283–290.
30. Henderson DL, Cromwell TA, Mes LG: Argon and carbon dioxide laser treatment of hypertrophic and keloid scars. Laser Surg Med 1984;3:271–277.
31. Sherman R, Rosenfeld H: Experience with the Nd:YAG laser in the treatment of keloid scars. Ann Plast Surg 1988;21:231–235.
32. Apfelberg DB, Smith T, Lash H, et al.: Preliminary report on the use of the neodymium-YAG laser in plastic surgery. Laser Surg Med 1987;7:189–198.
33. Abergel RP, Dwyer RM, Meeker CA, et al.: Laser treatment of keloids: A clinical trial and an in-vitro study with Nd:YAG laser. Laser Surg Med 1984;4:291–295.
34. Lask GP, Glassberg E: 585 nm Pulsed dye laser for the treatment of cutaneous lesions. Clin Dermatol 1995;13(1):63–67.
35. Alster TS, Kurban AK, Grove GL, et al.: Alteration of argon laser–induced scars by the pulsed dye laser. Laser Surg Med 1993;13:368–373.
36. Goldman MP, Fitzpatrick RE: Cutaneous Laser Surgery. St. Louis: Mosby–Year Book, 1994.
37. Dierickx C, Goldman MP, Fitzpatrick RE: Laser treatment of erythematous/hypertrophic and pigmented scars in 26 patients. Plast Reconstr Surg 1995;95:84–90.
38. Alster TS, Williams CM: Improvement of hypertrophic and keloidal median sternotomy scars by the 585 nm flashlamp-pumped pulsed dye laser: A controlled study. Lancet 1995;345:1198–1200.
39. Alster TS, McMeekin TO: Improvement of facial acne scars by the 585 nm flashlamp-pumped pulsed dye laser. J Am Acad Dermatol 1996;35:79–81.
40. Topol BM, Lewis VL Jr, Benveniste K: The use of antihistamines to retard the growth of fibroblasts derived from human skin, scar, and keloid. Plast Reconstr Surg 1981;68:231–232.
41. Narurkar V, Haas A: The efficacy of the 585 nm flashlamp pumped pulse dye laser on striae distensae at various locations and etiologic factors. J Am Soc Laser Med Surg 1997(Suppl)9:35.

16

HAIR REMOVAL

Donna Ko
Gary P. Lask
Nicholas J. Lowe

Initial interest in laser hair removal began when patients being treated with the ruby laser for tattoo removal also noted that the laser had an effect on their hair follicles. Many laser systems and techniques have been introduced and the technology of laser hair removal has expanded rapidly and significantly.

Laser hair removal is based on the principle of selective photothermolysis. This theory, proposed by Anderson and Parrish, holds that the thermal injury is confined to a specific target if there is preferential absorption of the light at an appropriate wavelength and the pulse duration or width is shorter than the thermal relaxation time of the target.[1] Thermal relaxation time is defined as the time it takes for the target to cool to 50% of its peak temperature.

Currently, the primary target or the chromophore for laser hair removal is (1) the melanin, which is mainly located in the hair shaft and in smaller amounts in the inner and outer root sheaths, or (2) an exogenous, pigmented topical lotion that is absorbed in the follicle. Theoretically, the laser energy directed primarily at the pigment of the hair shaft melanin or the lotion is absorbed and transferred to the surrounding follicle and perifollicular tissue, causing conductive thermal damage to the follicle. Adequate damage is required to cause long-term hair removal. Better understanding of hair biology in the future should also produce other targets that may more efficiently cause hair removal.

There are three key elements in achieving effective laser-assisted hair removal: wavelength, pulse duration, and fluence.

Wavelengths between 700 to 1000 nm are appropriate in targeting melanin, since these wavelengths are selectively absorbed by melanin. Oxyhemoglobin, a competing chromophore, absorbs less energy at these wavelengths. The currently available lasers for hair removal utilize these wavelengths.

The optimal pulse width for hair removal is in order of tens of milliseconds. This pulse duration is shorter than the thermal relaxation time of the hair follicle (40–100 msec for terminal hair follicles with 200–300 μm in diameter), yet longer than that of the epidermis (3–10 msec), allowing some preservation of the epidermis from thermal damage.[2, 3]

The fluence determines the efficacy of the laser system to cause follicular damage. Significant energy must be delivered at the appropriate wavelength and pulse duration in order to induce adequate follicular destruction. Insufficient energy may merely heat the hair shaft causing temporary epilation without causing long-term hair loss.

With most of the current hair removal laser systems, histologic assessments have shown that the thermal damage is confined to the follicular epithelium and that the coagulative follicular epithelial destruction appears to correlate with clinical efficacy.

Currently, permanent or long-term hair reduction is defined as a lasting reduction in terminal hairs for a period of time greater than the complete hair cycle of hairs in a given body site.

It is important, then, to understand the hair cycle in order to plan an efficient strategy of hair removal with laser systems. Hair follicles undergo asynchronous repeated sequences of growth (anagen) and rest (telogen) phases called the hair cycle.[4] In the active anagen phase, melanocytes transfer melanin to the matrix cells in the lower portion of the hair bulb. The matrix cells then give rise to the hair shaft and the inner and outer root sheaths as they move into the upper part of the hair bulb. At the end of anagen, the follicular bulb moves up to the superficial portion of the dermis as melanization is completed. Telogen then follows, which appears to be a relatively consistent period given a specific body site. Because of the rich concentration of melanin in the anagen hair, the laser energy is better absorbed.

The duration of anagen varies owing to multiple factors, including the body location, age, gender, genetics, hormonal effects, and season.[5–9] This may be significant in that the anagen hairs are especially sensitive to any insult, including physical, chemical, or inflammatory. This has been proven by mouse model studies by Lin and coworkers where only the actively growing anagen hairs were significantly sensitive to hair removal by a ruby laser.[10]

Multiple experiments have also shown that the location

of the damage to the follicle may be important in determining the efficacy of hair removal. Initially it was thought that the matrix cells and the dermal papilla were the only important sites in preserving hair follicle regeneration. More recent transection experiments of Kim and Choi have observed that the isthmus of the follicle is also needed for hair follicle regeneration.[11] These results and future research may allow for more efficient hair removal by targeting specific sites of the follicle for destruction other than those utilized today.

There are four main wavelength type lasers available for hair removal: the ruby (694 nm), alexandrite (755 nm), the diode (800 nm) and the neodymium:yttrium-aluminum-garnet (Nd:YAG; 1064 nm). Some of these lasers are described below and summarized in Table 16–1.

Long-Pulsed Ruby Laser

There are several ruby lasers with varying parameters of pulse width, fluence, and spot size. These units emit 694 nm wavelength of light, which is strongly absorbed by melanin and only slightly by hemoglobin. The efficacy of these lasers for hair removal has been demonstrated in several publications.[3, 12–14] See Figs. 16–1 to 16–3.

The first pilot study was done with a long-pulsed ruby laser (LPRL) by Grossman and coworkers.[3] In this study, 13 patients received a single treatment on the thigh or the back at fluences ranging from 30–60 J/cm^2. They were followed at 1, 3, and 6 months with manual terminal hair counts. At 6 months, four subjects had <50% regrowth (two with <50% regrowth and two with no regrowth). Follow-up observations of 7 of 13 patients at 2 years showed four patients with significant sustained hair growth arrest. Fluence-dependent hair loss was also noted for long-term effects. Histologically, heterogeneous injury to the follicular epithelium was noted initially after treatment followed by the subsequent development of vellus-like hairs.

An additional trial by Dierickx reported that 72% of 100 patients achieved long-term hair loss when fluences of 30 J/cm^2 or more were used (personal communications, 1998). These patients were also followed for long-term effects at 6, 9, and 12 months and were found to have sustained hair loss. Adverse effects included immediate erythema and edema that lasted less than 24 hours and transient dyspigmentation that was inversely related to skin type. No scarring was noted.

The Epilaser offers a 3 msec pulse width, 5 Hz repetition rate, and fluence ranging between 10–40 J/cm^2. A 7 or 10 mm spot size can be used. The epidermis including its melanin is cooled, allowing preservation from thermal injury by a sapphire cooling handpiece that is directly applied to the skin.[3, 16] This crystal has a high thermal conductivity that provides cooling of the epidermis before, during, and after the laser energy is delivered. This reduces the patient discomfort during the procedure, which affords higher fluences to be delivered. The concomitant direct pressure applied with the cool tip also flattens the epidermis, decreasing the distance that the laser light energy has to traverse in the dermis to target the lower portion of the hair follicle. It also temporarily blanches the blood vessels underlying the tip, which displaces the oxyhemoglobin, the competing chromophore. The tip must be routinely cleansed during the treatment to minimize collection of debris on the lens, which can cause epidermal injury. The area to be treated also must be closely shaven to lessen the singeing accumulation of the hairs on the lens surface.

Epitouch is another ruby laser effective for hair removal (Table 16–2).[13] The highest fluence is 40 J/cm^2 with spot size options of 4–6 mm. The pulse duration is 1.2 milliseconds. A pretreatment of a water-based gel is applied to cool the skin. Using fluences of 18–25 J/cm^2 on arms, Lask and associates noted 40–80% hair regrowth at 12 weeks.[14] Nestor treated arms, legs, and bikini areas once at 25 J/cm^2 and reported 60% regrowth at 3 months; with two treatments, a 25% regrowth occurred.[13] After a third session, less than 10% regrowth was noted at 1 year follow-up. The same fluences in the moustache and beard areas at 1 month yielded regrowths of 55%, 40%, and 25% after 1, 2, and 3

Table 16–1. Some Lasers Used for Hair Removal

LASER TYPE & WAVELENGTH	PULSE DURATION (msecs)	SPOT SIZES (mm)	MAXIMUM FLUENCE J/cm^2	CHROMOPHORE TARGET
Alexandrite lasers 755 nm				
Apogee	5, 10, 20	7, 10, 12.5	50	Melanin
Epitouch	1.2	5, 10	25	Melanin
Gentlelase	3	8, 10, 12, 15	100	Melanin
Photogenica	5, 10, 20	7, 10	40	Melanin
Diode lasers 800 nm				
Lightsheer	5 to 30	9 × 9	40	Melanin
Nd:YAG 1064 nm				
Softlight	10 μsecs	7	3	Topical carbon dye
Ruby lasers 694 nm				
Chromos	1.2	7, 10	20	Melanin
Epilaser	3	7, 10	40	Melanin
Epitouch silk laser	1.2	5, 6	40	Melanin
Epilight light source	Variable	10 × 45, 8 × 35	65	Melanin

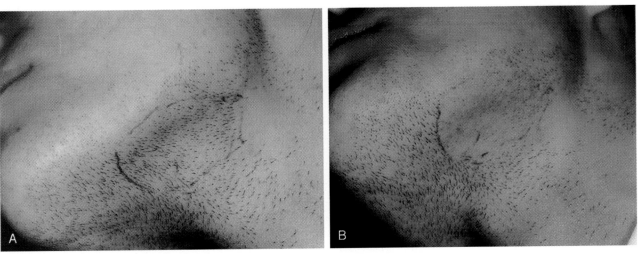

Figure 16–1. Hirsutism in a female patient before *(A)* and 4 weeks after *(B)* long-pulsed ruby laser.

treatments, respectively. However, there has not been longer-term follow-up in these patients.

A third ruby laser is the Chromos 694, which at the present time does not have adequate data on its efficacy.[13, 17]

Alexandrite

The long-pulsed Alexandrite laser systems currently available are the long-pulsed infrared lasers (LPIR), Gentlelase

and Epitouch. They emit wavelengths at 755 nm with varying spot sizes and fluences. Theoretically, the epidermal melanin absorbs this wavelength less than that of the ruby laser (694 nm), which may allow for a safer therapy in dark-skinned patients.[18] These lasers utilize a cooling mechanism to minimize the risk of thermal damage to the superficial melanin-containing epidermis. Pretreatment shaving further protects the epidermis from undesirable thermal injury.

LPIR has reported in its promotional data that 80–100% hair reduction can be achieved with three to four treatments

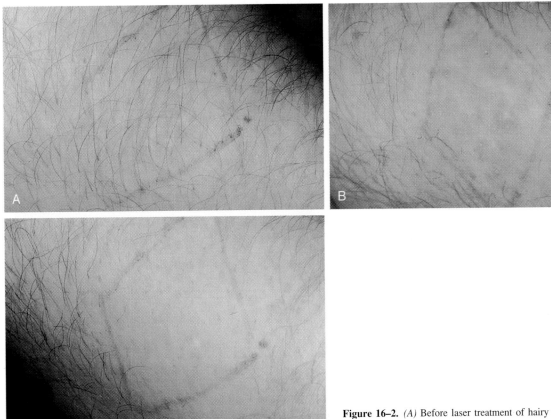

Figure 16–2. *(A)* Before laser treatment of hairy forearm skin. *(B)* Immediately after treatment with a long-pulsed ruby laser delivering 70 J/cm². Note follicular erythema. *(C)* Three weeks after laser.

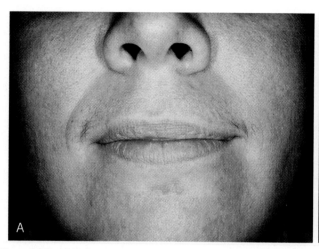
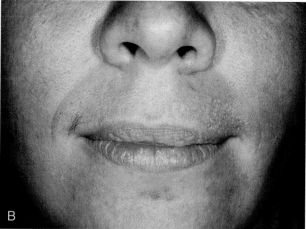

Figure 16–3. *(A)* Before treatment for upper lip hair. *(B)* After treatment with a long-pulsed ruby laser, 30 J/cm^2, 694 nm, 3 msec pulse. Left side of upper lip treated.

4–6 weeks apart, using fluences up to 40 J/cm^2.[17] It has a cool tip handpiece and offers 1–40 J/cm^2 fluence; 5, 10, 20 msec pulse duration, and a 7 or 10 mm spot size.

Gentlelase offers fluences of 10–100 J/cm^2 at 3 msec pulse width, and optional 8, 10, and 12 mm spot sizes.[19] It has a novel Dynamic Cooling Device, which consists of a burst of cryogen spray that protects the epidermis.

The Epitouch 5100 performs at 2 msec pulse duration at 5 Hz with a 5 or 10 mm spot size. It also offers a scanner with high repetition rates for rapid treatments. It uses a water-based gel that serves as a "heat sink" to cool the epidermis to decrease the risk of injury. Finkle and associates reported 5–15% regrowth of hair at 3 months after three treatments using 20–40 J/cm^2 at 1–2.5 month intervals.[18]

Comparable clinical efficacy and adverse effects were observed for these laser systems and the ruby lasers. The adverse effects of these lasers are few, including post-treatment erythema and edema lasting less than 4 hours, transient discomfort during the procedure, and epidermal changes in up to 10–15% of patients (dark-skinned or tanned individuals).[18, 19]

Diode

The Lightsheer diode laser emits a wavelength of 800 nm and also causes hair removal by effectively targeting melanin while deeply penetrating the dermis.[17] It offers a pulse duration of 5–30 msec, which is comparable to that of the follicle. Fluences range from 10–40 J/cm^2 and the spot size is 9 cm^2. A contact cooling sapphire tip as described for the Epilaser is also employed to effectively cool the epidermis. This has many advantages already discussed previously. Clinical studies have shown that higher fluences could be better delivered with less adverse effects using this cooling mechanism. This may allow a safer treatment in dark-skinned individuals.

In a personal communication in 1998, Dierickx reported a study of 100 subjects using a combination of fluences and pulse widths in 8 test sites mostly on the back and thighs. Patients were followed at 1, 3, 6, 9, and 12 months. Results showed that all patients had temporary epilation that lasted up to 1–3 months at all fluences used. Eighty-nine percent of the patients had long-term hair loss at 1 year follow-up, fulfilling the criteria for long-term hair reduction described

Table 16–2. Ruby Hair Removal Laser (Epitouch) Study: Results Summary

Multicenter study groups of >100 patients
One-year follow-up, multiple treatment sessions
  First treatment results
    Average 60% growth, 3 months after treatment: arms, bikini, legs
    Average 55% growth, 1 month after treatment: upper lip, chin
  Second treatment (performed on hair growth) results
    Average 24% growth, 3 months after second treatment: arms, bikini, legs
    Average 40% growth, 1 month after treatment: upper lip, chin
  Third treatment results
    Less than 10% growth 3 months after third treatment: arms, bikini, legs
    Average 25% growth 1 month after third treatment: upper lip, chin

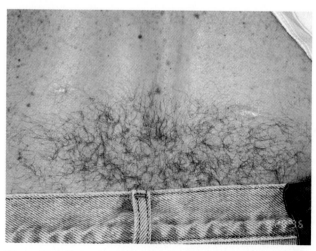

Figure 16–4. Lower back hair before softlight (Thermolase) treatment.

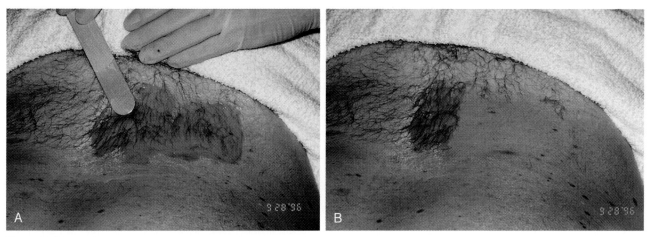

Figure 16–5. *(A)* Application of wax. *(B)* Removal of hair with waxing.

earlier. The efficacy was also fluence dependent. Patients who did not respond adequately had blonde hair, which intrinsically has less melanin and, therefore, less chromophore. These subjects, in addition to having decreased absolute number of hairs, had lighter and thinner regrowing hairs that added to the apparent miniaturization of hair follicles and granulomatous degeneration of follicle epithelium with consequent fibrotic event. In the study, a fixed parameter of fluence pulse duration combination was employed regardless of the patient's skin type, which may not have been well matched for each patient. This probably created a higher incidence of adverse effects. Six percent epidermal change and 3% textural change (mostly at higher fluences) were noted, both of which resolved at 3 months. Transient dyspigmentation was noted in 10%, mostly in dark-skinned and tanned individuals.

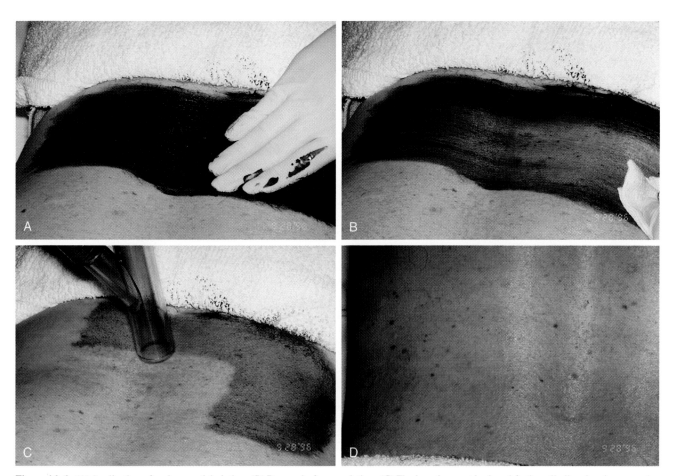

Figure 16–6. *(A)* Application of carbon-particle lotion. *(B)* Removal of excess lotion. *(C)* The laser is swept back and forth until all carbon is removed. *(D)* Posttreatment appearance shows mild erythema.

Clinical efficacy of the diode laser was also confirmed by observations of Adrian who reported that in 125 patients treated with the diode laser, most had <60% long-term (6 months) hair reduction after two to three treatments (personal communication, 1998). The treated areas included the lip, face, neck, axilla, and back. Subsequent treatments were given when significant clinical regrowth of hair was noted, which ranged from 1–3 months.

Nd:YAG

The Q-switched Nd:YAG laser produces light at 1064 nm in the near infrared spectrum. Water, hemoglobin, and melanin are poorly absorbed at this wavelength.[20] Because of this, the laser was employed in combination with a topical pigmented carbon-based suspension as an exogenous chromophore.[2, 18, 21] This method provides a selective target that is independent of the color of the hair shaft. This potentially permits effective treatment of even light-haired individuals who lack significant hair melanin, the main chromophore for other laser systems.

Softlight (Thermolase) was the first FDA approved laser-assisted hair removal system. It provides fluences of 2–4 J/cm^2 at 10 nsec pulse duration and a rapid 10 Hz repetition rate with a 7 mm spot size.[17] The original technique of treatment required the skin to be first waxed, theoretically allowing the carbon-rich lotion to be placed into the "empty" follicles.[18, 21] The carbon is then targeted with the laser beam causing a photomechanical and photothermal injury to the follicle as the carbon particle is vaporized (Figs. 16–4 to 16–6). This produced a 40–70% hair loss at 3 months in 35 patients after a single session, but the patients had full regrowth of hair at 6 months.[18] This process also proved to be time-consuming.

Nanni and Alster reviewed the efficacy of the treatment parameters.[22] While they observed adequate delay in hair regrowth in all the patients, they noted that neither the pre-therapy waxing nor the carbon-based lotion significantly determined the efficacy of the laser treatment at 3 months after a single session. At this time, further studies that better predict the parameters and the efficacy of this laser are needed.

REFERENCES

1. Anderson RR, Parrish JA: Selective photothermolysis: Precise microsurgery by selective absorption of pulsed radiation. Science 1983;220: 524–527.
2. Wheeland RG: Laser-assisted hair removal. Dermatol Clin 1997;15: 459–477.
3. Grossman MC, Dierickx C, Farinelli W, et al: Damage to hair follicles by normal-mode ruby laser pulses. J Am Acad Dermatol 1996;35:889–894.
4. Olsen EA: Disorders of hair growth: Diagnosis and treatment. New York: McGraw-Hill 1994;1–19.
5. Seago SV, Ebling FJG: The hair cycle on the human thigh and upper arm. Br J Dermatol 1985;113:9–16.
6. Randall VA, Ebling FJG: Seasonal changes in human hair growth. Br J Dermatol 1991;24:146–151.
7. Eaton P, Eaton MW: Temperature and the growth of hair. Science 1937;86:354.
8. Saitoh M, Uzuka M, Sakamoto M: Human hair cycle. J Invest Dermatol 1970;54:65–81.
9. Trotter M: The cycle of hair in selected regions of the body. Am J Phys Anthrop 1924;7:427–437.
10. Lin TY, Manuskiatti W, Dierickx CC, et al: Hair growth cycle affects hair follicle destruction by ruby laser pulses. J Invest Dermatol 1998;111:107–113.
11. Kim J-C, Choi Y-C: Hair follicle regeneration after horizontal resectioning: Implications for hair transplantation. In Stough DB, Haber RS (eds): Hair Replacement: Surgical and Medical. St. Louis: Mosby–Year Book; 1995 p. 358–363.
12. Dierickx CC, Grossman MC, Farinelli WA, Anderson RR: Permanent hair removal by normal-pulsed ruby laser. Arch Dermatol 1998;134: 837–842.
13. Nestor MS: Laser hair removal: Clinical results and practical applications of selective photothermolysis. Skin Aging 1998;1:34–40.
14. Lask G, Elman M, Slatkine M, et al: Laser-assisted hair removal by selective photothermolysis. Dermatol Surg 1997;23:737–739.
15. Alster TS, Nanni CA: Laser-assisted hair removal with long-pulsed ruby and alexandrite lasers. In Keller TS (ed): Lasers in Facial Plastic Surgery. New York: Thieme Publishers, 1998.
16. Olsen EA: Methods of hair removal. J Am Acad Dermatol 1999;40: 143–158.
17. Nanni CA, Alster TS: A practical review of laser-assisted hair removal using the Q-switched Nd:YAG, long-pulsed ruby, and long-pulsed alexandrite lasers. Dermatol Surg 1998;24:1–7.
18. Finkle B, Eliezri YD, Waldman A, Slatkine M: Pulsed alexandrite laser technology for noninvasive hair removal. J Clin Laser Med Surg 1997;15:225–229.
19. Dover JS, Arndt KS: Illustrated cutaneous laser surgery: A practitioner's guide. Stamford, CT: Appleton & Lange, 1990.
20. Goldberg DJ: Topical suspension-assisted Q-switched Nd:YAG laser hair removal. Dermatol Surg 1997;23:741–745.
21. Goldberg DJ: Topical solution assisted laser hair removal. Lasers Surg Med 1995;7:47.
22. Nanni CA, Alster TS: Optimizing treatment parameters for hair removal using a carbon-based solution and a 1064 nm Q-switched neodymium:YAG laser energy. Arch Dermatol 1997;133:1546–1549.

Table 16–3. Nonlaser Treatments for Hair Removal

METHOD	COMMENTS
Depilatory cream	Limited duration of effect, significant risks of skin irritation and allergy
Waxing	Limited duration of effect, frequently painful, risks of folliculitis and follicle infection
Shaving	Temporary; risk of hair follicle infection
Electrolysis	When skillfully and properly performed, can permanently remove hair. Painful, very time consuming, not universally effective, as adequate destruction of a susceptible hair follicle is necessary to treatment success

Appendix
CUTANEOUS LASERS AND LIGHT SOURCE SYSTEMS

NAME	TYPE	NAME	TYPE
Candela		**Luxor**	
Sclerolaser	Pulsed dye	Novapulse	CO_2
ScleroPLUS	Pulsed dye	**MDLT**	
Skinlight	Er:YAG	Quadralaz	QS alexandrite
SPTL-1B	Pulsed dye		QS Nd:YAG
YAGlazr	QS Nd:YAG		532-nm
			Er:YAG
Coherent			
UltraPulse	CO_2	**Mehl/Biophile**	
VERSAPulse	QS Nd:YAG	Chromos 585	Pulsed dye
	QS alexandrite	Chromos 694	Long-pulsed ruby
	Pulsed 532-nm	**Optomed**	
VPW	Pulsed 532-nm	Unilaser	Flashlamp
Continuum Biomedical		**Palomar**	
CB Diode	Pulsed 532-nm	Epilaser	Long-pulsed ruby
Medlite	QS Nd:YAG	RD-1200	QS ruby
CB Erbium	Er:YAG	Tru-Pulse	CO_2
Cynosure		**Polytec**	
PhotoGenica LPIR	QS alexandrite	Lase-Away	QS ruby
PhotoGenica V	Pulsed dye		
PhotoGenica LSV	Pulsed dye	**SEO Medical**	
PhotoGenica T	QS alexandrite	CLR2940	Er:YAG
		Trilase	QS alexandrite
ESC			QS Nd:YAG
PHOTODERM VL/PL	Flashlamp		532-nm
EpiLight	Flashlamp		
Derma-20	Er:YAG	**Sharplan**	
		Silk/Feather Touch	CO_2
HGM		Surgilase	CO_2
Erbium	Er:YAG	Epitouch	Long-pulsed ruby
Krypton	Krypton	Erbium	Er:YAG
Laserscope		**Thermolase**	
Aura	Pulsed 532-nm	Softlight	QS Nd:YAG & carbon lotion
Orion	Nd:YAG		
	Pulsed 532-nm		
Paragon	CO_2		

LASER ORGANIZATIONS

American Society for Laser Medicine and Surgery
2404 Stewart Square
Wausau, WI 54401
(715)845-9283
Fax: (715)848-2498

American Board of Laser Surgery
2722 W. Oklahoma, Suite 202
Milwaukee, WI 53215
(414) 643-1066
Fax: (414) 643-5219

British Medical Laser Association
Dr. S.G. Bown
School of Medicine, University College London
The Rayne Institute
University St
London WC1E 6JJ, England

International Society of Cosmetic Laser Surgery, Inc.
415 Pier Ave
Hermosa Beach, CA 90254
(310) 372-8802
Fax: (310) 318-6369

Laser Nursing Magazine
Mary Ann Liebert, Inc.
1651 Third Ave
New York, NY 10128
(212) 289-2300

Medical Laser Industry Report
One Technology Park Dr.
Westford, MA 01886
(508) 692-0700

Occupational Safety and Health Administration (OSHA)
Bureau of National Affairs
1231 25 th St. NW
Washington, DC 20037
(202) 452-4200

MANUFACTURER'S LASER TREATMENT GUIDELINES*

Candela

Candela ScleroPLUS: Physician's Treatment Experience

Treatment guidelines are currently under clinical development. Anecdotal evidence to date is listed below. Follow the approved test spot protocol outlined in the operator's manual prior to treating. Always start with lowest recommended settings and *evaluate patient response* before additional treatment.

LESION	SPOT SIZE	ENERGY	WAVELENGTH	RE-TREAT	COMMENTS
Telangiectasia:	5 mm	8–9 J/cm^2	595 nm	4–6 wk	Use spot that best covers
Facial	7 mm	4–6 J/cm^2	595 nm	4–6 wk	vein
	2 × 7 mm	10–12 J/cm^2	595 nm	4–6 wk	
Leg*	2 × 7 mm	15–25 J/cm^2	595 nm	6–10 wk	Red, more superficial leg veins†
	2 × 7 mm	18–25 J/cm^2	600 nm	6–10 wk	Larger, bluer, deeper leg veins†
Matting	5 mm	10–12 J/cm^2	595 nm	6–10 wk	Red, superficial veins
	5 mm	12–14 J/cm^2	600 nm	6–10 wk	Blue, leg veins
Scars	5 mm	10–12 J/cm^2	595 nm	4–6 wk	
	7 mm	5–7 J/cm^2	595 nm	4–6 wk	
Striae	7 mm	4–4.5 J/cm^2	585 nm	6 wk	Look for LIGHT pink purpura
	7 mm	4–5 J/cm^2	595 nm	6 wk	
Port wine stain (head/neck)‡	5 mm	10–15 J/cm^2	595 nm	8–12 wk	
	7 mm	7 J/cm^2	595 nm	8–12 wk	Infants
	7 mm	8 J/cm^2	595 nm	8–12 wk	Adult macular facial or trunk/extremities
					Child hemangioma
	7 mm	9 J/cm^2	595 nm	8–12 wk	Adult hypertrophic PWS
	10 mm	6 J/cm^2	585,590,595 nm	8–12 wk	If need to increase, change to 7 mm. Optimal treatment varies

Table continued on following page

*The information provided in this section is current as of the date of publication; but as new research and clinical experience broaden our knowledge, changes become necessary or appropriate. Readers are advised to check the product information currently provided by the manufacturers.

133

LESION	SPOT SIZE	ENERGY	WAVELENGTH	RE-TREAT	COMMENTS
Hemangiomas	5 mm	10–12 J/cm²	595,600 nm	2 wk infants, 8-12 wk adults	**Use caution with neonates§** 2 wk interval for *proliferative* hemangiomas
	7 mm	6–8 J/cm²	595,600 nm		
	10 mm	6 J/cm²	585 nm		
Angioma or spider angioma	10 mm	8 J/cm²	595 nm	4–6 wk	May double pulse on raised angioma
Warts¶	5 mm	4–5 J/cm²	595 nm	4–6 wk	
	5 mm	12–14 J/cm²	595,600 nm	2–3 wk	Test with both wavelengths & spot sizes
	5 mm	20 J/cm² **single pulse**	585/590 nm		
	7 mm	8–10 J/cm²	595,600 nm	2–3 wk	
Poikiloderma of Civatte	2 × 7 mm	10–12 J/cm²	595 nm	6–10 wk	Use of hydrogel dressing increases patient comfort. Recommended at higher energy.
	7 mm	4–6 J/cm²	595 nm	6–10 wk	
	5 mm	8–9 J/cm²	595 nm	6–10 wk	
Vulvodynia	7 mm	4.5–5 J/cm²	595 nm	8 wk	Look for LIGHT purpura

*Deliver energy through a hydrogel dressing for settings >13 J/cm².

†Skin types >III may blister at higher fluences, producing a characteristic epidermal snap. If so, decrease fluence or postpone treatment until tan has faded.

‡PWS on the extremities may require higher energy but TEST first.

§Previous experience treating hemangiomas is important to prevent scarring.

¶Pretreatment, pare down wart, and double or triple pulse depending on patient tolerance.

ADDITIONAL SUGGESTIONS:

⇒ When changing settings, increase energy in 0.5 J/cm² increments until the desired response is achieved.

⇒ Above suggestions are based upon adult responses. No treatment guidelines are yet available for children.

⇒ The suggested end point is a reddish discoloration, DARK PURPURA, WHITE or GRAY DISCOLORATION is not a desirable end point.

⇒ If hyperpigmentation/hypopigmentation occurs, do not re-treat until this resolves (can be 2–3 months).

⇒ With suntanned patients, do not treat until the tan fades. Inform patient that treatment of tanned skin may result in hypopigmentation, which is generally transient and should resolve in 2–3 months.

Candela SPTL Treatment Guideline

This guideline sheet does not take the place of the operator's manual or physician's companion book but is a summary of the information listed in these references. For more details, please refer to these manuals or the references listed next to each type of lesion. It is highly recommended that ALL patients receive test pulses BEFORE a complete treatment is initiated for a more efficacious and safe treatment result.

LESION	SPOT SIZE	ENERGY DENSITY	PULSE	RE-TREAT	REFERENCE/COMMENTS
Port wine stain	5 mm	Adults: 5.5-7.5 J/cm^2 Children: 5.0-7.0 J/cm^2 Infants: 5.0-6.25 J/cm^2	Single	8-12 wk	Physician's Companion or Operator's Manual
	7 mm	Adults: 4.5-6.5 J/cm^2 Children: 4.0-6.0 J/cm^2 Infants: 4.0-5.25 J/cm^2	Single	8-12 wk	Operator's Manual
	10 mm	Adults: 5.0 J/cm^2 Children: 4.0-5.0 J/cm^2 Infants: 4.0-4.5 J/cm^2	Single	8-12 wk	Operator's Manual
Facial telangiectasia	2 mm 3 mm or 5 mm 7 mm 10 mm	8.5-9.5 J/cm^2 5.5-7.5 J/cm^2 4.75-6.5 J/cm^2 3.0 J/cm^2	Single	6-8 wk	Physician's Companion or Operator's Manual
Angiomas Hemangiomas	3 mm or 5 mm 5 mm or 7 mm 10 mm	5.75-7.5 J/cm^2 5.5-9.0 J/cm^2 4.5-5.0 J/cm^2	Single or multiple Single	2-3 wk 2-3 wk	Physician's Companion or Operator's Manual Physician's Companion or Operator's Manual: Garden J: Treatment of cutaneous hemangiomas by the flashlamp pumped PDL*: Prospective analysis J Pediatr 1992. 120, No. 4, Part I:555; Geronemus RG: PDL* treatment of vascular lesions in children. J Dermatol Surg Oncol 1993; 19:303-310. After growth controlled, treat as for PWS.
Rosacea	5 mm	6.0-7.5 J/cm^2	Single	6-8 wk	Lowe NJ, et al.: Flashlamp PDL* for rosacea-associated telangiectasia and erythema. J Dermatol Surg Oncol 1991; 17:522.
Scars	5 mm	6.0-8.0 J/cm^2	Single	6-8 wk	Physician's Companion; Operator's Manual; Alster T: Improvement of erythematous & hypertrophic scars by the 585-nm flashlamp-pumped PDL* Ann Plastic Surg 1994; 32:186-190
Warts	5 mm	6.0-9.0 J/cm^2	Single or multiple	2-3 wk	Physician's Companion; Operator's Manual; Tan OT: PDL* treatment of recalcitrant verrucae: A preliminary report. Lasers Surg Med 1993; 13:127-137, or Borovoy M et al. PDL:* Effective for plantar verrucae. Clin Laser Monthly, May 1994. Except on face, pare warts down before treating.

7-mm or 10-mm spot recommendation: If no suggested energy above, when using the 7-mm or 10-mm spot size, both test spots and a reduction of energy (1.0-2.0 J/cm^2) are recommended. (from Operator's Manual).
2 × 7 mm elliptical spot: Guideline has not been established. Start at same energy as 5-mm and adjust as needed. *PDL = Pulsed Dye Laser
Revised 10/96

Candela Pigmented/Tattoo Lesion Treatment Guideline

This guideline sheet does not take the place of the Operators Manual or Physicians Companion book but is a summary of the information listed in these references or that listed with each type of lesion below. For more details, please refer to these references. Only the lasers that are applicable for treatment of the specific lesions listed will be mentioned.

LESION	Q-SWITCHED LASER	SPOT SIZE	ENERGY DENSITY	RETREAT	COMMENTS/RFFERENCE
Lentigines, age spots, freckles, cafe au lait	PLDL (510 nm)	3 mm 5 mm	1.5–3.0 J/cm² 2–4.0 Jcm²	6–8 wk	Day TW: Preliminary experience with a flashlamp-pulsed tunable dye laser for treatment of benign pigmented lesions. Fitzpatrick RE, et al.: Laser Treatment of benign pigmented epidermal lesions using a 300 nsecond pulse and 510 nm wavelength. J Dermatol Surg Oncol 1993; 19:341–347; Alster TS: Complete elimination of large café-au-lait birthmarks by the 510 nm PDL. Plastic Reconstr Surg 1995; 96 1660–1664.
	Nd:YAG (532 nm)	2 mm	2–4.0 J/cm²	4–8 wk	Kilmer SI et al.: Treatment of epidermal pigmented lesions with the frequency-doubled Q-switched Nd:YAG Laser. Arch Dermatol 1994; 130:1515–1519. Lask GP, Glassberg E: Neodymium: Yttrium–aluminum-garnet laser for the treatment of cutaneous lesions. Clin Dermatol 1995; 13: 81–86.
	Alex (755 nm)	2 mm 3 mm 4 mm	10–12 J/cm² 5–6 J/cm² 3–4 J/cm²	4–6 wk	Operator's Manual:
Nevus of Ota	PLTL/Alexandrite (755 nm)	3 mm	6.0–8.0 J/cm²	12 wk	White paper: A Clinical Test Report: Treatment of Nevus of Ota and Other Pigmented Lesions Using the Candela Q-switched Alexandrite Laser, Hayashi, H., 1994.
	AlexLazr (755 nm)	3 mm 4 mm	4.75–7 J/cm²	8–12 wk	Alster TS, Williams CM: Treatment of nevus of Ota by the Q-switched alexandrite laser, Dermatol Surg 1995; 21: 592–596.
Blue/black/green tattoos	PLTL/Alexandrite (755 nm)	3 mm	6.0–8.0 J/cm²	8–12 wk	Fitzpatrick RE, Goldman MP: Tattoo removal using the alexandrite laser. Arch Dermatol 1994; 130:1508–1514; and Amir N: Alexandrite laser offers tattoo removal without scarring or skin texture changes. J Clin Laser Med Surg 1993; 11:263–266.
Blue/black/green/red or purple tattoos	AlexLazr (755 nm)	3 mm 4 mm	5–10 J/cm² 4–5.5 J/cm²	6–8 wk	Operators Manual: Alster TS: Q-switched alexandrite laser treatment (755 nm) of professional and amateur tattoos. J Am Acad Dermatol 1995; 33:69–74 or Stafford TJ, et al: Removal of colored tattoos with the Q-switched alexandrite laser. Plastic Reconstr Surg 1995; 95:313–320.
Blue-black tattoos Red/green tattoos	Nd:YAG (1064 nm)	2 mm 3 mm	10–12 J/cm² 6.0 J/cm²	6–8 wk	Lask G, Glassberg E: Neodymium: yttrium-aluminum-garnet laser for the treatment of cutaneous lesions. Clin Dermatol 1995; 13:81–86.
Red tattoos	Nd:YAG (532 nm) PLDL (510 nm)	2 mm 3 mm, 5 mm	4–5.0 J/cm² 3.0–3.75 J/cm²	6–8 wk	Grekin RC, et al.: 510 nm Pigmented lesion dye laser: Its characteristics and clinical uses. J Dermatol Surg Oncol 1993; 19:380–387.

Note: It is recommended that all new patients receive test pulses, using the *lowest* recommended fluences first, until the post-op results show a safe and effective treatment. If pinpoint bleeding occurs when treating tattoos with alexandrite laser, reduce energy 0.5 J/cm² and test again. Continue to lower energy until little to no pinpoint bleeding present.

SkinLight Treatment Guideline

This table represents conservative and basic parameters. It is recommended to start with basic parameters, and then if necessary, modify the parameters to achieve the desired tissue effect.

LESION TYPE	ENERGY/PULSE (MJ)	SPOT DIAMETER (MM)	ENERGY DENSITY (J/CM²)	NO. OF LASER PASSES NEEDED FOR LESION PER SESSION	NO. OF PATIENTS	TOTAL NO. OF LESIONS	NO. OF TREATMENTS REQUIRED	FOLLOW-UP MEAN (MONTHS)	FOLLOW-UP RANGE (MONTHS)	DEGREE OF LESION CLEARANCE (%)
Seborrheic warts	300–500	3–5	4–5	3–10	6	18	1	8	1–15	100
Senile lentigo	250–500	3–5	4–6	2–5	5	10	1–2	10	1–15	100
Epidermal nevi	250–300	3–5	3–4	3–5	6	15	1	6	3–15	100
Chloasma	350–500	5–7	1.3–1.7	2–5	2	2	5	6	1–9	80
Milia	100–300	2–3	3–4	2–5	3	60	1	8	6–14	100
Xanthelasma palpebrarum	450–550	3–5	5–7	5–15	6	25	1	3	1–10	100
Hydroadenoma	400–800	3–5	5–7	5–10	3	45	2–3	5.5	2–11	70–95
Plantar warts	350–500	3–5	4–5	3–5	6	8	1	8	4–12	100
Actinic keratosis	300	4	2.4	2–4	5	5	1	13.5	12–15	100
Fibroepithelial papillomata	300	4	2.4	2–5	3	21	1	4.3	3–7	100
Tattoos	500–900	2–5	10–30	1–4	3	3	1–2	3	2–5	70–100
Hypertrophic scars	500–900	2–5	10–30	5–15	6	20	3–4	5.3	1–9	50–95
Acne scars*	100–500	3–7	0.5–1.5	1–3	2	2	1–2	8	5–11	30
Wrinkles*	300–500	3–8	1.5–5	1–2	6	6	1	6	3–15	30–50

*Coagulation mode, for all others, use ablation mode (see energy density sheet).

Energy Density Table

ENERGY (mJ)	ENERGY DENSITY (J/cm^2)			
	1.5 mm spot	*3 mm spot*	*5 mm spot*	*7 mm spot*
100	5.8	1.4	.52	.27
200	11.6	2.9	1.0	.53
300	17.3	4.3	1.6	.79
400	23.1	5.8	2.1	1.06
500	28.9	7.2	2.6	1.33
600	34.7	8.7	3.1	1.59
700	40.4	10.1	3.6	1.86
800	46.2	11.6	4.2	2.12
900	52.0	13.0	4.7	2.39
1000	57.8	14.4	5.2	2.65

Ablation/coagulation modes: Energy densities just below ablation threshold result in a combination of ablation and coagulation modes. Therefore it is recommended for the beginning practitioner to start with the basic energy densities which are:
Ablation mode: Basic energy density in ablation mode = 2.5 J/cm^2.
Coagulation mode: Basic energy density in coagulation mode = 1 J/cm^2.
According to the effect on tissue with the basic energy density settings, adjust energy until the desired effect is achieved.
ref. Fotona Medical Laser Report, Dermatology and Aesthetic Surgery Vol. 1.2.

Continuum Biomedical*

Treatment Parameter Update: CB Diode/532 Diode Pumped Nd:YAG

Facial Telangiectasias

The preferable spot size for treating facial telangiectasias is 400 microns. The 800 micron spot can be used, but increases the pain factor and will often times require a longer exposure time. This in turn can cause increased epidermal damage (i.e., whitening and subsequent scabbing)

INITIAL SETTINGS

400 micron spot size—20–25 milliseconds "on" time repetition rate—4 Hz or 10 Hz—depending on user's comfort. (It is preferable to use 10 Hz if the user can handle it, because 10 Hz yields a smoother treatment technique).

If the vessel disappears at this setting without "whitening" of the epidermis, the treatment is complete. If there is "whitening" then shorten the exposure time by 2 milliseconds and continue treating. Again observe the treatment. If you again see "whitening" shorten the exposure and repeat as above. Conversely, if you do not see the vessel disappear, increase the exposure time by 2 milliseconds until you see the vessels disappear with little or no "whitening."

Most facial vessels can be treated with 35 milliseconds or less. If the user is unsuccessful in his treatment, he is most likely missing the vessel. Treating with the 800 micron spot enables the user to "hit" the vessel easier. The treatment regimen for the 800 micron spot size is exactly the same as for the 400 micron spot size except you will need to start at 25 to 30 milliseconds and will usually treat at

*From Continuum Biomedical, a Medical Division of Continuum Electro-Optics, Inc., Dublin, CA.

longer "on" time exposures than with the 400 micron spot. This is due to the significantly higher energy densities available with the 400 micron spot size.

Pigmented Lesions

The successful treatment of pigmented lesions with the diode laser is a result of carefully controlling the deposition of light on the pigmented lesion in order to in turn, control the heating of the lesion. The clinical end point that is desirable is a "graying" or "darkening" of the lesion. Consequently, there are many possible settings to choose from. Working with the 1.2 mm spot size hand piece is more desirable than the smaller spot sizes. An "on time" of approximately 30 milliseconds should work fine because the user will treat repeatedly until the appropriate color change occurs.

Some users have experimented with adding an additional chromophore to the pigmented lesion (such as marking the lesion with a black surgical marker) to increase the absorption. This works well because the lesion literally peels off after treatment. Again, the parameters are the same as above.

Leg Veins

Visible blood vessels of the lower extremities are the most difficult vascular lesions to successfully treat. The underlying pathological problems which lead to the appearance of these vessels are varied and this adds to the complexity of the treatment scenarios. The CB Diode/532 laser should not be viewed as a primary treatment source for leg veins, but plays an adjunctive role for the treatment of these vessels.

Standard therapies include: microvascular surgery and sclerotherapy. Both of these procedures have advantages and drawbacks but have been recognized to reduce the amounts of vessels present. The additional use of the CB Diode/532 Laser enhances the overall effectiveness of the final result. The typical settings used are very similar to the settings used for facial telangiectasias, except a longer exposure time is usually chosen. Exposure times of 35–45 milliseconds will deliver more energy to these leg veins. Although the thermal relaxation time of vessels on the face and legs may be similar if they are of similar size, the added problem of hydrostatic pressure (gravity, etc.) adds significantly to the leg vein treatment limitations.

Consequently, the complexity of treating leg veins increases and requires a combined therapeutic approach. Most commonly, the CB Diode/532 Laser is used in conjunction with injection sclerotherapy. There exists no exact protocol to follow. The treatment seems to be most effective if the laser is used to treat remaining vessels after sclerotherapy has been completed. Clearly, as in standard sclerotherapy, the best results are attained after repeated treatments.

There has been some interesting information gathered on using the laser first and then doing the sclerotherapy within 7–10 days. When using the laser first, some apparent damage is done to the endothelial lining of the vessel wall, which in turn, enhances the sclerotherapy's effectiveness. Again, repeat therapies are necessary, but there seem to be fewer treatments necessary.

Another recommendation is to cool the surface of the leg before treating. Because the exposure times for treating leg veins are longer than those used for treating facial vessels, the patient will feel increased pain due to the increased heating of the skin. The use of a simple icepack (Ammonium Chloride—"crush" packets available at pharmacies for use by sports teams) work very well, with no mess. Applying the cold pack in the area to be treated prior to treatment and then moving it along as you commence treatment, significantly reduces pain. As is commonly done, reapplying an ice pack after treatment also is helpful.

Overview and Update: Treatment Parameters & Techniques

Following the completion of protocol studies, four years of further clinical experience has led to the revision and fine tuning of several treatment parameters and techniques. An overview of current treatment methods is outlined.

I. Medlite Q-Switched Nd:YAG Laser Treatment Parameters*

A. TATTOO TX @ 1064NM

1. Indicated for black, dark blue, and difficult-to-treat inks.
2. Turn the power all the way up, then lower power by ¼ to ½ turn and take test pulse. Look for a crisp, bright white spot.
3. If bleeding or fragmentation of the skin is noted, turn

the power down. If the spot is not bright white (i.e., if it seems yellowish), increase the power.
4. Usually begin treatment at 5–6 J/cm^2 with the 3mm spot size; and with 3–4 J/cm^2 when using the 4mm spot size.

B. TATTOO TX @ 532NM

1. Indicated for red, orange, and purple inks.
2. Turn the power all the way up. Then lower power by ¼ to ½ turn and take test pulse. Look for a crisp, bright white spot.
3. If bleeding or skin fragmentation is noted, turn the power down. If the spot is not bright white (i.e., if it seems yellowish), increase the power.
4. Usually begin treatment at 3–4 J/cm^2 with 3mm spot size, 2–3 J/cm^2 with 4mm spot size.

C. PIGMENTED LESION TX @ 532NM

1. Indicated for freckles, solar lentigos, cafe-au-lait macules, liver spots, etc.
2. Usually begin at 2–3 J/cm^2 with the 3mm spot size (or 1–2 J/cm^2 with the 4mm spot size) and adjust power up or down according to tissue effect. Look for the same bright white spot as with tattoos.
3. Lighter lesions require more power.
4. Use lower power on darker complexions.
5. Black or very darkly pigmented skin should not be treated with 532nm. Try 1064nm first, and only use 532nm if no clearing occurred with first treatment.

D. VASCULAR LESION TX @ 532NM

1. Telangiectasia (small veins), angiomas, hemangiomas, some port wine stains (not children).
2. Usually begin at 3–4 J/cm^2 with the 3mm spot size and adjust power up or down according to tissue effect. The vessel must be obliterated in order to clear it, so expect to see some bleeding.

E. DERMAL MELANOCYTOSIS TX @ 1064NM

1. Indicated for Nevus of Ota, aberrant Mongolian spot.
2. Using the 3mm spot size, recommended start treatment value is 5–6 J/cm^2. Using the 4mm spot size, begin treatment at 3–4 J/cm^2. (Note: recommended energy settings are similar to those used in tattoo treatment.)
3. Expect to see whitening at first, followed by punctate hemorrhages within a few minutes.
4. Treatment intervals should be at least 8–12 weeks. Multiple treatments required.

II. General Guidelines for Q-Switched Lasers

A. Pulses should be overlapped slightly in order to cover the entire area.

*Sections I and II have been edited by David J. Goldberg, M.D., The Skin Laser Center of New Jersey, Westwood, NJ.

B. Patients should be treated at 8 week intervals for tattoos, and 4–6 weeks for pigmented and vascular lesions.

C. Most tattoos require at least 4–8 treatments (some more, some less). Pigmented and vascular lesions usually require only one treatment, occasionally two.

D. The power will probably need to be increased from the initial settings in most applications, but better to start low.

E. Remember the importance of cleaning the handpiece optics, thoroughly, yet gently. Use only methanol (available at pharmacies) and lense tissue on the optics. Both harsh and insufficient cleaning will damage the optics. Never use an optic with a damaged lens coating. This will cause back reflection, which will in turn burn mirrors in the articulated arm.

III. Post-Operative Care*

A. TATTOO TREATMENT

1. Apply anti-bacterial ointment (Mycitracin+, Bacitracin, Polysporin).
2. Cover with Telpha or Vigilon or Spenco Second Skin dressing.
3. Keep the site moist with ointment for the first ten days. Do not let the area dry out or scab. This is especially important during the first 48 hours.
4. Patient may shower, but should not scrub the area until healed.
5. Patient should avoid scratching the area during the healing process.
6. Patient may feel discomfort for the first 24 hours and may need non-aspirin pain medication.
7. The skin should heal normally within 10–14 days.
8. The tattoo will look foggy and begin its fading process over the next month. Fading is typically 30 to

*Section III has been contributed by Milton Waner, M.D., University of Arkansas School for Medical Science Little Rock, AR.

50% with each treatment. The total fading process can take up to 8 weeks after each treatment. Green inks fade slower and can take up to 16 weeks for maximum fading.

9. Sunscreen is recommended until healing is completed.

B. PIGMENTED LESIONS

1. An immediate post treatment dose of antibiotic ointment should be adequate for 90% of patients.
2. If slight bleeding or blistering should occur, apply a thin film of antibiotic ointment (Mycitracin+, Bacitracin or Polysporin) for 3–5 days.
3. Patient may shower, but should not scrub the area until healed.
4. Patient should avoid scratching the area during the healing process.
5. The skin should heal normally in 7–12 days.
6. After the redness subsides, the pigment may still be present. It will gradually lighten over the next 3–4 weeks. It is very important that the patient avoids direct sun exposure within 8 weeks of treatment. A sunscreen with a high protective rating should be used to prevent recurrence.
7. Large treatment areas (cafe au lait, etc.) will require post operative care similar to tattoo treatments.

C. VASCULAR LESIONS

1. For slight bleeding or blistering, apply a thin film of antibiotic ointment (Mycitracin+, Bacitracin or Polysporin) for 3–5 days.
2. Patient may shower, but should not scrub the area until healed.
3. Patient should avoid scratching the area during the healing process.
4. Purpura will clear and the skin should heal normally in 7–12 days.

PhotoDerm VL Treatment Parameters

TREATMENT INDICATION	SKIN TYPE	BUTTON	PULSE TYPE	PULSE DURATION (MSEC)	PULSE DELAYS (MSEC)	FLUENCE J/CM²	FILTER	GEL TEMPERATURE
Port wine stain	Light	PWS/L	Single	2.5		20	515	Room temp.
Child-type	Dark	PWS/D	Single	3		22	550	Room temp.
Hemangiomas	Light	H/L	Double	3.0, 2.0	10	30	550	Cold
	Dark	H/D	Triple	3,0, 2.0, 1.7	10, 10	38	570	Cold
Facial telangiecta-sia	Light	Face/L	Single	3		22	515	Room temp.
	Dark	Face/D	Double	2.6, 1.8	10	30	550	Room temp.
Leg veins (<0.4 mm)	Light	LV1/L	Single	3		22	515	Room temp.
	Dark	LV1/D	Double	2.4, 2.4	10	35	550	Room temp.
Leg veins (0.4 ~ 1.0 mm)	Light	LV2/L	Double	2.4, 2.4	10	37	550	Cold
	Dark	LV2/D	Double	2.4, 2,4	10	37	570	Cold
Leg Veins (>1.0 mm)	Light	LV3/L	Triple	3.8, 3.1, 2.5	20, 20	50	570	Cold
	Dark	LV3/D	Triple	3.8, 3.1, 2.5	30, 30	50	590	Cold

TREATMENT INDICATION	VESSEL SIZE	SKIN TYPE	PULSE TYPE	PULSE DURATION (MSEC)	PULSE DELAYS (MSEC)	FLUENCE J/CM²	FILTER	GEL
Telangiectatic matting	<0.4 mm	Light	Double	2.7, 3.2	10	37	550	Room temp.
		Dark	Double	3, 2	10	35	570	Room temp.
Adult-type port wine stain	>0.4 mm	Light	Triple	3.2, 2.6, 2.1	20, 20	44	550	Cold
		Dark	Triple	3.2, 2,6, 2.1	30, 30	44	570	Cold
Facial/truncal telangiectasia	0.4 mm	Light	Triple	3.2, 2.6, 2.1	20, 20	45	570	Cold
	1.0 mm	Dark	Triple	3.2, 2.6, 2.1	30, 30	45	590	Cold
Hemangiomas	>0.4 mm	Light	Triple	3.2, 2.6, 2.1	30, 30	45	570	Cold
		Dark	Triple	3, 3, 3	30, 30	60	590	Cold

PhotoDerm PL Treatment Parameters

CLINICAL INDICATION	SKIN TYPE	FILTER	FLUENCE (J/CM²)	PULSE MODE	PULSE DURATION (MSEC)	PULSE DELAYS (MSEC)
Epidermal	I, II	515	25	Single	3	
	III, IV	570	25	Single	3.5	
	V	590	25	Single	3	
Junctional	I, II	570	35	Double	3/3	10
	III, IV	590	35	Double	3/3	20
	V	615	35	Double	3/3	20
Dermal nevi and hemosiderin stain	I, II	590	40	Triple	2.5/2.5/2.5	20/20
	III, IV	615	40	Triple	2.5/2.5/2.5	20/20
	V	645	45	Triple	2.5/2.5/2.5	20/20
Tattoos	Yellow/Red	515	25	Single	3	
	Green	570	25	Single	3.5	
	Blue	590	25	Single	3.5	
	Black	590	25	Single	3.5	

Laserscope
Luxor

Parameter Settings

CUTANEOUS LESIONS	ORION/AURA STARPULSE PARAMETERS	FLUENCE (J/CM²)	PULSE WIDTH (MSEC)	FREQUENCY (PPS)
Port wine stain	SmartScan			Various Sizes
Pink		15	5	
Purple		15–20	3–5	
Red		15	3	
Venous lake	1-mm Dermastat	15–20	10–15	1–3
	2-mm Dermastat	9–15	10	1–3
AVM	1-mm Dermastat	15	30	1
	2-mm Dermastat	6–10	30	1
Facial telangiectasia—distinct linear,	250 μm Dermastat	45–70	10–20	4–5
or arborizing	1-mm Dermastat (female)	14–18	10–20	1–5
	1-mm Dermastat (male)	15–20	10–20	1–5
2-mm Dermastat	12–16	10–20	1–5	
Facial telangiectasia—matted	SmartScan	12–14	8–10	Various sizes
Leg veins (superficial)	1-mm Dermastat (<1-mm lesion)	26–28	15	2–3
	2-mm Dermastat (1–2 lesion)	14–20	15	2–3
Leg veins (very superficial)	1-mm Dermastat (<1-mm lesion)	26–28	10	2–3
	2-mm Dermastat (1–2-mm lesion)	14–20	10	2–3
Spider angioma	SmartScan	20	10–15	KTP
Syringoma	1-mm Dermastat	20	10	1
Café-au-lait spot	1-mm Dermastat	18–20	3–5	2–3
	2-mm Dermastat	8–10	3–5	2–3
	SmartScan	18–20	3–5	Various sizes
Warts	1-mm Dermastat	30–40	20–30	1–3
Nevus spilus	SmartScan	15	10	KTP
Solar lentigo	SmartScan	12–18	2–10	KTP (treat twice)
	2-mm Dermastat	7–12	2–10	2–3, KTP (treat twice)
Posttraumatic	1-mm Dermastat	12–19	3	2–3
Hyperpigmentation	2-mm Dermastat	10–16	3	2–3
Cherry angioma	1-mm Dermastat	16–20	15	1–2
	2-mm Dermastat	8–10	15	1–2

Always use ultrasound or KY jelly and always keep the Dermastat perpendicular to the skin.
The chart above indicates a Laserscope Delivery Device (instrument) and laser parameter(s) (settings) by lesion type as reported to us by clinicians successfully treating a variety of cutaneous lesions.

Superpulse Programs in Repeat Exposure

	MSEC	HZ	% ON	PROGRAM	AVERAGE POWER (W)				
					2	4	6	8	10
Light Ablation	10	2	2	A1	.04	.08	.12	.16	.20
with increasing repetition	10	5	5	A2	.01	.2	.3	.4	.5
rate for faster manual	10	10	10	A3	.2	.4	.6	.8	1.0
scanning	10	15	15	A4	.3	.6	.9	1.2	1.5
A1–A6	10	20	20	A5	.4	.8	1.2	1.6	2.0
	10	30	30	A6	.6	1.2	1.8	2.4	3.0
Medium Ablation	15	2	3	A10	.06	.62	.18	.24	.30
with increasing repetition	15	5	8	A11	1.6	3.2	4.8	6.4	8.0
rate for faster manual	15	10	15	A12	.3	.6	.9	1.2	1.5
scanning	15	15	23	A13	.46	.92	1.38	1.84	2.30
A10–A14	15	20	30	A14	.6	1.2	1.8	2.4	3.0
	15	30	45	C1	.9	1.8	2.7	3.6	4.5

Superpulse Programs in Repeat Exposure Continued

	MSEC	HZ	% ON	PROGRAM	AVERAGE POWER (W)				
					2	4	6	8	10
Heavy Ablation	20	30	60	C2	1.2	2.4	3.6	4.8	6.0
or Cutting	25	30	75	C3	1.5	3.0	4.5	6.0	7.5
C1–C3	50	2	10	P21	.2	.4	.6	.8	1.0
	50	10	50	P22	1.0	2.0	3.0	4.0	5.0
	100	2	20	P23	.4	.8	1.2	1.6	2.0
	100	5	50	P24	1.0	2.0	3.0	4.0	5.0
	200	2	40	P25	.8	1.6	2.4	3.2	4.0
	500	1	50	P26	1.0	2.0	3.0	4.0	5.0

Exposure Programs—NovaScan "E"

SCANS PER SECOND	ON TIME (MSEC)	PROGRAM	1	2	3	4	5	6	7	8	9
2	60	E2	.1	.2	.4	.5	.6	.7	.8	1.0	1.1
3	60	E3	.2	.4	.5	.7	.9	1.1	1.3	1.4	1.6
4	60	E4	.2	.5	.7	1.0	1.2	1.4	1.7	1.9	2.2
5	60	E5	.3	.6	.9	1.2	1.5	1.8	2.1	2.4	2.7
6	60	E6	.4	.7	1.1	1.4	1.8	2.2	2.5	2.9	3.2
7	60	E7	.4	.8	1.3	1.7	2.1	2.5	2.9	3.4	3.8
8	60	E8	.5	1.0	1.4	1.9	2.4	2.9	3.4	3.8	4.3
9	60	E9	.5	1.1	1.6	2.2	2.7	3.2	3.8	4.3	5.0
10	60	E10	.6	1.2	1.8	2.4	3.0	3.6	4.2	4.8	5.4
11	60	E11	.7	1.3	2.0	2.6	3.3	4.0	4.6	5.3	5.9
12	60	E12	.7	1.4	2.2	2.9	3.6	4.3	5.0	5.8	6.5
13	60	E13	.8	1.6	2.3	3.1	3.9	4.7	5.5	6.2	7.0
14	60	E14	.8	1.7	2.5	3.4	4.2	5.0	5.9	6.7	7.6
15	60	E15	.9	1.8	2.7	3.6	4.5	5.4	6.3	7.2	8.1
16	60	E16	1.0	1.9	2.9	3.8	4.8	5.8	6/7	7.7	8.6
2	120	E22	.2	.5	.7	1.0	1.2	1.4	1.7	1.9	2.2
3	120	E23	.4	.7	1.1	1.4	1.8	2.2	2.5	2.9	3.2
4	120	E24	.5	1.0	1.4	1.9	2.4	2.9	3.4	3.8	4.3
5	120	E25	.6	1.2	1.8	2.4	3.0	3.6	4.2	4.8	5.4
6	120	E26	.7	1.4	2.2	2.9	3.6	4.3	5.0	5.8	6.5
7	120	E27	.8	1.7	2.5	3.4	4.2	5.0	5.9	6.7	7.6
8	120	E28	1.0	1.9	2.9	3.8	4.8	5.8	6.7	7.7	8.6

MilliJoules Per Scan

	1W	2W	3W	4W	5W	6W	7W	8W	9W
E2–E16	60	120	180	240	300	360	420	480	540
E22–E28	120	240	360	480	600	720	840	960	1080

Sharplan*

Exposure Programs—Novascan "F"

MSEC	NUMBER OF SCANS	PROGRAM
60	1	F1
120	2	F2
180	3	F3
240	4	F4
300	5	F5
360	6	F6
420	7	F7
480	8	F8
540	9	F9
600	10	F10
660	11	F11
720	12	F12
780	13	F13
840	14	F14
900	15	F15
960	16	F16
1020	17	F17
1080	18	F18
1140	19	F19
1200	20	F20
1260	21	F21
1320	22	F22
1380	23	F23
1440	24	F24
1500	25	F25
1560	26	F26
1620	27	F27
1680	28	F28
3000	50	F50

*From Sharplan Lasers, Allendale, NJ.

Safe Start Settings for Laser Procedures

SKIN RESURFACING WITH CO_2 SILKLASERS

FeatherTouch 200-mm HP	36–40 W
FeatherTouch 260-mm HP	65–70 W
SilkTouch 200-mm HP	14–16 W
150XJ DM Scanner Pulse Mode	350 mJ–20% density
150XJ DM Scanner Flash Mode	65 W–10% density

HAIR TRANSPLANT RECIPIENT SITES WITH CO_2 SILKLASERS

SilkTouch Mode 0.6-mm hole	45 W/0.1 sec on time
SilkTouch Mode 0.9-mm hole	70 W/0.1 sec on time
SilkTouch Mode 1.2-mm hole	110 W/0.1 sec on time

HAIR REMOVAL WITH RUBY SILKLASER

EpiTouch Long-Pulse Mode	25 J

TATTOO REMOVAL WITH RUBY SILKLASER

EpiTouch Q-Switch Mode	6–10 J

NOTE: The above parameters are based on average patient conditions and skin types; these are general guidelines and in no way substitute for clinical training on the various procedures and in-servicing on the operation of the equipment. Effective settings may change over time as technology and clinical experience evolve.

PATIENT INFORMATION AND PATIENT RELEASES: SOME EXAMPLES USED BY THE EDITORS

Flashpump Dye Laser Therapy of Vascular Skin Lesions

Nicholas J. Lowe

What Is a Port Wine Stain or Hemangioma?

A port wine hemangioma is an abnormal collection or network of blood vessels present beneath a layer of otherwise normal skin. This dense network of vessels is a reminder of extra blood vessel tissue that was present during the first month of embryologic life. Port wine hemangiomas are so named because the skin appears as though a red, pink, or purple liquid has been poured over it.

What Is the Natural History of a Port Wine Hemangioma?

Port wine hemangiomas are present on the skin at birth and appear to grow at the same rate as the surrounding tissue. In other words, they keep pace with the normal adjacent skin as far as size is concerned. In the third, fourth, or fifth decade of life, however, they may become thicker or spongier than the adjacent normal skin. Furthermore, the surface of the hemangioma, which may have been quite smooth during the first decades of life, may develop an irregular and lumpy "cobblestone" appearance by the time the patient is in his or her 40s, 50s, or 60s. Fortunately, port wine hemangiomas are neither dangerous nor malignant.

What Treatments Are Available for Port Wine Hemangiomas?

Many forms of therapy have been used on port wine hemangiomas in the past; most have been abandoned because they create another deformity that is as undesirable as the port wine hemangioma itself. Surgeons have removed these areas and then reconstructed the defect with flaps or skin grafts. Such procedures entail a substantial amount of surgery, and the scars that result are often objectionable. X-rays, used in the past, are known to be potentially dangerous and are no longer used to treat port wine hemangiomas. A variety of agents have been injected into the involved skin but without any considerable success. Also ineffective has been the use of dry ice and carbon dioxide. Tattooing has been tried to camouflage these hemangiomas, but this method of treatment appears to be temporary and merely camouflages the birthmark.

Spider Veins

Spider veins are prominent and dilated (widened) blood vessels that are frequently present on the head and neck as well as the legs.

Treatment for Spider Hemangiomas, Spider Veins, or Telangiectasia

These blood vessels frequently increase with age, and a variety of treatments have been attempted, including cauterization, injections of sclerosing solutions into the vessels, and different forms of lasers.

For dilated vessels on the head, neck, trunk, and thighs, the flashpump dye laser is an effective treatment in many patients. For dilated blood vessels and veins on the lower leg, sclerosing vein injections are considered to be superior. Some of these veins can also be treated with a combination of sclerosing vein injections and flashpump dye laser therapy.

Laser Therapy

Two currently used lasers are the flashpump dye laser and the argon laser. The flashpump dye laser has major advantages in that it produces less pain and less risk of scarring than the argon laser.

145

Can the Flashpump Dye Laser Be Used for Children?

The flashpump dye laser is ideally suited to the treatment of port wine hemangiomas in children. In general, the earlier the port wine stain is treated, the better the results. Some children and infants are able to tolerate this procedure extremely well. Other children are disturbed by any procedure, and the use of sedation is often necessary. General anesthesia can be used if they are unable to tolerate the laser therapy.

How Does the Flashpump Dye Laser Work?

The dye laser generates a very powerful yellow light. It carries enormous energy that can be finely focused. When this light contacts the skin, the red color of the birthmark absorbs the light, which then releases its energy as heat. The heat coagulates, or cauterizes, the small vessels under the skin. In theory, the overlying skin is not affected by this laser. As a practical matter, however, some of the laser energy is absorbed by the outer layer of skin (epidermis), which can result in temporary scale, crust, and pigmentation.

What Will the Laser Treatment Feel Like?

The flashpump dye laser produces much less pain or discomfort than argon or carbon dioxide lasers. However, a small amount of discomfort does result from this treatment. It has been likened to the flicking of an elastic band against the skin. Most patients find this to be tolerable. Others require cream or injection of an anesthetic into the skin area to be treated (local anesthesia). Ice can also help reduce the discomfort.

A small skin area will be used as a test site, and a decision will be made about the need for local anesthesia.

What Is the Sequence of Healing After a Laser Treatment?

The immediate effect of the laser treatment is that tiny blood vessels under the skin are coagulated, which causes the area to turn a much darker color. These changes usually persist for approximately 1 to 2 weeks. During the time, the patient should apply antibiotic ointment (Polysporin), especially at night, to prevent the scab from forming. The area should be kept as clean as possible. The scab or crust must not be picked or scratched, since this can increase the chance of scarring or permanent pigment change. Improvement, fading of the treated skin, can take between 8 and 12 weeks to reach its maximum. This laser therapy should not result in scarring, but some patients have increased or decreased pigment (skin color) for several weeks or months. Rare cases of pigment changes have lasted up to 2 years. Extremely rare cases of permanent pigment change have been reported.

What Are the Hazards, Complications, and Limitations of Laser Treatment?

There are several potential hazards and limitations in this treatment program. It is important to realize that the laser may not completely eliminate a hemangioma. At best, the laser may cause a marked lightening of the birthmark, so that birthmarks that are deep purple may become lighter in color and birthmarks that are deep red will become light pink. Usually, patients are able to switch from a thick, heavy makeup, such as Covermark or Dermablend, to one that is more normal and easier to apply. Although extremely rare with laser therapy, the possibility of scarring does exist.

Finally, there is no way of predicting what long-term, undesirable, or unusual side effects may occur as a result of laser treatments. Every new treatment method raises the possibility that unsuspected effects may be created that will not become evident for many years after treatment. However, many types of lasers have been used in medicine for more than 15 years, and so far there is no evidence of unsuspected side effects. This finding does not guarantee that they will not occur or be discovered at some time in the distant future. We also are not completely certain whether some treated hemangiomas could return years after treatment.

Costs of Treatment and Insurance Coverage

There is no guarantee that medical insurance will cover the costs of laser treatments. Some insurance companies consider the treatment purely cosmetic. Each patient or patient's family should check with the insurance carrier to determine whether treatments will be covered. Treatment fees will be discussed with each patient at the time of consultations, and questions about such fees are welcome.

We do not guarantee results. We guarantee only that this office and physicians will use their best efforts and best judgment on your behalf.

I confirm that I have read the information provided in the Flashpump dye laser therapy of vascular skin lesions consent form. I have discussed this with my physician and understand the information provided.

I hereby authorize Dr. _____ and his/her delegated associates to perform and assist in the laser procedure.

_____

Patient's Signature/Date

_____

Witness/Date

Laser Therapy for Pigmented Lesions and Tattoos

Nicholas J. Lowe

Now there are safer and more effective treatments for tattoos, brown birthmarks, age (or liver) spots, freckles, nevi of Ota, and other benign cutaneous pigmented lesions of the skin. The Q-switched ruby laser is a medical breakthrough that allows selective treatment of the melanosomes of a benign lesion while leaving surrounding tissue relatively *unharmed*. In fact, the laser is not only safer for treating brown birthmarks in infants but is also more effective in treating very difficult lesions, such as age spots, in adults.

What Is a Benign Pigmented Lesion?

Benign pigmented lesions are caused by an excess of pigment in the skin, usually as a result of ultraviolet light exposure and congenital factors. In the skin, there are melanin-producing cells called melanocytes that package melanin into sacs of melanosomes. An abnormal increase in either the melanosomes or melanocytes results in pigmented lesions.

What Is the Pigmented Lesion Laser?

The Q-switched ruby laser is a device that produces an intense but gentle burst of laser light that is especially optimized to treat pigmented lesions. The system's unique combination of parameters creates a thermal effect, called photothermolysis, on the excess pigment in the epidermis or dermis. The wavelength (694 nm) of the laser is optimized to be absorbed by melanosomes while minimally affecting the surrounding healthy tissue. The delivery of high peak power allows adequate power for destruction of the melanosomes, while confining the thermal effect to the targeted cells. Because of the short pulse width, there is no heat transfer and little damage to adjacent tissue.

Why Is the Laser a Safe Laser Treatment?

The laser is safer and more effective than other lasers because of its unique ability to selectively treat the melanosomes of a pigmented lesion without adversely affecting the surrounding tissue. Thus, it will eliminate many lesions while leaving the surrounding skin and skin pigment intact.

What Pigmented Conditions Are Treated With This Laser?

The most commonly treated conditions are solar lentigines, also known as age spots or liver spots, café-au-lait birth-

marks, freckles, and nevi of Ota. What all these lesions have in common is that they are made of an overabundance of melanosomes in the skin. They vary, however, in appearance. Age spots can appear as enlarged light freckles on the face and hands. Café-au-lait birthmarks can appear as light brown markings anywhere on the body and can be quite large. Freckles can also be treated, if desired. Any questionable moles, of course, require biopsy to verify that they are benign.

Why Should Someone Have a Pigmented Lesion Treated?

Many people are uncomfortable with unsightly pigmented lesions. Young adults may be embarrassed by age spots, and the lesions may affect their self-confidence. Young children or infants may suffer psychologically from teasing by other children often associated with café-au-lait birthmarks. With a safer and more effective means of treatment such as the Q-switched ruby laser, there is simply no reason to live with a pigmented lesion at any age.

What Does Treatment Involve?

Treatment with the laser varies from patient to patient depending on the type of lesion, size of the affected area, color of the patient's skin, and depth to which the abnormal pigment extends beneath the skin's surface. In general, these steps will take place:

1. The patient is asked to wear eye protection consisting of an opaque covering or goggles. Occasionally, protective contact lenses are used in treating immediately around the eye.
2. The skin's reaction to the laser is tested during the first visit to determine the most effective treatment.
3. Treatment consists of placing a small handpiece or "wand," against the surface of the skin and activating the laser. The laser is pulsed rather than continuous in its action. As many patients describe it, each pulse feels, for a fraction of a second, like the snapping of a rubber band against the skin.
4. Some lesions, such as lentigines, require only a few pulses, but others, such as café-au-lait birthmarks, require many more. Other lesions require repeated treatment, necessitating multiple patient visits.
5. Most patients do not require anesthesia. In some cases, however, depending on the nature of the lesion and the patient's age, the physician may elect to use some form of anesthesia.

Is Treatment With the Laser Painful?

The laser is more comfortable and requires less recovery time than some other treatment methods. Most adults tolerate the treatment without anesthesia, but treatment of larger lesions may be less comfortable. Children, who have a lower pain threshold, may tolerate the procedure better with sedatives or anesthesia. Parents of young patients should discuss these options with their physician.

Is It Possible to Have a Lesion Treated That Was Previously Treated by Another Modality?

Patients with previously treated pigmented lesions are often candidates for the Q-switched ruby laser. Pigmented lesions that have not been effectively removed by other treatments may respond well to the Q-switched ruby therapy, providing prior treatment did not cause excessive scarring or skin damage.

How Many Treatments Are Necessary?

The number of treatments necessary is highly variable. It is difficult to predict this number in advance. Some lesions take several treatment sessions to achieve maximum improvement. Lesions such as amateur tattoos may require 4 to 8 sessions. Professional tattoos may require 6 to 12 sessions. Some tattoos, such as multicolored ones, may not clear completely.

Are There Precautions That Should Be Taken After Treatment?

Immediately after treatment, some patients find the application of an ice pack to be soothing to the treated area. Some patients require the application of a topical antibiotic cream or ointment. It is best to apply this nightly, keeping the area moist. Care should be taken in the first few days after treatment to avoid scrubbing the area, and abrasive skin cleansers should be avoided. A bandage or patch can help to prevent abrasion of the treated area. If a scab forms, it must not be picked or scratched, since this can increase the chance of scarring or permanent pigment changes (either increased or decreased).

Are There Any Side Effects?

Unlike other methods of treatment, this laser greatly reduces the potential for scarring or changes in skin texture. However, about 5% of patients experience mild scarring. All patients experience some temporary discoloration or reddening of the skin at or around the treatment site; this can last from 5 to 7 days, depending on the skin type. Also, a scab will form at the treatment site and drop off within 7 to 10 days. Some patients also experience a lighter or darker discoloration of the skin for a few months after treatment. This usually resolves, leaving normal pigmentation, but it is rare but possible for this to persist. Rare cases of increased pigment (hyperpigmentation) have lasted up to 2 years. Rare cases of decreased pigment (hypopigmentation) can last a year. It is important to follow the recommendations of the treating physician for proper posttreatment skin care.

What Tattoos Can Be Helped?

Blue, green, and black tattoos clear most effectively. Amateur tattoos clear more completely than professional tattoos.

What Are Older and Other Ways of Removing Tattoos?

Surgery, dermabrasion, freezing, and the laser are other ways of treating pigmented lesions. All are associated with a risk of scarring.

What Are the Hazards, Complications, and Limitations of Laser Treatment?

There are several potential hazards and limitations in this treatment program. It is important to realize that the laser may not completely eliminate a pigmented lesion or tattoo. At best, the laser may cause a marked lightening of the area. Finally, there is no way of predicting what long-term, undesirable, or unusual side effects may occur as a result of laser treatments. Every new treatment method raises the possibility that unsuspected effects may be created that will not become evident for many years after treatment. However, many types of lasers have been used in medicine for more than 15 years, and so far there is no evidence of unsuspected side effects. This finding does not guarantee that they will not occur or be discovered at some time in the distant future. We also are not completely certain whether some treated problems could return years after treatment.

We do not guarantee results. We guarantee only that this office and physicians will use their best efforts and best judgments on your behalf.

I confirm that I have read the information provided in the laser therapy for pigmented lesion and tattoos consent form. I have discussed this with my physician, and understand the information provided.

I hereby authorize Dr. _____ and his/her delegated associates to perform and assist in the laser procedure.

_____

Patient's Signature/Date

_____

Witness/Date

Patient Photography Consent And Release Form

You, the undersigned, voluntarily consent to the taking, copyright, publication, and use (as indicated below) of your picture and likeness by _____ .

You agree to the following uses of these photographs (please check the categories for which you give consent):

☐ = For education or informational purposes

☐ = For general advertising, publicity, and promotional purposes

You hereby release _____ and _____ from any claim, demand, cause or action, or proceeding of whatever nature arising out of the publication and distribution of the said photographs in accordance with the terms of the release.

_____

Signature/Date

_____

Printed Name

_____

Parent/Representative Signature/Date

_____

Witness Signature/Date

We do not guarantee the results. We guarantee only that this office and physicians will use their best efforts and best judgment on your behalf.

Informed Consent and Authorization for Laser Treatment of Tattoos and Other Lesions

I understand that the procedure planned is the treatment of a decorative or traumatic tattoo or other lesion (e.g., brown spots, pregnancy mask) with the Q-switched neodymium: YAG laser using local, topical, or no anesthesia. The goal and purpose of the procedure is to attempt removal of the tattoo or lesion or to make the pattern or lesion as unrecognizable as possible by lightening the pigment.

Alternative methods include camouflage with makeup or tattooing, abrasive treatments, acid treatments, treatment with different lasers, surgical excision (cutting out) with or without tissue expansion, and skin grafting. If no treatment is performed, there is no adverse consequence to my health.

I understand the risks of this laser procedure are like for any other surgical procedure and include pain, bleeding, infection, scarring, drug reactions, and inconvenience to me during the recovery phase. The risk of scarring despite proper laser treatment exists in all cases but can be reduced by carefully following my aftercare instructions and by notifying the office if a problem develops.

In addition, I understand that there is a risk of accidental eye injury by the laser beam. This is unlikely since complete eye protection is provided at all times during the laser treatments. There is also a risk of patchy residual pigmentation or persistence of the original pigment pattern (a ghost-like appearance), change in skin texture, permanent lightening or darkening of the treated skin, hair loss at the treated site, or easy bruising of the skin after laser treatment.

I understand that, in some cases, laser treatment occasionally fails to remove all pigment, especially from professionally applied tattoos, and may not be effective on certain pigments, such as green or yellow, and may make a white tattoo darker. Multiple treatments are generally required for maximum fading or clearing.

Improvement may not be seen in the tattoo or lesion for up to 6 weeks. Laser treatments can be repeated at 4- to 6-week intervals. Continued improvement can occur for several months after treatment.

I understand that this procedure is considered cosmetic and is not covered by my health insurance. This office will not bill my insurance for this treatment. My insurance may or may not cover treatment of any complications should they arise.

I agree that any pictures taken of my treatment site can be used for publication or teaching purposes, but my name will not be disclosed.

I have discussed my proposed laser surgery in detail with the doctor or his/her assistant. I understand that all photographs I have seen are for illustration only and do not predict the result I can expect. I have been asked at this time if I have any questions about this procedure, and I do not have any. I understand the goals, alternatives, risks, and possible complications and request the laser treatment be performed on me by the doctor or his/her assistant. I understand that no guarantees or promises have been made as to the expected results or outcomes.

_____

Patient Signature/Date

_____

Physician or Assistant Signature/Date

Laser Skin Resurfacing

Gary P. Lask

What Is Laser Resurfacing?

The carbon dioxide (CO_2) laser has been used for the treatment of various conditions for more than 30 years. It emits an intense beam of light that heats and vaporizes skin tissue instantaneously; its limitation in treating skin has always been the unwanted side effect of scarring. Recent advances in technology, however, have allowed the CO_2 laser to be refined; it now works so precisely that normal surrounding tissue is hardly affected. The CO_2 laser is now the main tool in the rapidly expanding field of laser resurfacing. This procedure is usually performed on the face to remove the superficial layers of skin, softening wrinkles and stimulating the growth of new skin cells. There is also evidence that the temporary inflammation induced by the resurfacing can produce new fibers of collagen, the skin's support network, thereby increasing the turgor and strength of the skin. Thus, the overall effect can be fresher, more supple, and youthful-looking skin.

Who Would Benefit?

Patients who can benefit from this procedure are those with one or more of the following:

Wrinkling
Dull, weathered skin
Freckling
Blotchy pigmentation
Sun damage (including signs of precancer)
Shallow or saucer-shaped acne scars

Because of the nature of this procedure, persons with darker skin tones, including those of Asian, Hispanic, and African-American background, may require additional preoperative and postoperative care; the treatment could produce unwanted pigmentary alterations. It may be necessary to treat such patients with a bleaching agent before any procedure can be done.

What Is the Procedure?

Laser resurfacing is basically a controlled mechanical removal of skin. The laser selectively heats and vaporizes the superficial layers of skin. Patients feel pain during treatment if no anesthetic is used. Therefore, a local anesthetic, either as an anesthetic cream or as a nerve block injection, is usually used to block pain during treatment.

A spot test is sometimes recommended in patients with darker skin tones to check for the possible unwanted pigmentary alterations. If the spot test does not produce adverse effects, a full resurfacing procedure can be performed at a later date.

The procedure is performed on an outpatient basis and usually takes about 30 to 60 minutes, depending on the number of areas treated. After anesthesia is given, the area of concern is treated with the laser. Once the procedure is complete, a special gel-like dressing is applied to ensure that the face stays moist and protected. Depending on the patient's medical history, it may be necessary to prescribe a few days of oral antibacterial and antiviral medication to prevent infection. Pain after the procedure is variable and is often well treated by Tylenol, Advil, or other over-the-counter pain medications.

What Results Can a Patient Expect?

The effects proceed in phases:

1. Redness and swelling
2. Oozing with crust formation
3. Reformation of new skin with redness (redness usually lasts about 6 to 8 weeks but may persist as long as several months)
4. Fresher, smoother skin

What Side Effects May Occur?

Possible side effects include failure to produce the desired effect, temporary or permanent hyperpigmentation, scarring, reactivation of cold sores (herpes infection), bacterial infection, and allergy to the ointments used after the peel.

What Special Instructions Must a Patient Follow After the Peel?

All special skin care instructions for immediately after resurfacing will be given in writing after the procedure. It is our office's routine to follow the patient closely after the procedure to ensure that healing is proceeding optimally. From the time the patient leaves our office until the healing process is complete, he or she should avoid exposure to the sun. All future sun exposure should be kept to a minimum to maximize the benefits of treatment and to prevent future skin damage.

Always remember to wear sunscreen.

Laser Skin Resurfacing Posttreatment Instructions

The laser treatment will create a superficial burn wound. You may develop blisters, crusts, or scabs within 24 to 72 hours, which may last 7 to 10 days. Do not pick at the scabs or allow the skin to become abraded, as this may result in infection and scarring. The treated area will be pink after the scab separates. Loss of or increase in skin pigment in the treated area can appear. However, it is usually temporary. Tylenol is usually all that is needed for discomfort (avoid aspirin or aspirin products). Do not apply any cream or medication not prescribed by our office for at least 5 days. Avoid sun exposure until healed, and then wear a sunscreen with an SPF of 30 for 6 months. The redness usually lasts several weeks, and you will be able to cover this with makeup.

1. Starting the morning after treatment, remove your bandage in the shower. It is okay to shampoo. Make sure you rinse your face well with cool water.
2. Starting after your first morning shower, soak your wound two or three times a day for 1 or 2 minutes with distilled white vinegar rinse (mix one to two capfuls into 1 pint of water). This will help clean the honey-colored ooze around the area.
3. After each soak and as needed, apply pure Crisco to the affected areas to keep it moist. Do not allow the areas to become dry.
4. Apply cool compresses three or four times a day for 7 to 10 minutes. This may provide some relief if the area is uncomfortable and will help reduce swelling.
5. Place Crisco and a nonstick Telfa dressing on areas when you sleep at night. This will help keep the area moist. In the morning, gently remove dressing and begin soaks.
6. You will be given an antibiotic to take to help prevent infection. If you have any allergies to antibiotics, please let us know. We usually prescribe Keflex 250 mg four times a day for 7 days.
7. If you have a tendency to get cold sores, we will also prescribe a medication to help prevent this—Acyclovir 400 mg twice a day for 5 days.

My posttreatment care has been explained to me, and I understand my responsibility for properly fulfilling the after care instructions.

All of my questions have been answered.

_____

Patient Signature/Date

_____

Witness Signature/Date

Carbon Dioxide Laser Surgery Patient Advisory and Consent

I hereby authorize and direct _____, MD, and assistants of his/her choice, to perform laser treatment of _____
_____ .

I further authorize the physician(s) and assistants to do any other procedure that in their judgment may be necessary or advisable should unforeseen circumstances arise during the procedure.

I understand that there can be no warranty, either expressed or implied, as to final results. Although a good result is expected, the following list of complications on rare occasions may occur.

Complications with the carbon dioxide (CO_2) laser may include the following:

1. *Pain and discomfort:* The level of pain and discomfort varies with an individual's tolerance, and both may be experienced during treatment when no anesthetic is used. Therefore, I consent to the administration of anesthesia, as needed and appropriate.
2. *Swelling:* Immediately after laser surgery, swelling or bruising may be present, especially when the cheek or nose area has been treated. This is temporary and usually subsides in 3 to 7 days.
3. *Healing:* CO_2 laser surgery causes a superficial to deep wound, which can take several weeks to heal. The treatment results in swelling, weeping, and crusting of the wound area, which can take 1 to 4 weeks to heal. After healing, the area treated is pink and may be sensitive to the sun for an additional 2 to 4 weeks. Deeper wounds, necessary to remove certain growths, will take a longer time to heal and may leave more of a scar.
4. *Scarring:* Although unsightly scarring is extremely rare, some scars may be more visible than others. The quality and appearance of scarring is variable and is related to an individual's genetic makeup. While good wound healing is expected, abnormal scars may occur both within the skin and deeper tissues. If you have any history of unfavorable healing, please report it before the procedure. To minimize scarring, you must follow all postoperative instructions carefully and notify the doctor if a problem develops.
5. *Skin color change:* The treated area may heal either lighter or darker in color than the surrounding skin. Any changes in pigmentation are usually temporary but occasionally may be permanent.
6. *Recurrence of lesion:* Some skin conditions may be affected partially or not at all by the laser and may require additional surgical or other treatment.
7. *Infection:* Any invasive procedure carries a risk of infection and may require treatment with antibiotics.

It may be necessary to return for multiple treatments of certain conditions to attain suitable results or to conclude that the laser treatments may not be fully effective for a particular condition. Therefore, the consent will be effective for the duration of laser treatments of the procedure named above.

The details of the operation or procedure, including anesthesia and its possible complications, have been explained to me in terms that I understand. Alternative methods of treatment have been explained to me, as have the advantages and disadvantages of each.

Pictures can be taken of the treatment site for record purposes. I understand that these photographs or video tapes will be the property of the attending physician. I do _____/do not _____ agree to allow these pictures to be used for publication or teaching purposes. If I agree, I understand that my name and identity will be kept confidential and protected.

The essential information necessary to make an informed decision has been given to me. All questions have been answered to my satisfaction.

_____

Patient/Date

_____

Witness/Date

I hereby certify that I have discussed all of the above with the patient. I have offered to answer any questions about the procedure and believe the patient fully understands what I have explained and answered.

_____

Physician/Date

High-Energy Ultrapulsed Carbon Dioxide Laser for Resurfacing Wrinkles, Lines, and Scars

Nicholas J. Lowe

PLEASE READ THESE INSTRUCTIONS CAREFULLY AND MAKE NOTES ON THE BACK IF YOU HAVE ANY QUESTIONS.

You have a right to be informed about your skin condition and treatment so that you can make a decision whether or not to undergo this procedure after knowing the risks and hazards involved. This disclosure is not meant to alarm or scare you. It is simply an effort to better inform you so that you can give or withhold your consent for the treatment.

In the past few years, scientists have developed a high-energy laser with a beam that pulses on and off in microseconds. All lasers generate heat. This laser is "too fast" to damage the surrounding area, rather like lifting your finger rapidly on and off a hot surface. It works by vaporizing tissue. The heat that is formed is carried away by steam.

History of the Carbon Dioxide Laser

Carbon dioxide (CO_2) lasers have been used effectively by dermatologists for many years to destroy or excise conditions such as warts, superficial skin cancers, and acne scars. The advantages of treating these conditions with a laser rather than a knife have been less pain, less bleeding, precisional control for the doctor, less infection, and in some cases faster surgery. However, these older lasers have the potential to scar as heat builds up in the surrounding healthy tissue, which may be damaged.

How Does This New High-Energy Ultrapulsed Laser Differ From Chemical Peels or Dermabrasion?

During a chemical peel, areas such as deeper wrinkles may be masked by the frosting effect of the chemical on the skin. Some skin surfaces may absorb the chemical peel at different rates, and the depth of the peel can be unpredictable, leading to a risk of scarring and some discoloration. During dermabrasion, the blood produced by the sanding effect reduces visibility. These missed areas will become apparent only after healing. Dermabrasion also carries a risk of infection from blood-borne diseases.

Laser surgery is virtually bloodless, because the high-energy laser seals blood vessels as it goes.

Will I Need an Anesthetic?

One hour before laser treatment, EMLA cream, a topical anesthetic, may be applied to the area to numb the skin. Ice may also be applied. Some patients prefer to have a local injection of anesthetic. Some prefer to have sedational anesthesia.

For full-face peels, you will need some sedational anesthesia. If you have any type of sedational anesthesia, it will be necessary for someone to collect you and take you home.

What Areas Can Be Treated?

Lines around the mouth (including the ones that cause lipstick bleed) and eyes, deeper scars, frown lines, and some acne or surgical scars can be treated with the CO_2 laser. It also allows newer advanced surgical techniques in lower eyelid blepharoplasty and for micrograft hair transplantation.

Will I Need to Have Any Pretreatment?

You may be prescribed Retin-A or a bleaching gel 3 to 4 weeks before the laser treatment. The day before the procedure, you will begin taking an antibiotic by mouth and Zovirax or Famciclovir (to prevent cold sores or fever blisters) for 5 days. The night before, you will take Dalmane (a short-acting sleeping pill), which will help you sleep. Photographs will be taken before and after treatment.

What Happens During the Laser Resurfacing Treatment?

The doctor will map out the area to be treated, with input from you on particular wrinkles or lines that bother you. He or she will then evenly "paint" those areas with the high-energy laser, making one pass. This area will be wiped and deeper lines retreated if needed. This laser provides excellent depth control even for deeper lines and wrinkles. The wrinkles are sculpted away by peeling down the high points or "shoulders" of the wrinkle. Skin is tightened by vaporizing excess water and stimulating collagen. Some deeper areas may need three or four passes. Other areas may be feathered and blended in using less power. The surgery is virtually bloodless because the laser sears and seals the walls of the surrounding vessels. If there is a lot of sun damage to the soft part of the lip (vermilion border), there may be some bleeding there. Deeper lines may need resculpting about 4 to 6 months after all signs of pink have disappeared. The procedure takes between 15 and 30 minutes for areas around the mouth or eyes, and 1 to 1½ hours for a full-face peel.

How Will I Look and Feel After Treatment?

Immediately after laser treatment, the skin will look white with an occasional yellow-brown area. The skin will feel hot and may sting for 4 to 6 hours. If you had intravenous sedation, you will be drowsy for at least 6 to 8 hours and sometimes the next day. In the next few days as healing occurs, a thin scab will appear, which will gradually be replaced by scaling and peeling. Camouflage makeup can be used after 10 days for local areas and after about 14 days for a full-face peel. The area will initially be red, fading to a light pink. This pink color sometimes lasts for up to 4 months and represents a new blood supply. It may also represent an increase in your own collagen, but more research is needed on this.

Posttreatment for Ultrapulsed Resurfacing

The patient must be seen the day after their Ultrapulse procedure. This is mandatory.

Please inform us of any medications you are taking on a regular basis. It may be necessary to stop these before the resurfacing, but we must be informed.

I am taking the following medications for

_____.

The last medication I took was

_____ for _____.

I am not taking any medications.
Initial: _____.

It is very important for you to take your antibiotics and Zovirax as prescribed by the doctor. Please complete the entire course of antibiotics even if you have no infection.

1. Please take your antibiotic twice a day starting the morning before your resurfacing. Take one the morning of your resurfacing and again after the treatment. Continue the antibiotics for 8 days in total.
2. Start the anti–fever blister (cold sore) medication the day before the resurfacing. Some patients will take one or two pills a day for 8 days total.
3. Some patients prefer to have light sedation during the resurfacing, especially around the eye area or during a full-face resurfacing. You will take a Dalmane, 30 mg, before bedtime (no later than 10:30 PM) and again just after you arrive in the clinic. You must be driven to and from the clinic if you elect to have light sedation. The doctor will discuss and advise you at your preoperative visit.
Initial:_____
4. You must arrive 1 hour before your appointment to have EMLA cream applied and to allow for the full benefit of this topical anesthetic.
5. Please do not drink coffee, alcohol, or strong tea for 24 hours before the resurfacing. Avoid all caffeine.
6. You will be required to wear a bandage for at least 24 hours, maybe longer, depending on your doctor's instructions. Please be prepared for this.
Initial:_____

Instructions for Post–Laser Skin Resurfacing Treatment

Please read these instructions carefully and make notes on the back if you have any questions.

1. The area treated by the laser will be crusted and will weep for up to 7 days. It may also feel tender. Small areas of skin may bleed slightly for a few days. As healing occurs, the skin may feel tight.
2. You may have special nonstick dressings applied for the first 24 hours to keep the area moist. You should reapply the moisturizing ointment under the dressing to any parts of the skin that feel dry. The mouth dries out rapidly because of movement, and careful attention should be paid to keep this moisturized. If there is any sign of infection, call the doctor immediately.
3. It is very important that you are seen on the second day. On this day the areas should be soaked two times a day, once in the morning and about 12 hours later, using diluted white distilled vinegar soaks. Dilute the white distilled vinegar 1 capful to 1 pint of warm water, and leave a soaked gauze pad on for 10 minutes. Continue to use the white distilled vinegar soaks until the area is healed or no longer feels tight.
4. Avoid any strenuous activity for 7 days, which can cause perspiration. Avoid excessive alcohol consumption.
5. Apply the ointment provided to the treated area until all signs of scabbing or peeling have disappeared. Apply at least six times a day. *Do not let the skin dry out* as this increases the risk of infection and scarring. If there is any sign of infection, call the doctor immediately.
6. Do not use makeup on crusted or scabbed areas until these are healed. It is all right to apply makeup to lightly peeling or scaling areas.
7. Stop using any other creams and lotions, such as glycolic acid or tretinoin, until the doctor advises you to continue.
8. **DO NOT GO OUT IN THE SUN UNTIL ALL SIGNS OF SCABBING HAVE GONE.** Wear the mask provided if you must be exposed to the sun. Once the scabbing has gone completely, start using the recommended sunscreens daily. *Avoid all sunbathing.*
9. We must stress how imperative it is that you be seen the day after the Ultrapulse procedure.

Some patients are extremely sensitive to various creams and lotions, a sensitivity that can manifest itself as an itchy rash or small white spots. Do not be alarmed as the normal skin barrier will return after healing is complete.

DO NOT PICK OR SCRATCH. THIS WILL CAUSE SCARRING OR DISCOLORATION.

Risks and Discomforts

The most common side effects and complications of this type are as follows:

Hyperpigmentation (increased skin color): This is more common in those with dark complexions but may occur with any skin type, it is usually temporary. It should respond to the use of hydroquinone cream and lotions and UVA sunscreens postoperatively. Any exposure to the sun without sunscreens must be avoided.

Hypopigmentation (decreased skin color): This is uncommon and appears to be related to the depth of the peel. It is also temporary.

Erythema (redness of skin): The laser-treated areas have a distinctive redness, which may well last 1 to 4 months beyond the time normally required to heal the skin surface (usually 7 to 10 days). This redness is thought to represent increased blood flow from healing as well as new growth of the superficial tissue. It fades gradually over the weeks. Exposure to sunlight, alcohol consumption, and perspiring can prolong the erythema.

Induration (hardening) and tightness: It is not uncommon for the treated area to feel tight, hot, and itchy for up to 10 days. The ointment recommended by your doctor should be used whenever the skin feels dry. If the skin around the mouth is swollen or tight, drink using a straw. Hydrocortisone cream or antihistamine pills can help alleviate itching and dryness.

Scarring: Scarring is not anticipated as a consequence of this procedure, but any procedure in which the surface of the skin is removed can heal with scarring. This usually occurs because of some secondary factor that interferes with healing, such as infection, irritation, scratching, poor wound care, or exposure to the sun. Scarring from infection, irritation, or scratching does blend and often disappears in a few months, but some scarring may be permanent. Hypertrophic reactions or keloids in susceptible people may suddenly appear. These should respond to injections or special creams.

Allergic reactions: Allergic reactions or irritation to some of the medications or creams may develop, especially to the antibiotic creams or ointments. This manifests itself as a redness, an itchy rash, or small white spots that may be painful to touch. An increased sensitivity to wind and sun may occur but is temporary and clears as the skin heals.

Drug Side Effects

The drugs that will be administered during and after this treatment have the following general side effects:

Local anesthetic creams: Possible skin irritancy or allergy.
Retin-A: Sensitivity to sunlight, including sun lamps.
Zovirax: Fever, headaches, pain, and peripheral edema. Serious allergic reactions (anaphylaxis) that can be life-threatening may occur.
Vicodin: Light-headedness, dizziness, sedation, nausea, and vomiting.
Valium: Drowsiness, fatigue, and defective muscular coordination (ataxia).
Antibiotics: Allergic skin rashes, nausea, vomiting, and diarrhea.

Alternative Treatments

Alternative treatments include chemical skin peels, collagen injections, fat transplantation, dermabrasion, and a facelift.

High-Energy Ultrapulsed Carbon Dioxide Laser for Resurfacing Wrinkles, Lines, and Scars Informed Consent

We do not guarantee results; we guarantee only that this office and physicians will use their best efforts and best judgment on your behalf.

I have read the information in this packet. I agree this constitutes full disclosure and that it supersedes any previous verbal or written disclosures. I certify that I have read and fully understand the above paragraphs, and that I have had sufficient opportunity for discussion and to ask questions.

I agree to allow Dr. _____ and his/her staff to photograph or video tape me before, during, or after the procedure. These photos and videos shall be the property of Dr. _____ and can be used for teaching, publication, or scientific research.

_____

Patient Signature/Date

_____

Printed Name

_____

Witness Signature/Date

Erbium Laser Skin Resurfacing Treatment

Nicholas J. Lowe

Preoperative Concerns

Before your erbium laser procedure, medication prescriptions will be phoned into your pharmacy. These are helpful to promote healing and are important for your results. Unless otherwise discussed, you should arrive 1 hour before your procedure. At this time, the nurse will apply EMLA (a topical numbing cream) and dispense your preoperative medications.

Remember to wear comfortable clothing—button-down or zippered loose clothing. Do not wear makeup or jewelry. Arrange to have someone drive you home unless otherwise specified.

Postoperative Concerns

You may leave with a dressing on the area treated. *Do not* remove it until the doctor says it is okay to do so. This dressing usually stays on about 3 days with daily checks to make sure it is intact. The night you go home, there will be some oozing from the sides. This is normal. Simply take a gauze pad or wash cloth and blot it dry. Other than this blotting, do not touch the dressing. Sleep on your back with your head elevated on two pillows. Do not eat anything hot, spicy, or hard. Minimal chewing is best. Soft foods and clear liquids are best for the first 2 days.

You will be seen in our office 1 day after the laser procedure. The nurses will give you full instructions. Do not scratch scabs. If the area becomes itchy, phone the office. There are special medications for this, if needed.

You will be shown how to apply ointment and do soaks. This is very important and also assists the skin with healing. The skin must be kept moist with ointment. Avoid sun and strenuous exercise for at least 7 days.

Do not use any products on these areas other than what has been given to you. Your skin may remain pink for the next few weeks. Once advised, you can cover with makeup. Make sure to use a hypoallergenic and noncomedogenic makeup to cover pink areas for the first few weeks. Dermablend is a good coverup. Ask the nurses for the list of recommended makeup.

Over the first 3 days you may experience superficial bleeding from the skin surface. This is usual with this laser and is not a problem.

Sunscreen is very important when the doctor says it is all right to start using it. It is extremely important the first few months postoperatively.

Make sure to follow these instructions. If you have any questions, please do not hesitate to contact the office.

Risks and Discomforts

The most common side effects and complications of this type are as follows:

Hyperpigmentation (increased skin color): This is more common in those with dark complexions but may occur with any skin type. It is usually only temporary. It should respond to the use of hydroquinone cream and lotions and UVA sunscreens postoperatively. Any exposure to the sun without sunscreens must be avoided.

Hypopigmentation (decreased skin color): This is uncommon and appears to be related to the depth of the peel. It is also temporary.

Erythema (redness of skin): The laser-treated areas have a distinctive redness, which may last 1 to 2 months beyond the time normally required to heal the skin surface (usually 7 to 10 days). This redness is thought to represent increased blood flow from healing as well as new growth of the superficial tissue. It fades gradually over the weeks. Exposure to sunlight, alcohol consumption, and perspiring can prolong the erythema.

Induration (hardening) and tightness: It is not uncommon for the treated area to feel tight, hot and itchy for up to 10 days. The ointment recommended by your doctor should be used whenever the skin feels dry. If the skin around the mouth is swollen or tight, drink using a straw. Hydrocortisone cream or antihistamine pills can help alleviate itching and dryness.

Scarring: Scarring is not anticipated as a consequence of this procedure, but any procedure in which the surface of the skin is removed can heal with scarring. This usually occurs because of some secondary factor that interferes with healing, such as infection, irritation, scratching, poor wound care, or exposure to the sun. Scarring from infection, irritation, or scratching does blend and often disappears in a few months, but some scarring may be permanent. Hypertrophic reactions or keloids in susceptible people may suddenly appear. These should respond to injections or special creams.

Allergic reactions: Allergic reactions or irritations to some of the medications or creams may develop, especially to the antibiotic creams or ointments. This manifests itself as redness, an itchy rash, or small white spots that may be painful to touch. An increased sensitivity to wind and sun may occur but is temporary and clears as the skin heals.

Erbium Laser for Resurfacing Wrinkles, Lines, and Scars Informed Consent

We do not guarantee results; we guarantee only that this office and physicians will use their best efforts and best judgment on your behalf.

I have read the information. I agree this constitutes full disclosure and that it supersedes any previous verbal or written disclosures. I certify that I have read and fully understand the above paragraphs, and that I have had sufficient opportunity for discussion and to ask questions.

I agree to allow the doctor and his staff to photograph or video tape me before, during, and after the procedure. These photos and videos shall be the property of the doctor and can be used for teaching, publication, or scientific research.

_____

Patient's Signature/Date

_____

Printed Name

_____

Witness Signature/Date

Botulinum Toxin Information and Consent

Nicholas J. Lowe

Background

Botulinum toxin (Botox) has been used for years to treat muscular problems, including eye deviation (strabismus), eyelid spasm (blepharospasm), facial spasms, and muscle spasm.

Aging is associated with the development of wrinkles and furrows on the face. These lines may develop as a result of weakened dermal collagen from sun exposure and gravity or as a direct result of facial muscle action of the skin.

Botox for Frown and Smile Lines

Botox, or *Botulinum* toxin, reversibly paralyzes muscle. Therefore, it may be used to treat facial lines caused primarily by the action of muscles on the skin. The ideal areas to treat are wrinkles caused by muscles that provide no true function. An example of this type of area is the glabellar furrow, the deep crease found between the eyebrows. Other areas that can be treated include crow's feet wrinkles, forehead lines, and persistently flared nostrils.

Injection of Botox into the glabellar furrows has been shown to be very successful. Good results can be obtained after a single session and can last from 2 to 4 months. Some patients have had excellent results for 7 months after injection. We may use an electromyelographic machine, which targets the exact muscle and delivers the injection at the same time. The injection can take between 3 to 5 days to have its effects. Some patients with very powerful muscles may not see a complete paralysis of the targeted area, but subsequent injections further weaken them.

Botox Combined With Line Fillers and Laser Resurfacing

Other available treatments for these furrows include injections of collagen and fat. There are also temporary fillers.

Botox may also be used prior to laser skin resurfacing for the lines around the eyes. While the muscle activity is reduced by the Botox, there is more efficient renewal of connective tissue in your skin, allowing better improvement of smile lines or crow's feet.

Botox for Hyperhidrosis

Botox has recently been found helpful for the reduction of excess sweating in places like the armpits and hands. It seems to last between 6 to 8 months. The only possible side effect is temporary weakness to the underlying muscle.

What Will I Look Like After Treatment?

Immediately after injection, there may be mild swelling that usually subsides in 24 to 48 hours. For best results, remember to use these muscles often in the first few hours after the injection. Do not lie down flat for at least 8 hours. Do not receive massages while lying flat on your stomach for 8 hours after your injections.

Side Effects

Side effects of this treatment are rare. Occasionally, temporary drooping of the eyebrow or eyelid may occur and last up to a few weeks. Rarely, numbness develops in the treated area. Patients also may rarely develop antibodies or allergies to the *Botulinum* toxin or experience double vision and tearing or watering of the eyes. A very rare side effect is generalized weakness and fatigue. In one study, only 3% to 4% of patients experienced any of these complications.

How Many Treatments Will I Need?

Repeated treatments are usually needed every 3 to 4 months over a 12-month period. It is being reported and observed that some patients who have had continued treatment over the 12-month period only need further treatments once or twice a year. These reports are being researched.

Note: It takes 3 to 5 days for the Botox to work.

Other Types of Reactions

Occasionally, you may experience a reaction to the injection itself. Mild bruising may appear. If you have a history of cold sores from herpes simplex at the injection site, treatment may bring out another eruption. Finally, any injection carries a small risk of infection.

Pregnancy

If you are pregnant or a nursing mother, treatment is not recommended.

Informed Consent

We do not guarantee results; we guarantee only that this office and the physicians will use their best efforts and best judgment on your behalf.

I have read the information in this packet. I agree that this constitutes full disclosure and that it supersedes any previous verbal or written disclosures. I certify that I have read and fully understand the preceding paragraphs and that I have had sufficient opportunity for discussion and to ask questions.

I agree to allow the doctor and his staff to photograph or videotape me before, during, and after the procedure. These photos and videos shall be the property of the doctor and can be used for teaching, publication, or scientific research.

_____

Patient Signature/Date

_____

Printed Name

_____

Witness Signature/Date

INDEX

Note: Page numbers in *italics* refer to illustrations; page numbers followed by (t) refer to tables.

161

ISBN 0-443-07639-1